The Psychedelic Renaissance

Reassessing the Role of Psychedelic Drugs in 21st Century Psychiatry and Society

Dr. Ben Sessa MBBS BSc MRCPsych

Consultant Psychiatrist in Addictions and Child and Adolescent Psychiatry and Senior Research Fellow at Bristol, Cardiff and Imperial College London Universities.

Second Edition — April 2017

Front cover artwork: *'The Meatery'* (2016) Acrylic and chalk on canvas. 100cm x 125cm.

Rear cover artwork: *'Around'* (2016) Acrylic and pencil on canvas. 21cm x 30 cm.

By Daniel TM Campbell.

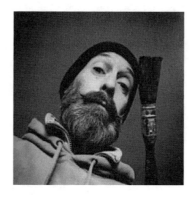

First published by Muswell Hill Press, London, 2017

© 2017 Ben Sessa

Ben Sessa has asserted his right under the Copyright, Design and Patents Act 1988 to be identified as the Author of this Work. All rights reserved. No part of this publication may be reproduced without prior permission of Muswell Hill Press.

www.muswellhillpress.co.uk

First edition published by Muswell Hill Press 2012

British Library CIP Data available

ISBN 978-1-908995-25-4

Printed in Great Britain

This book is dedicated to my darling little children Huxley, Kitty and Jimi. May your beloved brains continue to respond to a host of endogenous mystical compounds forever more, giving rise to a lifetime of spontaneous, organically, non-drug induced spiritual experiences.

Contents

Foreword for
The Psychedelic Renaissance (Second Edition)

I am delighted to be writing this forward for the second addition of Dr Ben Sessa's book *The Psychedelic Renaissance*. Ben has been a dear friend for over 10 years. We met in Basel, Switzerland, in 2006, at the International Symposium on LSD, a landmark event in the renaissance of psychedelic science, and a landmark also for Albert Hofmann, the discoverer of LSD, who was celebrating his 100th year. Ben had travelled from the UK with his nephew, Jamie McCutcheon, and I had befriended another couple of Brits, Luke Williams and Roland Neal. In the 3 or so days we spent together in Basel, we struck up quite a friendship. It felt mutually invigorating to share thoughts and ideas with like-minded souls who could appreciate the special wonder of psychedelics. I was only 6 months into my PhD in Professor David Nutt's Psychopharmacology Unit in Bristol, and had felt somewhat of an outsider there; the nervous kid with his Freud books and peculiar interest in psychedelics. Meeting Ben and the gang was affirming on a number of levels. After the day's lectures, we would sit in cosy Swiss pubs drinking Weiss beer and eating Rosti, while discussing receptor profiles and Rankian birth trauma – it was such a welcome and expansive space. We spoke about setting up a web-forum for discussions on topics of psychology, philosophy, and pharmacology – and named ourselves 'the Basel club'.

While the Basel Club would eventually fizzle out, the enthusiasm that drove its creation was symbolic of the spirit of that meeting in 2006. Ben and I continued our friendship as he became a visiting member of the Psychopharmacology Unit in Bristol. Ben would sometimes stay over, or I would visit him at his home in the Somerset countryside and together we devised plans for an ambitious project to test psilocybin with adjunctive spiritual support, for alcohol dependence. Sometime in 2007, Ben presented these plans to the Psychopharmacology Unit during a weekly meeting. To say they fell on deaf ears would be an understatement! They were actively desecrated by the resident alcohol dependence expert, while others lunged in to ensure the prey was dead. An uncharacteristically quiet presence in the room that day was Professor Nutt. "What are you and Sessa up to?" he would say to me in the corridor, when learning of our impending presentation.

In hindsight, it was too much too soon, but I look back fondly on our initiative. In our despondency after the meeting, among laments of "they just don't get it", I remember saying to Ben "in 10 years, we'll be doing this work, it's inevitable, it just needs time." It's so satisfying to know that this has turned out to be true.

The Psychedelic Renaissance is about taking stock of where we've been, where we are now, and what might be possible in the future. It builds on the highly commendable first edition by incorporating some of the impactful recent developments in psychedelic science, including the important work on psilocybin for end-of-life psychological distress, ayahuasca and psilocybin for depression, and brain imaging with LSD. To say this work has been impactful, is justified: our LSD and psilocybin for depression papers both made it into the top 100 'most immediately impactful' scientific papers of 2016 as judged by *Altmetrics* and *Inverse magazine* voted our LSD paper the most important scientific publication of the year. These achievements are symbolic of a more general zeitgeist, in which psychedelics are firmly transitioning back into mainstream science and society; *The Psychedelic Renaissance* captures this spirit, and may prove a definitive text on these times.

As Ben expertly discusses throughout *The Psychedelic Renaissance*, psychedelics are uniquely polarizing. One could characterise the key challenge for psychedelic science as navigating between the antagonistic forces of 'magic' (psychedelics are all-powerful) and 'moralism' (psychedelics are all-bad). Ben is as conscious of the pitfalls of a magical worldview, as he is critical of the righteous moralism that has so impeded this work in the past. But as we step forward into the exciting unknown, empowered by a growing knowledge-base, and confidence in our methods and tools, it is important to better understand *who* may wish to challenge us and *why* they might wish to do so. In this way, we may be able to better understand our own position; its strengths and weaknesses. Psychedelic science need not strive to temper itself, nor to please anyone. It needn't strive for anything, except truth.

Good science is about *daring* and *discipline*; it is combination of these things that sets it apart as a method of learning, defining its unique explanatory power and potential. It is *daring*, as it endeavours to *test* its ideas, rather than rest on assumption, and it is *disciplined* because it recognises that scepticism and attention to detail are necessary if we are to refine our inferences and so, advance our learning. In time, I hope that science can serve as a bridge to moderate extreme views, by informing on the beliefs that motivate them. It is difficult to see how such a development could be anything but positive.

So onward, intrepid explorer, keep your wits, while allowing them to be tickled (it won't be hard), as Dr Sessa leads you into a world of remarkable wonders! There are few as charismatic as Ben; his company is always a joy, pleasure and privilege. You are in for a real treat!

Dr Robin Carhart-Harris, PhD
Research Associate and study lead of the Beckley-Imperial Psychedelic Research Programme. Robin is at the forefront of UK contemporary research studies with LSD, psilocybin, DMT and MDMA.

Endorsements For The Psychedelic Renaissance Second Edition

Ben Sessa is one of a new rising generation of psychedelic drug research-ers and clinicians, one of the chief organizers of Breaking Convention, an important UK conference of ideas that does just that: break conventions! But his contributions to this field are not limited to that. In his work as a clinical psychiatrist working with Professor David Nutt's group at Imperial College, London, Dr. Sessa has been author or co-author on over 20 peer reviewed papers on psychedelic research. In this engagingly written mani-festo, Dr. Sessa shares his story and narrates the events in his personal life and professional career that led him to commit to a lifetime of clinical and basic research with psychedelics. He makes a strong and passionate case for the re-introduction of psychedelics into psychiatric therapies, and in the process provides illuminating background on the checkered (and often maligned) history of psychedelics in medicine. His book also includes helpful chapters on both the phenomenology of psychedelic experiences, as well as the chemistry and pharmacology of different members of the psychedelic pharmacopoeia, useful for those who are not specialists but who may be curious about the many different psychedelic substances and their sometimes not so subtle differences. All in all, Dr. Sessa's book is a succinct, entertaining overview of the emerging "Psychedelic Renais-sance" written by an insider, and one of the brightest young architects of this new emerging paradigm.

Dr Dennis J. McKenna, Ph.D.
Assistant Professor, Center for Spirituality & Healing
University of Minnesota, USA

No-one in the UK knows more about the burgeoning psychedelic renais-sance than Ben Sessa. He has, by virtue of his profession, legally ingested an alphabet soup of psychedelic drugs and is fully aware of their power to change consciousness. Moreover, Ben is cognisant of the potential these drugs have to enhance 'traditional' psychotherapy in order to heal the damage caused by PTSD and many other kinds of emotional turmoil as well as addictions and other afflictions of the mind.

With intelligence, fact-based optimism and compassion Ben throws open the doors of perception and guides the reader through the complexities of the history, pharmacology, legality and potential of MDMA and LSD among other psychedelic drugs. Ben's clarity of vision is underpinned by personal experience of these substances, both socially and medically and tempered with the insights of someone who cares about the human condition and who wants to change people, and the world, for the better via the agency of these miraculous molecules.

Andy Roberts
UK psychedelic historian, co-curator the Psychedelic Museum and the author of two contemporary books on LSD in the British Isles, *Albion Dreaming* **and** *Acid Drops***. He also sells T-shirts at Breaking Convention.**

Psychedelic drugs are arguably the most important drugs for neuroscience. They have been used by different human societies for millennia. But currently, there is limited use of them in science because of the intense regulations that control their production and use. We now have a great range of new neuroimaging scanning techniques for exploring brain function. This new edition of Sessa's book, *The Psychedelic Renaissance*, will encourage researchers to work in this field, to the benefit of our understanding of how the brain works and, in the longer term, to the development of new approaches to psychiatric disorders.

Professor David Nutt
Emeritus Professor of Psychopharmacology at Imperial College London

Dr. Ben Sessa's insightful and comprehensive resource, *The Psychedelic Renaissance*, arrives at just the right time, when the general public is being increasingly informed by the media of the advances in psychedelic research taking place around the world. *The Psychedelic Renaissance* is a book that deserves to be widely read. Dr. Sessa prescribes a way forward for the mainstreaming of psychedelics and the many benefits they can offer when used carefully and cautiously, for a world in deep need of healing, spirituality and inspiration.

Rick Doblin Founder and Executive Director of the Multidisciplinary Association of Psychedelic Studies (MAPS)

As each year brings forth more breakthroughs in the exciting field of psychedelic science, Ben Sessa's energetic review of the research and cultural use of psychedelics provides a unique perspective from a British psychiatrist working within this fast-moving field. Taking us on an entertaining journey through the rise and fall and subsequent resurrection of psychedelics within psychiatry and medicine, he highlights the tremendous therapeutic potential of these compounds and the ways in which historical events and political expediency have obstructed their development. As the research moves forward, Sessa draws attention to the urgent need for a pragmatic and thorough review of global drug policies, backed by science and ethics, so that new treatments can be developed and made available for those suffering from a wide range of mental health disorders. The way forward is clear: we urgently need more scientific research, and a rational reform of drug policies.

Amanda Feilding
Founder and Executive of *The Beckley Foundation*

Dr. Ben Sessa's Psychedelic Renaissance is a clearly and concisely written historical overview of the clinical and social psychological literature on psychedelic plants, fungi and drugs. Covering people and projects all the way back to the fifties and early sixties, it includes projects in the US, the UK and other European countries and brings the story up to date on the most promising applications of these mysterious and alluring substances – in medicine, addiction treatment, trauma psychotherapy and others. The reader cannot fail to be impressed by the remarkable results obtained with these substances, as Ben Sessa describes them. This book will inevitably and rightlybe seen as an important marker of their assimilation into the cultural mainstream. I highly recommend it.

Ralph Metzner, Ph.D.
Researcher on the Harvard Psilocybin Project with Dr Timothy Leary
Author of Allies for Awakening.

Dr. Sessa skilfully chronicles important developments, perhaps a turning point, in psychiatry and in the understanding of psychedelics in the wider culture. This new updated edition of The Psychedelic Renaissance is informative, entertaining and timely.

Michael Mithoefer MD, Psychiatrist
Lead Clinical Investigator for MDMA-Assisted Psychotherapy for PTSD

Introduction

Apocalypse, Now and Then

These are interesting times. Some may say apocalyptical. While every generation flatters itself by imagining this, our own moment in history does feel particularly special. Humanity is witnessing the unprecedented convergence of major crises and threats to its way of life: global warming, intercontinental religious conflict, constantly impending nuclear threat, wars for oil, wars for water, societal meltdown and the potential collapse of capitalism in the wake of global financial crisis. Half the world is withering in starvation while the other half — just a click of a mouse away — die from obesity. You couldn't make it up.

New technologies bombard us with profound alterations in consciousness, simultaneously shrinking our world and expanding our minds. Culture is homogenised into an unstoppable snowball of uniformity fuelled by television campaigns pushing for obligatory global democracy. We apathetically update our Facebook statuses as archaic dictatorships are pushed aside to make way for exported TV talent shows and celebrity dictators peddling the politics of exclusion, xenophobia and other symbols of alleged progress.

In the centre of all this turbulence and uncertainty, stands the contemporary Western individual; overweight, spoilt, media-obsessed and bored, searching as ever for answers to the perennial questions of human life. Of course, there is no single agent, political solution or religious creed that will save us from this seemingly inevitable march. Rather, a united multidisciplinary effort is required. But while we sit and wait for the political strategists in the hallowed corridors of power to come up with the answers, what can we do as individuals?

Shall we just simply be ourselves? This is easier said than done. Who are we, after all, but our complex bundles of experiences, genes, childhoods, conditioning environments and wishes for the future? Amidst the cacophony of divergent influences pulling us to and fro, we can easily lose track of where we are going. Not to mention why.

If only there were a magical elixir to illuminate the way! Something to provide answers to our multitude of questions, both profound and banal.

Regrettably, of course, there is not. Had this book been written 50 years ago in 1967's Summer of Love an enthusiastic social commentator might have inserted those three little letters here; L, S and D, but, alas, no mere drug will save humanity or the planet.

But What *Can* Psychedelics Offer Us?

Maybe not salvation, but perhaps these fascinating psychoactive compounds *do* possess some important qualities which Humanity 2.0 may be foolish to ignore. Psychedelic drugs are the subject of this book, and although they will not teach us everything we need to know about ourselves, they may offer an innovative angle from which to help us approach afresh the same age-old questions.

Psychedelics are uniquely placed to assist us with our queries; partly because of the fundamental qualities of the psychedelic experience itself, and partly because of the place they occupy in the development of our culture. There is, at the core of the psychedelic experience, an unavoidable drive to explore our fundamental human questions. To quote a famous psychedelic folk band, '*What is it that we are part of? And what is it that we are?*'[1] from which stems a peculiarly curious element of developed consciousness; spirituality. From here we dive into religion, mysticism, anthropology, culture and politics. Not to mention, as I will be doing at length, neuroscience. It seems those prehistoric plants, anilmals and mushrooms may have a lot to answer for.

As a medical doctor, with a traditional education and methodical approach rooted in objective, evidence-based scientific rigour, I have a profound distaste for pseudoscience. The very word *healing* used to infuriate me. Throughout my medical career it has been a word I associated with that hoax homeopathy, and other fringe elements of the New Age movement. Because, strange though it may seem speaking as a modern doctor, I have not been taught how to *heal*. Rather, my education trained me to recognise, categorise and adjust the pathology before me. My job was to overcome and eradicate the pathogens as they appear.

But then things changed for me when I learned about psychedelic medicine. And, for the record, I am *not* talking about a eureka moment of hippy-fuelled personal drug use in which I embraced psychedelics as a magical panacea to all and sundry. On the contrary, my epiphany came slowly and gradually — in line with my methodical clinical approach. Psychedelics taught me how best to conduct science. But might they, I wonder sometimes, have taken me to the same place as the hippies?

My hope is that this book can have a similar effect on the reader: judiciously presenting the argument that science and medicine *need* psychedelics. And this means we must place that word, '*science*' in quotation marks for the same reason that I used to shrink from my nemesis, '*healing*'. Through learning about the potential role for psychedelics in medicine, I have inevitably examined the current role of science in my profession, psychiatry, and the human condition at large. Reformation of these phenomena is long overdue.

We are today at a place in psychiatry where general medicine was 100 years ago. In the late 19th century patients were dying from infectious diseases, but the medical profession was yet to discover the miracle cure of antibiotics. We knew all about smallpox, tuberculosis and post-operative infections, but Victorian physicians were powerless to stop them. Then in the 20th century antibiotics transformed the face of general medicine. Once this discovery was made, humans, for the first time in the history of physical disease, began winning the battle against morbidity.

Today in modern psychiatry we are similarly expert at the diagnosis, classification and categorisation of our common mental diseases. We know childhood psychological traumas are at the heart of most chronic mental disorders. But our current best treatments are unsuccessful at effecting a lasting cure. Instead we provide a wide pharmacopeia of medications, from antidepressants to mood stabilisers to antipsychotics and hypnotics, willingly marketed to doctors by a profit-driven pharmaceutical industry, all of which do little more than mask the symptoms of the underlying psychological problems — leaving the trauma grumbling away beneath the surface. Psychiatry is still, sadly, a palliative care intervention for many people, whose intractable mental illnesses require long-term maintenance therapies but see little opportunity for curing or eradicating their problems.

Why is this? The answer is that we have been lacking an effective treatment to help patients tackle their long-standing unresolved memories. And this is where psychedelics come in. Modern psychiatry's equivalent of the early 20th century's antibiotics, psychedelic agents, get to the heart of the psychological problem and offer patients an opportunity to address their trauma. If modern psychiatry can wake up to this realization we could be looking at a major renaissance of psychiatric practice; a Psychedelic Renaissance.

Defining Psychedelic Drugs

What is it that fascinates people about psychedelics? And how can we best define them? A clue comes from the various words we have given these molecules through the ages.

Brain Toxins

Mainstream psychiatrists define psychedelics as drugs that cause an 'acute confusional state'; exogenous agents, coming from outside the body, producing profound alterations in consciousness and perceptual distortions, with the classical hallmarks of an organic psychosis. This definition is reflected in the medical term *hallucinogen*, a name often rejected by modern psychedelic researchers. *Hallucinogen* not only carries negative societal connotations, but it is also phenomenologically incorrect. The perceptual distortions induced by psychedelics are rarely true hallucinations ('a perception in the absence of an physical stimulus'), but, rather they are more often *illusions*; perceptual distortions of a genuine stimulus. Further descriptions of some of these medical terms will be given later in the book as we explore the individual effects of the major psychedelic drugs. One way or the other, the doctors' definition of psychedelics is one of pathology: they are toxins mangling the brain.

Sacraments

Another definition is afforded by the cross-cultural dimension. For many people from non-Western cultures psychedelics are sacred spiritual tools used as part of their religious practice. In this context the word *entheogen* ('that which creates god within a person') may be preferable to *psychedelic*. There is a vast range of naturally occurring psychoactive plants, fungi and animal products including ayahuasca, psilocybin, ibogaine, mescaline and bufotenin. Ancient humans likely knew of many more than we do today. Some scholars claim entire civilisations developed in symbiotic cohabitation with these naturally occurring compounds; spawning their religions, with the psychedelic experience validating and informing their spiritual beliefs. We shall explore later in the book the role these drugs have played in almost all societies on the planet. Long before the 'turn on, tune in and drop out' days of the 1960s, our culture, creativity and the arts have been inspired and shaped by psychedelics.

Alien Visitors Sent to Save Humanity

Crazy though it may seem, many stalwart psychedelic enthusiasts — those starry-eyed hippies (about whom we will hear a lot as I betray my ambivalent conflict with their values) — neither question nor criticize the psychedelic drugs. Leary called LSD the key, the philosopher's stone, the chalice and the Holy Grail.[2] The ably verbose commentator Terence McKenna postulated that psilocybin 'magic' mushrooms are alien spores scattered throughout the universe on meteorites in a deliberate act of propagation by a higher intelligence; by imbibing the mushroom one can communicate with wider extra-terrestrial culture[3]. Growing communities of online followers hold their mushrooms aloft as the only hope we have to reconnect with our pre-technological roots and save ourselves from destruction. For many the magic mushroom experience is a return to nature, a communion with the trees, an opportunity to eschew modern living. Whilst for others, psychedelics represent the ultimate post-modern tool; embracing ultra-high tech computers, artificial intelligence and cyber culture to finally transcend our monkey bodies and emerge into a 21st century of interplanetary exploration.

Dangerous Drugs of Abuse

For most lay people, psychedelics are nothing more than illegal and dangerous drugs of abuse; addictive compounds, no different than cocaine and heroin. Many police, politicians and parents believe cannabis, LSD and Ecstasy are basically the cause of individuals', if not the whole of society's, ruin.

The current position of drug prohibition carries important implications for the topic of medical research. The infamous 'War on Drugs' will be discussed in detail in later chapters alongside the ludicrously simplified question: 'Are drugs good or bad?' (One may as well ask 'are knives good or bad?', and then try slicing a loaf of bread without one.) In discussing The War we are forced to examine fundamental questions about our society, and issues of personal and religious freedoms. To what extent can we possibly continue with an approach to drugs that criminalises the majority of the world's population, and furthermore funds and maintains morally unsustainable social systems? There appears to be a tremendous rift in what the authorities are prepared to say in private and do in public. Few subjects besides the legalisation of drugs call into question more vividly the conflict between evidence-based politics and the emotional response of timid politicians.

We have seen the recent emergence in the UK of the Psychoactive Substances Act (2016)[4]. In the wake of the growing problem of Legal Highs, the UK government, without adequate consultation, drew up this draconian legislation making all compounds with psychoactive properties illegal. The old favourites caffeine, alcohol and nicotine are exempt, of course, but everything else is effectively banned. The short-sightedness of this move is evident to those of us working in the field of addictions. Simply banning a substance does not make it magically disappear from society. If it were that easy, then why have cocaine and heroin not been eradicated?

Rather, these substances are pushed underground, their users are criminalized and the process of education and harm minimization hampered, whilst the criminal gangs that profit from the black-market distribution and supply of the drugs thrive.

It remains to be seen how society will react to the Psychoactive Substances Act. The issue of drugs supplied by the internet will be discussed in greater detail later in the book. But one thing is for certain; gone are the days of recreational users getting their drugs from shady face-to-face liaisons in dodgy pubs. Today's technologically savvy psychonaut is far more sophisticated. And an approach that simply blanket bans all drugs in an attempt to manage their use, misuse, and harms is folly in the extreme.

Research and Clinical Tools

I would most like to convey one final definition of psychedelics, which must be emphasized with utmost importance, is that they are clinical tools to improve the plight of patients suffering with mental and physical disorders, and have an important role as agents to inform our understanding of neuroscience and human consciousness.

In some respects the historical association of psychedelics with recreational abuse is a tiresome irritation. LSD and MDMA began their lives in medicine, which is where they should belong. But trying to convince politicians and medical researchers of this can be an uphill battle. Many people who would normally have no interest in the rather stolid process of medical research throw themselves into this debate with pseudoscientific arguments, which threaten to undermine what should be the simple presentation of robust, evidence-based data. My general medical colleagues, for example, when developing new lines of treatments for liver, heart or

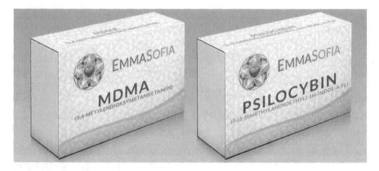

Picture 1: How long before we see these products appearing as licensed medicines on our shelves? (Picture courtesy of Emma Sofia, the Norwegian organisation campaigning for psychedelic research).

endocrine disorders, rarely stimulate the kinds of hot-headed debate we see in psychedelic research. As a doctor, this is most frustrating. And in this respect, the hippies, with their wanton advertisement of chemically-induced utopia with psychedelics, have almost (albeit inadvertently) ruined the party for psychiatric research. For this reason, at times I feel inclined to distance myself from them in my scientific work with psyche-delic drugs.

The Joy of Hippie Culture

On the other hand, (there is always another hand), as recreational drug users go, the psychedelic community is completely unlike any other group. Psychedelic conferences, those niche festivals, get-togethers and scien-tific meetings on the subject, are not hedonistic events. Rather, they are a colourful celebration of all the best aspects of reflective communalism, ecological thinking and harmony of shared differences. Since 2010, along-side several other like-minded academics, I have set-up and run the UK's *Breaking Convention* conference, to which we will return later.

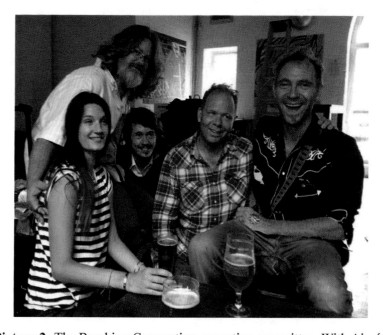

Picture 2: The Breaking Convention executive committee. With Aimée Tollan, Cameron Adams, Dave King and Dave Luke. This was on Monday morning after the weekend conference in July 2015. Smiling faces of relief, extreme exhaustion and a well-earned afterglow.

And the reason why such gatherings work on an academic and intellectual level is that most serious psychedelic users are uniquely respectful and understanding of their drugs' powers and dangers. They use the substances for healing (there's that word again); to search for a deeper personal understanding of their internal and external worlds, and to bring themselves and their communities closer. Psychedelic users are often linked with wider societal and global issues — especially those pertaining to preventing the abuse of nature. Frequently displaying a mixture of liberalism, a conservative appreciation of nature and a tangible humility regarding the human's place upon the planet, a gathering of psychedelically inclined individuals is a colourful celebration of the art, music and creative expression that flows from the psychedelic experience. It is hard to imagine a similarly enlightened mind-set emerging from an annual conference of cocaine or heroin users — or even alcohol, for that matter, which, at best, would be a chaotic festival of self-serving egocentricity and, at worst, involve serious casualties and death. The reasons for the differences between these groups of drug users are complex and encompass many aspects of our cultural development of the last fifty years. But the chief explanation is the fundamental nature of the drug experience itself. And it is this, that, as a neuroscientist, interests me the most.

There are, then, many ways to view psychedelics in these special and interesting times. Faced with so many conflicting environmental influences it takes a willingness to go both outside and inside our heads, as it were, to help us to come up with some new answers to old questions. In these fascinating times, we are now seeing many disparate elements of society glancing 'back to the future', looking again at psychedelics. Whether one aligns oneself with the doctors, the politicians, police, artists, the ravers, the hippies or the worried parents influenced by a dynamic but fragile popular media, we are clearly amid a *Psychedelic Renaissance.*

CHAPTER 1

Personal Reflection

The literary world of psychedelic drugs is peppered with pseudo-scientific personal reflections. This is understandable: the experience itself is such a massive departure from everyday life — perhaps *the greatest* departure imaginable — that, once glimpsed, it is hard not to talk about it and attempt to radicalize others. In this respect the experience has a lot in common with reports of other 'born-again' experiences. Unfortunately, the inherent ineffability of one's first psychedelic experience renders any meaningful attempt at description redundant for the listener. For this reason, I will try to avoid boring the reader with too many personal trip accounts. On the other hand, what I cannot say is 'I will stick entirely to the scientific point'. Because the truth is, from a scientific as much as from an epistemological point of view, these substances are as yet far from adequately understood by any discipline. So, to justify why I am willing to base my judgment partly on subjective and unproved descriptions of these drugs, I would like to begin with a brief description of the journey that brought me to the study of psychedelics as a medical doctor.

Just Missed the Sixties

Apart from the occasional dose of cough medicine, no drugs of any kind featured in my childhood. Born just after the sixties, the youngest of six, I looked up to a family of older siblings who had lived through the height of the hippie counterculture. My parents were teachers and Quakers: my father a headmaster and English teacher who had emigrated from America, and my mother English. The household was liberal, and I was brought up surrounded by the middle-class intellectual left-wing values of peace, pacifism and protest. From my older brothers and sisters, I inherited an abundance of music: particularly Dylan, The Stones and The Beatles. Through my father I was exposed to Hardy, Lawrence, Kerouac, Huxley, Koestler and Kafka — and through them in turn to Ginsberg, Kesey, Laing and

Leary. My mother gave me unconditional love, taught me to play music and inspired a passion for creativity, providing channels for personal transcendence and a boundless confidence to be myself. There was always a stimulating combination of live music, art and performance throughout my childhood. Little attention was paid to the television, with far more interest in communal activities such as making things and discussing ideas.

At 15 years old, I almost died in a climbing accident in Scotland, falling 60 feet off a cliff, breaking both my legs and lying on the rock face for three hours before being winched away by helicopter. I spent the next year in and out of hospitals, and in a wheelchair. Thereafter, I developed a tremendous zeal for life, absorbing every precious moment of experience, fuelled with a sense of having been given a second chance that was not to be squandered. That near-death experience also cemented my ambition to become a doctor; the first in my family of teachers, artists and musicians. In response to the pain I had suffered, I was determined, moreover, to be the first doctor who was nice to children.

From a Pair of Crutches to a Pair of Turntables

By the time I left school in 1990, rave music had well and truly emerged into the forefront of contemporary culture, even in my locale, rural Oxfordshire. My friends and I spent that extraordinary summer with gangs of other long-haired, baggy trousered kids at Oxford's embryonically emerging rave hot spots; *Spectrum* at the Co-Op Hall club and *The Set*. Clues given out at the local record shop, or coded messages from pirate radio stations, would produce a cavalcade of cars and rendezvous in lay-bys and petrol stations. From Cheltenham to Chelmsford gatherings sprang up that summer to take us to forbidden parties in farmers' fields and disused barns. We followed the young DJs who have since become household names in this wonderful developing cottage industry, run by and for entrepreneurial space cadets. We danced till dawn. When the music petered out a bucket would be passed around for people to throw in their 50ps for more diesel for the generators and the beats would kick back into life. The scene thrived on a diet of cannabis, ecstasy and LSD, but it was the communal cohesiveness of those parties that gave the greatest high. The early UK raves provided an enlightening experience of dissolution of class, race and social status; everyone united under a bassline. The summer of 1988 was dubbed the 'second summer of love'. They were experiential and enlightening times; my generation's version of the cultural shifts of the 1960s. Screw Thatcher. Screw the system. Just give us White Doves and a beat.

Leaving the raves behind, after school I took my guitar and set out on a six-month trip with two like-minded, wannabe-hippies to tread the path of well-known locations around the world: San Francisco, Hawaii, Australia, Bali, Thailand, Nepal. I read voraciously, and learned of the role psychedelics played not only in the formation of the drug culture of psychedelia, but in terms of cultural history before the sixties with the Beat poets and pioneers like Kesey, Grof and Leary. I could see clearly that LSD and MDMA were much more than simply hedonistic playthings for ravers or hippies; rather, they were tools for psycho-spiritual development and, crucially, for medicine.

Medical Student with a Penchant for Rave

On return to England in 1991, I entered University College London and Middlesex Hospital School of Medicine. Situated in the centre of London, at that time the school was still rooted in its dusty past; with traditional professors teaching hands-on medical examination to tiers of students in oak-lined Victorian lecture theatres. We talked to patients and prodded for clinical signs of pathology amongst the rows of beds on vast hospital wards that have since been demolished or turned into luxury Bloomsbury flats. Studying to become a doctor was a dream come true. I dissected the human body and mind both literally and metaphorically throughout six years of medical training. This was coupled with the freedom of living in central London with other young people; playing in bands, partying and DJ-ing. The old-school-tie brigade of heavy drinking rugby songs, a staple of many medical students' experience through university, held little interest. And besides, I knew alcohol was overly toxic and cognitively impairing as an accompaniment to serious academic and philosophical studies. For me the raves continued between the lectures and clinical learning; no longer in fields, now in abandoned city basements and suburban warehouses. I didn't know anyone who arrived at a party without a bag of records in those days of the early 1990s.

Studying medicine is, of course, a deeply privileged pursuit. Countless hours were spent with my head in books in the Rockefeller Library at UCL; looked down upon by the bronze busts of the school's illustrious alumni. But it was the being alongside patients that I loved most; collecting their stories to elicit and unravel their symptoms. Employing physiological detective work, we assigned diagnoses and formulated bespoke management plans. Medicine became a craft, not a science. And as the years progressed I became more interested in my patients' recitations of their personal lives, their relationships, their wishes, failed desires, psychological pains and misfortunes than the broken bone or obstructed bowel that had put them in the bed before me.

In 1993 I took time out of medicine to complete an intercalated BSc in psychology, which meant studying all three years' worth of the degree course in a single year. The psychology department at UCL was a hot-bed of revolutionary anti-psychiatry and I loved it. Taught to question, if not entirely obliterate, the medical model, I hoovered up Tzasz, Illich, Cooper and Laing and developed a deep respect for psychotherapy. After qualifying as a psychology graduate I returned to complete the medical course; now armed with an understanding of how *not* to practice medicine. In the final years of the medical course I immersed myself in psychiatry; took on a psychotherapy patient as a member of the UCL student psychotherapy programme, attended extra-curricular neuropsychiatry clinics at Queens Square, and family therapy sessions at the Tavistock centre in Hampstead. Eventually, in 1997, I graduated as a medical doctor.

My first house job in general medicine was at Chase Farm in North London. Like my colleagues, I had just 48 hours to learn the essential tricks to survive as a junior doctor: How to cannulate and catheterise inaccessible veins and withered penises, how to write long streams of numbers shouted down a phone line without looking at the page and how to switch

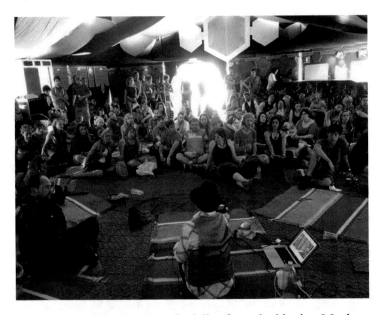

Picture 3: Learning about psychedelics from the hippies. Much more fun than talking to doctors. Presenting at Sunrise Festival, UK. Summer 2013. Photograph by James Jackman, hippie.

seamlessly between just three limited mental states: alert at work, asleep and extreme unwindingness. And then on to Stirling Royal Infirmary in Scotland for six months on a surgical team, where I absorbed the unique hospitality of the Scots and got even less sleep. Those years of raving had been good groundwork for life as a junior surgical house officer.

But I was now faced with making a decision about what branch of medicine I was going to follow for the rest of my career. My supervising surgical consultant made the decision for me. Reviewing one of my clerkings, he remarked on the scanty few lines I had used to describe the patient's presenting complaint (that of a gangrenous foot) in comparison to what was, in his view, the superfluous pages of writing dedicated to my patient's home life and relationships. "You," he said, "are going to be a psychiatrist. I suggest you go and get on with it." He was right. I decided to specialise in psychiatry. Besides, I always looked better in corduroy than scrubs.

Mind Over Matter

General medicine cannot compete with the infinitely more fascinating subject of studying the brain (which Woody Allen calls his second favourite organ). To me at that time physical medicine seemed too easy, mere mechanics; whether it be blockages to tubes, breakages to bones or even chemical and metabolic imbalances in the organs and tissues. Even pure neurology, which certainly piqued my interest at first, was not close enough to what I wanted to be studying. I felt that to be a neurologist was to be a masterful piano tuner, but never listen adequately to the music. No, the psychological world, and the human encounters its breakdown created, was the area that held the greatest appeal. Starting work as a junior psychiatrist at St. Luke's Hospital in Muswell Hill, North London, nothing else came close to the fascination of meeting people who had literally gone out of their minds.

Psychosis is always a big attraction for young psychiatrists, and initially I, like my trainee colleagues, thought this was the area in which I wanted to work. It is easy to be seduced by the curiosity of patients who believe their brain waves are transmitted to Venus by the CIA. But I soon found myself increasingly attracted to the plight of patients with anxiety and depression, and particularly those entrenched by earlier traumatic childhood experiences that had effectively stagnated their psychological development. Child abuse in all its forms cropped up again and again in almost every adult patient I met. I spoke to 90-year-olds who told me about their lifelong struggles with relationships that began with their abuse at three years old. Such memories had never left them and had coloured every aspect of their life since. It is well known how those crucial early months and years of bonding between baby and caregiver set the scene for attachment with others for the rest of one's life.

I began to see little point in administering treatments to sick adults without first understanding as much as possible about the beginnings of their pathologies, rooted in childhood where the personality itself forms. Every book I read, from Freud to Laing, alluded to it. So, after twelve years of studying medicine and psychiatry in London, I made the decision to return to Oxford to specialise in child and adolescent psychiatry. I believe every adult psychiatrist should work for at least five years as a child and adolescent psychiatrist. The developmental perspective of mental disorder one gains by doing so is invaluable for the work of any psychiatrist.

Throughout my general training, I became increasingly involved in studying the history of psychedelics in medicine. I read everything I could find on the subject and pestered my tutors incessantly for the benefit of their experience and wisdom. Alas, no one I asked could tell me about the potential for psychedelics as medical treatments. Some of the more wizened, bearded professors recalled a time when LSD gave a brief glow of light to clinical psychiatry in the 1950s and 1960s, but everything since then had been lost or forgotten. Whenever I picked up a psychiatric textbook I always went to the index to see what they had to say about psychedelic medicine. Most books had no mention at all. Some would say simply: 'LSD: Dangerous drug of abuse with no medical uses', or there might be a chapter on 'How to treat a medical emergency when someone has consumed a hallucinogen: Restrain the patient and inject with a high dose sedative'. It was all about the dangers, and never anything about the therapeutic potential of psychedelics.

Where Did All the Flowers Go?

But I knew from my private study that there was a rich history of psychedelic research and that these drugs could be used safely. I devoured papers by the British psychiatrist Ronald Sandison and books by the Czech psychiatrist and researcher Stanislav Grof. But these names never appeared in any of my mainstream texts and, of course, even the well-known Timothy Leary, who I had always appreciated foremost as a clinician, was never to be found in the medical sections of the bookshops I frequented, though he could be unearthed — together with Grof and Laing — on the philosophy, popular psychology or even religion shelves. Frustrated at what looked like a deliberate whitewash, an attempt to eradicate this fascinating piece of medical history, I made it my intention to educate my contemporary psychiatric colleagues about the role LSD had played, not merely as the drug that influenced 'flower-power', but as a vital part of mainstream psychiatry in the not-so-distant past. For a brief time in the early 1960s the medical profession truly believed psychedelics could be the next big thing in mental healthcare. I decided people needed to know about this part of our medical heritage.

Meanwhile, I was learning the trade of clinical psychiatry and frequently saw populations of patients for whom treatment with traditional methods was often ineffective. I diligently followed the evidence-based algorithms specified by the textbooks and the National Institute for Clinical Excellence (NICE) that stipulated treatments with this drug and that. Many interventions worked satisfactorily for a large proportion of people. But many others, no matter what drugs or psychotherapy we recommended, remained unable to connect with the cause of their problems, especially when it involved unresolved past trauma. Their ego and personality structures were too well defended, too strong for their own good to allow themselves to break through and stare their childhood traumas in the face.

I looked at what Sandison and Grof were saying about this kind of resistance. They had talked about the same population of patients I was meeting; people whose traumas were leaving them psychologically and existentially stuck. When LSD came along in the 1950s, these pioneering clinicians of their day had found, much to their surprise, that this peculiar new substance seemed to allow a special access to traumatic repressed memories. And, when combined with careful and diligent psychotherapy, the patient could be carried through the resistance to find some peace and resolution.

Ronald Sandison stumbled across LSD serendipitously while visiting the Sandoz laboratories in Basel in 1951. A year later he was giving his psychologically stuck patients the drug, alongside their traditional psychotherapy. He found LSD increased access to their repressed experiences, opening childhood memories, allowing the patients to explore traumatic events of their past and providing associated emotional release. Prior to being treated with LSD, many of Sandison's patients had been sidelined as hopeless cases, having had extensive electro-convulsive therapy (ECT), and destined for psychosurgery if LSD didn't work. Despite their previous treatment-resistance, LSD was a tool that enabled them to progress. The drug provided access to a unique mental state, the *non-ordinary state of consciousness*, that under the supervision of their doctor allowed traumatic material to be worked through in clear, waking consciousness. LSD produced in its users an intense flood of internal visual imagery, pictures in the mind's eye of both archetypal and highly personal recollections, a Technicolor route to the unconscious. Furthermore, there was often a spontaneously felt sense of divine experience that allowed for spiritual growth and self-realization.

Discovering the Lost History

Why, I wondered, had my profession turned its back on this apparently miraculous treatment? And why, forty years on, and with a dizzying pool of new medications available to the 21st century psychiatrist, were so many patients from my own caseload not progressing? I knew Leary and colleagues were now seen as quacks by the orthodox psychiatric community, but there were elements of their approach that attracted me and I wanted to bring their methods back into the spotlight.

At the same time as I was learning from the history of psychedelic medicine, I had also been following the beginnings of new research occurring in the States. In 1995 the Food and Drug Administration (an important American regulatory body that approves and monitors medical research) had granted permission for the first human study with a psychedelic drug since the 1970s[1]. Increasing numbers of aging psychiatrists were emerging from the shadows to support revisiting research into the drugs psilocybin and LSD. And an American organisation, The Multidisciplinary Association for Psychedelic Studies (MAPS), which had been set up in 1986 in the wake of the banning of MDMA, was now pushing vigorously for a new study to test MDMA's ability to assist trauma-focused psychotherapy[2]. All this looked like the verge of something new and vibrant in psychiatry, and a million miles away from the mainstream safety of my medical practice in Oxford.

I looked up Ronald Sandison and went to meet him several times at his home in Herefordshire. By now he was in his late 80s, and told me he was thrilled to learn that a UK psychiatrist was interested in taking up the mantle of psychedelic research which he had begun in this country half a century earlier. He showed me old photograph albums of suited doctors and formal-looking nurses dispensing LSD to patients in the 1950s[3]. Although Sandison's work had attracted some interest within the hippie community, until now no doctors had expressed an interest in rekindling his early research.

Turn On, Tune In and Disseminate

It was only a matter of time before I came across the Beckley Foundation and Amanda Feilding, who was conducting consciousness research from her rural setting near where I worked in Oxford[4]. Then in 2003, while still a trainee in child psychiatry, I wrote a brief report of what I had learned about this fascinating subject, which resulted in the first published paper about clinical psychedelic therapy in the British medical press since the 1960s[5].

What happened next took me by complete surprise. Some of my colleagues advised me against getting involved in this whacky subject, warning of 'career suicide'. They urged me instead to choose more mainstream research topics, such as antidepressant or antipsychotic drug therapies. In this context, I didn't expect much support for what I had written. But to my astonishment, on publication I made contact with a resonant community of people interested in psychedelics, and received invitations to talk at medical schools and academic gatherings up and down the country. I sent my paper to Albert Hofmann, the discoverer of LSD, who replied with a positive letter of support and a photograph of him with his wife. I had discovered a considerable network of non-medical psychedelic followers who, far from lying dormant, had been actively involved in propagating the message of these substances since the end of the sixties. But within British psychiatry I still felt like a lone voice — until, that is, I was contacted by two doctors from the Royal College of Psychiatrists Spirituality Special Interest Group, Nicky Crowley and Tim Read, both trainees of Stanislav Grof's transpersonal therapy. We put together a symposium for the college, entitled 'Psychosis, Psychedelics and the Transpersonal Journey', which was warmly received in 2006 and put me in touch with an even wider network of like-minded people[6]. This network was further expanded when I attended my first psychedelic conference in 2006, in celebration of Albert Hoffman's 100th birthday, in Basel.

Validation from Senior Figures

On finishing training in child psychiatry, I moved with my young family to rural Somerset to take up my first consultant post at an in-patient adolescent unit. I saw a steady stream of young people with, among other diagnoses, treatment-resistant post-traumatic stress disorder. Meanwhile, I continued to publish further peer reviewed editorials on psychedelics. Professor David Nutt, the respected national lead for psychopharmacology, read my papers and invited me to talk to his psychopharmacology unit at Bristol University. Nutt was challenging the British government to review the outdated classification scheme for illegal drugs that had been in place since 1971. He had just published an influential paper on the subject, which highlighted the relative safety of psychedelic drugs[7]. Encouraged by my risk-averse child psychiatry colleagues in Somerset to not continue publishing on psychedelics under their NHS trust's name, I joined Nutt's department as a research associate. Around this time the British government's Advisory Committee on the Misuse of Drugs (ACMD), which Professor Nutt chaired, was preparing a report about Ecstasy. David Nutt asked me to contribute on the therapeutic applications for MDMA. After extensive consultation with experts in the field, Nutt's 2009 publication of the ACMD review stated that, given its relative harm and safety profile, MDMA was inappropriately placed in Class A and ought to be moved to Class B of the Misuse of Drugs Act[8]. An overwhelming wealth of evidence, including the potential role for MDMA therapy, supported this outcome.

However, the British government distanced itself from the advice of its own committee. Professor Nutt objected to this blatant disregard of experts' unbiased opinions and subsequently published protestations in the scientific and popular press. In a semi-serious editorial he wrote about the dangers of *Equasy* — an addictive condition (horse riding). He reflected that Equasy is a legal risky pursuit enjoyed by approximately the same number of people who use Ecstasy every weekend. However, in comparison with Ecstasy use, Equasy is associated with approximately 350 times more deaths per year, thousands of cases of permanent brain damage and, of course, the release of a lot of environmentally harmful methane. Yet Equasy is legal and Ecstasy is not. 'Why is this?', asked David Nutt[9].

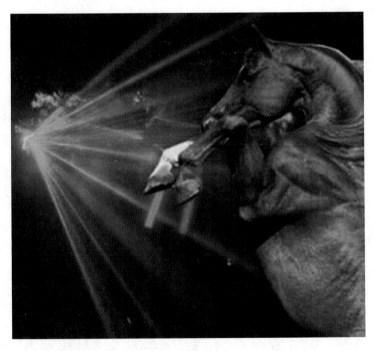

Picture 4: A Raving Horse. (Artist Unknown)

His efforts upset the British Home Secretary and resulted in him being sacked from chairmanship of the ACMD. In a published open letter, the Home Secretary, Alan Johnson, stated that the then Labour government objected to Nutt, 'lobbying for a change of government policy' and that, 'it is important that the government's public message on drugs is clear'[10]. Nutt rightly protested that the scientific, evidence-based truth *is* the clearest message for the public. Undeterred, David's sacking cemented his position with the media as a crusader who stood up to a government prepared to disrespect scientists who dared to clash with their pre-conceived, non-evidence-based, political agenda.

The camaraderie of David's loyal department in Bristol was tangible and I struck up a friendship with a young PhD student, Robin Carhart-Harris, whom I had first met a few years earlier at Hofmann's LSD conference in Basel. Carhart-Harris was planning the UK's first human psychedelic

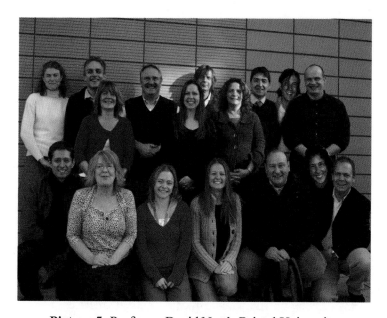

Picture 5: Professor David Nutt's Bristol University Psychopharmacology Unit in 2009. Left to right: Lindsay Sinclair, Ben Watson, Jayne Bailey, David Nutt, Alison Cobb, Neil Rich, Ann Rich, Simon Davies, Andreas Papadopoulos, Robin Tyacke, Robin Carhart-Harris, Sue Wilson, Claire Durant, Louise Paterson, Andrea Malizia and Jaci Paniker. It was an exciting moment of pioneering psilocybin research. Many of these scientists followed David to Imperial College London when he moved in 2010 and still work with him today.

drug trial since the sixties — and the first ever using the drug psilocybin, the active component in magic mushrooms. I got involved, helping as the study doctor with some of the sessions and co-authoring the paper[11]. But more excitingly, I agreed to be the first subject in the study, which meant that when David Nutt injected me with intravenous psilocybin in Clinic 17 at the Bristol Royal Infirmary in 2009, I became the first person in the UK to be legally given a psychedelic drug for over thirty years. We all knew it was a historic event that day, but as he plunged the syringe into my arm, I think David was more anxious than me[12].

Over the last twelve years I have immersed myself into this unique area of medical research and played a grateful part in many of the UK-based psychedelic research projects, either as a study doctor administering psychedelics to healthy volunteers and patients, or through volunteering as a healthy subject myself. Thus, I have had the marvellous opportunity to be given pure, clinical-grade LSD, psilocybin, ketamine, DMT and MDMA on various occasions, in a legal setting as part of studies exploring the mechanistic and clinical effects of these drugs. All in the name of science, of course.

Closure of the Past, Foundation for the Future and Acknowledgments to the many who have made it so much fun

Becoming part of the vibrant international community of psychedelic research has brought me close to a lot of influential figures through the years – many of whom have become good friends and are listed later in this book. In the last twelve years, since starting my academic and clinical interest in psychedelics, we have seen an explosion of psychedelic research throughout the world, which includes an impressive group of UK scholars and clinicians stretching in a line from UCL and Imperial College in London, through Bristol and on into Cardiff — not to mention the off-shore developments emerging on the Isle of Mann and on Guernsey.

Personally, I feel a great sense of closure in that my fringe interest in psychedelic drugs, which started, as for most people, with an eye-opening experience of wonder and awe, has now matured to connect so many aspects of my own personal history with my chosen profession. The psychological stuckness I see in many of my patients, just as Sandison had described, and my glimpse of the clinical potential of psychedelic therapy, are too much for me to disregard. As we steam ahead into the 21st century, psychiatry is desperately in need of a reawakening. Too many psychiatric disorders are unnecessarily labelled as 'treatment-resistant'. But the psychedelic therapies represent a new way of working alongside patients ensnared in intractable psychological conditions. Furthermore, developments in modern techniques for neuroimaging that provide not only an anatomical picture of the brain, but also a real-time demonstration of its functional workings, have transformed psychiatry into a cutting-edge field of medicine and neuroscience. Today we have tools in contemporary brain science that were undreamt of in the 1960s when psychiatrists first discovered the psychedelics. These technologies provide a tremendous opportunity to revisit those studies of the 1950s and 1960s with new eyes.

I am currently in the fortunate position of taking three years out of full-time clinical work to concentrate primarily on psychedelic research. As part of my work at Imperial College London, under the supervision of David Nutt, I am putting together two UK-based MDMA studies; one in Cardiff using fMRI neuroimaging in patients with PTSD and one in Bristol using MDMA-assisted psychotherapy as a treatment for alcohol dependence. I am gratefully indebted to the generosity of the funder who has made this work possible and fully intend to use these years to progress the subject. I have a determination to see psychedelic drugs researched as potential developments for clinical practice.

Despite my personal and evidence-based clinical conviction about the potential value of psychedelic drugs, those of us in the field are acutely aware that a large portion of the general public still consider this subject deeply controversial. An important part of the future of psychedelic research, therefore, involves providing medical education on psychedelics to the new generation of doctors, other healthcare professionals and the public at wide. In view of this, in 2015 I published (with the Royal College of Psychiatrists) a teaching module on psychedelic medicine[13]. Trainee doctors can now access these materials and learn about the history and practice of clinical research in this field, and we continue to use the media wisely to disseminate to the public the overwhelming safety and benefits profile of psychedelic drugs.

Above all it is my patients' plights that continue to drive my practice. Post Traumatic Stress Disorder (PTSD), which arises from psychological trauma and haunts the sufferer thereafter, is a devastating condition. Its prevalence is rising following the recent wars in Iraq, Afghanistan and Syria. I have seen too many valuable people lose their battles with PTSD and take their lives because of psychiatry's inability to provide an effective intervention for their trauma. Similarly, in my work as an addictions psychiatrist I understand how feeble our current treatments are for those patients trapped in a cycle of substance misuse. Addiction arises primarily not from a simple dependence on drugs, which are best seen as a catalyst. Rather, the difference between drug use and drug misuse comes from the preceding psychological and social distress of people whose childhood memories and ongoing social environment is intolerable. This is a well-established fact for those of us in the field. It was illustrated beautifully by the famous 'Rat Park' experiments of the late 1970s carried out by Bruce Alexander. Alexander demonstrated that when rats are kept in cramped, unnatural conditions in small cages they tended to self-administer with the drugs provided and display all the signs of dependence. But when they were free to roam, play, and, crucially, have sex with other rats, they showed little interest in taking drugs[14]. So, addiction is a complex field. But at the heart of it is rigidity. Our patients' inability to break out of the stuckness traps them into a cycle of abuse.

Psychedelic drug therapies offer addicts a new approach to tackling the rigid personality traits that maintain their addictions. This is the cutting edge of modern psychiatric research. And an area, perhaps more so than anywhere else in medicine, where innovative approaches are in desperate need. Even with the best current treatments the rates of relapse of alcohol, cocaine, nicotine and opiate dependence are staggeringly high. If psychedelics can inform our practice of addictions, then this is vital research that needs to happen without delay.

The psychedelic drugs are not a panacea, and not without their risks. But I truly believe they represent an extra level of treatment that can be safely harnessed to help people who are unable to make progress with established forms of therapy. And that potential should not be ignored.

Undreamt of Possibilities for Therapy

In London in 1938, a year before his death, and the same year Hofmann first synthesised LSD, Sigmund Freud wrote:

> The future may teach us how to exercise a direct influence, by means of particular chemical substances, upon . . . the neural apparatus. It may be that there are other still undreamt of possibilities of therapy[15].

Freud was a neurologist prior to developing modern science's first systematic approach to the psychology of the unconscious. I believe, had he known about them, he might have been a supporter of psychedelic therapies; recognising the vital marriage between psychotherapy and psychopharmacology, utilising a physical approach to directly improve his 'talking therapy'.

There remain barriers to the acceptance of this concept. A cornerstone narrative of psychotherapy is that it is supposed to be hard work and lengthy. Drugs offering a quick fix or an easy pathway are deemed wrong. Carl Jung, who did not die until 1961, certainly knew about psychedelics, particularly mescaline and, later, LSD. But he rejected them, saying the flood of repressed material in psychoanalysis was already sufficiently fast, and there was no need to increase it with drugs. It is ironic then, in my opinion, how warmly Jung is embraced for his theory of the collective unconscious (and Freud is rejected) by so many in the psychedelic community. This dogma — that psychotherapy ought to be delivered only to the sober patient — has persisted.

I wonder to what extent traditional psychotherapy is a legacy of traditional Christian values that tell us there is something inherently wrong or immoral about the intoxicated state? As we shall see in later chapters, we in the West are obsessed with being in control and, with traditional psychotherapy, assume access to the unconscious is best achieved only with an abstemious brain. But this emphasis on consciousness control is a culturally bound phenomenon, dependent on one's geography and specific to consumerist modernity. It is merely a matter of opinion and certainly worth challenging if we are to explore all facets of the human experience.

Indeed, there are many misconceptions to be challenged. It is *not* career suicide to do this work (as some of my more risk aversive colleagues warned me as a junior doctor entering the field of psychedelic medicine), but rather a ticket to an exciting future in clinical research. Psychedelic medicine may be considered an offbeat subject to those people unable to detach themselves from the stereotypical images of stoned hippies at Woodstock. But for neuroscientists at the world's leading research organisations, psychedelic drugs can no longer be ignored. They are increasingly recognised as important tools to further our understanding of the brain. I encourage any young and enthusiastic clinician or researcher to enter this field, which is an important part of the future of psychiatry.

CHAPTER 2

The Experience and the Drugs

Why Do They Do It and What's It Like?

What does a psychedelic experience feel like? This is a difficult question to answer — especially given that the experience itself is, by definition, ineffable. And why do people want to do it? The answer to this is, perhaps, easier to define, and is associated with an individual's and society's needs. After all, one person's cognitive impairment is another person's party[1]. There will always be good reasons for leaving all *this* behind and taking a sideways glimpse at life. Why limit oneself to just one normal waking state of consciousness? Many worthy commentators consider it highly irresponsible for a person *not* to experience the psychedelic state; as grave a mistake as limiting oneself only to jazz or rock and not even daring to listen to rap, opera or dubstep. (OK, granted, one can probably do without dubstep.)

Many artists, poets, musicians and literary folk, far more erudite than I, have attempted to describe the psychedelic experience and failed, so I will not venture an aesthetic appreciation of it here. Besides, I could probably play it better on the trumpet better than I could explain it in words.

Personally, I like Ford Prefect's description of another ineffable experience, hyperspace travel, to his friend Arthur Dent in *The Hitchhiker's Guide to the Galaxy*:[2]

Prefect: You should prepare yourself for the jump into hyperspace; it's unpleasantly like being drunk.
Arthur: What's so unpleasant about being drunk?
Ford: Just ask a glass of water.

Nothing can prepare one for an experience that defies definition. One can read sentences like 'one becomes the essence of nature itself' or 'one becomes in touch with every living, breathing cell in the universe' but what on earth (or elsewhere) does that even mean?

Many researchers and voyagers have tried to develop systematic schemes for describing the psychedelic experience. Psychiatric phenomenology provides a number of central defining features of the experience, listed below. And although no descriptions come close to understanding what it actually *feels* like, the medical model demands that we at least try to know what one might expect to occur after ingesting a 'classical' psychedelic drug:

1. Physiological effects:

Most classical psychedelics do very little physiologically; mild fluctuations in pulse, blood pressure and dilatation of the pupils are about all one can expect. MDMA is slightly different, with notable bodily changes. But essentially, the LSD experience is a *mental* experience. However, intense mental experiences can have *very* physical implications. For example, after ingesting LSD you can *imagine* that your heart has left your body or that your brain is physically leaking. It isn't, of course, but it may feel so. Tim Leary provides an excellent description of this phenomena in his book *High Priest*, as he experienced a trip vicariously through a dog, in February 1961[3].

2. Heightening or distortion of perceptions in all sensory modalities:

Sounds and colours appear more vivid. The corners of the room no longer meet at right angles. The walls undulate and breathe; flowing with magnificent liquidity. Objects have an iridescent halo and everything pulsates as if alive. Tactile sensations are heightened so that a massage on the skin's surface feels as if the bare bones themselves are being palpated. Furthermore, sensory perceptions do not stay neatly in the modality in which they ought to belong. Sights become sounds. I have had the experience on LSD, for example, of a red flower giving a different tone of a ringing bell than a blue flower. This phenomenon, called synaesthesia, was employed by Owsley Stanley, The Grateful Dead's sound engineer and LSD chemist, who could see the waves of sound flowing across the stage and so knew best where to position the band's speakers[4].

3. Altered sense of space and time:

Time can move forwards, backwards or stay still. A lifetime can be lived watching the ignition of a match, or six hours can pass with a turn of the head. Boundaries waver and dissolve, eventually disappearing altogether. One's hand can be ten thousand miles away from one's face and then all at once one is standing on the silvery surface of a grain of sand. Identity and sense of self dissolves. Clothes are meaningless, amusing rags, as are the skin, the bones, organs and brain. Existence becomes simply a thought, a notion. Along with this, systems of politics and social hierarchies are obliterated, prompting novel observations and new directions for thought.

4. Emergent Emotional Material and Memories:

Every experience one has ever had is available for scrutiny. The entirety of one's past is recorded, stored and waiting to get out. Under the influence of the psychedelic, as in dreams, the emergent material may not present in an obvious form, but rather as a display of latent and abstract images. Rapid fluctuation of thoughts and emotions might link the past experiences with the here and now. Through practiced psychotherapy with a skilled facilitator, this material can provide opportunities for self-discovery.

5. Increased sensitivity to the feelings of others:

The high dose psychedelic experience can undoubtedly be harrowing, characterised by traumatic death-rebirth phenomena as described by Stanislav Grof or Christopher Bache. But at lower doses there is usually an inherent peacefulness to the psychedelic state. This is certainly the case with MDMA, in which many users describe intense feelings of closeness to other people and an enhanced understanding of others' points of view. Empathy is one of the major therapeutic aspects of clinical MDMA. So too, with LSD, which was dubbed 'the love drug' in its day, and became for the hippie generation a validation of a peaceful way of life. However, as Stan Grof describes them, psychedelics are 'non-specific amplifiers', such that any emotion, good or bad, benign or destructive, can be magnified to dramatic proportions.

6. Religious or spiritual experience:

The spiritual aspects of the psychedelic experience have been studied extensively and will be revisited throughout this book. Psychedelic drugs undeniably induce feelings of connectivity accompanied by an otherworldliness. Psychedelic spirituality has been tested empirically on numerous occasions, from Walter Pahnke's famous Marsh Chapel Experiment in 1963 to Roland Griffiths' psilocybin studies, starting in 2006[5,6]. The role that various psychedelics have played in the formation of most of the world's religions is well documented.

7. Being at one with the universe:

Often called 'oceanic boundlessness', psychedelics can induce the experience of expansion beyond the traditional boundaries of personhood. One no longer defines oneself as simply a doctor, a father or mother, a husband or wife, a friend, neighbour or citizen; rather, one is a leaf on a tree, a drop of water in a lake, a breath on the wind. One can feel part of a plethora of vibrating energy moving like electricity through all things, stretching back in time to the very origin of the universe. Paradoxically (to the rational mind), one may be simultaneously as large as the universe and as small as the most elemental particle: everywhere and nowhere, inside and outside, alive and dead. Timothy Leary described the psychedelic trip as a cellular experience that connects us consciously with our DNA, allowing an 'upload' of information from inherited genetic 'databanks' in order to relive memories of our ancestors[7]. Leary believed information encoded in DNA's double-helix goes right back to the earliest amoebas swimming in a cosmic primordial soup, and that consuming LSD taps into this intergenerational connectivity. With our present knowledge about DNA, Leary's theory — though beautiful — is conjecture rather than science. But it is intuitively attractive and Grof's research presents a similar view, as does Terence McKenna's description of his 'hyperspace', in which all space and time are stored and accessible through the use of psychedelics[8].

8. Psychotic/delirious changes:

To many readers, much of the above may sound mad, incomprehensible and confusing. Maybe the entire psychedelic state is pure suggestibility or merely delusion, illusion and hallucination? A dangerous organic psychosis with no meaningful value, and certainly not at all therapeutic — especially for someone with a pre-existing mental illness. However, someone else may say the same about the rigid values and social structures we blindly follow, which to many appear equally mindless and ill-thought-through.

There is no doubting that the misuse of psychedelic drugs can cause harm (by definition). The psychedelic experience can certainly be frightening and disorientating for ill-prepared users. Feelings of panic and losing control can become overwhelming. For some people with pre-existing mental illness, especially those with psychosis, psychedelic use can trigger severe reactions. The concept of the 'bad trip' is well documented by both users and non-users of psychedelics. The issues that increase or decrease the likelihood of having a good or a bad trip are discussed in greater detail in coming chapters.

As a Neuroscientist, What Does All This Mean?

With all the diversity and range described above, one thing is for certain: the psychedelic experience gives one an entirely new way of looking at

THE EXPERIENCE AND THE DRUGS 29

the day. From a neuro-scientific point of view, what interests me is that imbibing a drug like LSD makes one at least *think* these peculiar, abnormal experiences are happening. And this reveals to us something fascinating about the brain. If instead of simply dismissing these experiences as illusions we take care to explore, map and understand the neural and personal roots of such an experience then they may have real therapeutic value.

An impressive attempt at describing the qualities of the classical psychedelic experience comes from Professor William Richards and Walter Pahnke in their 1966 paper 'Implications of LSD and Experimental Mysticism'[9]. Bill, who, from his position as senior psychologist at Johns Hopkins Bayview Medical Center, Baltimore, remains at the forefront of psychedelic research today, described the following features of the psychedelic state:

1. **Unity**: The sense of merger: Inside merges with outside, self merges with others, the Earth merges with the universe and so forth.
2. **Objectivity and reality**: One's existence is genuine and valid. For the duration of the experience one can reliably answer that eternal question 'What am I?' with great lucidity.
3. **Transcendence of space and time**: Losing the sense of physical boundaries, one's ego and one's place in time. Time and space become meaningless 'games' (as Leary called them), laughable distractions, as one merges with a wholeness greater than one's self.
4. **Sense of sacredness**: Being overwhelmed by feelings of awe and reverence, one is standing in 'the *white light* of absolute purity'. Such experiences shed light on the links between psychedelics and the historical development of religion.
5. **Deeply felt positive mood**: Euphoria, delight, rapture and sensual love. The psychedelic experience is a Maslowian peak experience; a life-transforming ultimate soaring through unbridled pastures of joyous ecstasy. Sound good?
6. **Paradoxicality**: My favourite on Bill's list, this describes peculiarly illogical states of contradictory thinking: 'I am everywhere and I am nowhere!' 'I am inside and I am outside!' 'I am an amoeba, I am the universe!' Such paradoxes make sense under the influence of a psychedelic drug.
7. **Alleged ineffability**: It cannot be described. It can only be known. One of those cruel twists of fate that polarises people into those who have and those who haven't. As Hendrix said: 'Are You Experienced?'[10]
8. **Transiency**: A sacred glimpse of the other world, after which one must return back to the normality of one's ordinary state of consciousness.

9. **Positive changes in attitude and/or behaviour:** An important aspect of the experience. Because although ineffable, transient and illogical, the psychedelic state can provide real and lasting positive developmental change for an individual.

The Importance of Set and Setting

During the Western world's experiments with psychedelics in the 1950s it became crystal clear that the totality of the user's psychedelic experience encompasses more than merely the choice of drug used or the dosage taken. Different laboratories and researchers produced wildly varying responses for the same chemicals, reasons for which seem obvious to us now. The essential concepts of 'set and setting', are coined by Leary in the 1964 book *The Psychedelic Experience*, where set refers to the user's mindset, and setting refers to the environment in which the drug is taken. Earlier psychonauts were aware of these influences, and engineered supportive environments and expectations accordingly; however the lack of connection of the clinical world with a living 'psychedelic community', and the emergence of LSD as a brand new substance, meant age old lessons had to be learnt anew.

Set includes a whole range of cultural attitudes, beliefs and expectations about what will happen. This includes whether the users bring religious expectations, their prior experience of a particular drug, what they have heard from others, what the media tells them and what they know of the drug's physiological effects. The user's preconceived mindset will influence and be influenced by their fears and fantasies about what might happen and what they wish to gain by taking the drug.

Setting includes the physical environment in which the drug is taken, including who users are with at the time, what music is played (if any), whether they know the place, how hot or cold they are, how physically active or recumbent they are during the session, whether they have things to do the next day and even broader issues such as what the social climate and attitude towards drugs is, in the environment in which they take them.

Set and setting have an important effect on the overall outcome of the psychedelic experience and they must never be disregarded. When one hears horror stories of 'bad trips' it is invariably because of a lack of attention paid to set and setting.

Much has been written and spoken about what are the best conditions for a psychedelic experience. Leary, Alpert and Metzner's *The Psychedelic Experience* of 1964, which uses the framework of *The Tibetan Book of The Dead*, provides many useful tips on how to pay attention to both the right

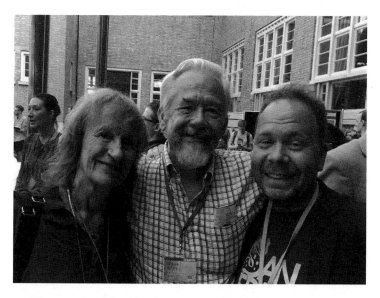

Picture 6: With Bill Richards and Amanda Feilding at the International Conference on Psychedelic Research, Amsterdam, June 2016.

mind-set and the physical settings to achieve the best outcomes for a psychedelic trip[11]. Countless writers have since expanded on getting the conditions just right. As a result, a certain clichéd genre surrounds psychedelic use that has, in my opinion, become familiar and, at times, overly rigid. The usual trappings of ethereal music and soft furnishing over which one can lounge are inevitable props but not all users are going to feel most at ease surrounded by Indian print throws and incense sticks. However, many users will say these props are genuinely helpful, as they provide external stimuli which matches their internal mental state. Similarly, many people choose to take psychedelic drugs outside in the countryside, or in city parks, surrounded by nature in order to emphasise their felt connection with the Earth.

Careful Planning, Due Care and Attention

The uniting feature of these settings is that the user must feel safe, free to express themselves and contained. Feeling unfettered by the annoying interruptions of everyday life is essential. Mobile phones or any other connections with the outside world are generally best avoided.

How to Take LSD Safely

It is important to engender a positive mindset before setting out on the trip. This is the case not just for the recreational use of these substances, but also when they are used medically. Indeed, it is something that all psychedelic researchers do. After all, when you go to your family doctor and she gives you a course of antibiotics, obviously she doesn't do so in a malicious or hopeless manner. You would not leave her consulting room believing the drugs she gave you may cause you harm or even kill you.

Similarly, if you take a drug like LSD without preparation and with the preconceived belief that it will cause you harm or ruin your life (a message one might get from the media) then the chances are you *will* have a miserable time. But if you have prepared well and take the drug in a relaxed and comfortable setting among people close to you who you trust, then not only are you very unlikely to come to any harm but you are also giving yourself the best opportunity to have a deeply profound experience. Indeed, when a drug such as LSD or psilocybin is taken safely and judiciously, there is every possibility it will be one of the most profound and meaningful experiences of your life.

In exploring psychedelics as clinical tools, the concepts of set and setting ought not be mere luxurious added extras or simple confounders. Rather, they are an active part of the experimental intention. The totality of the psychedelic experience is a combination of pharmacological and psychological factors interacting together in a synergistic fashion; set and setting are essential components of the psychedelic experience that *must* be attended to, in order to achieve a maximum positive response.

Personal Opinion, Matter of Judgment and Disclaimer

Before I go any further, at this point in the book I want to be clear that I am not encouraging, supporting or condoning anyone reading this text who intends to go out and take drugs, especially if that means breaking the law and even more so if one suffers with any serious medical condition, including a personal or family history of severe mental illness. But what I am clear about is that if people are going to choose to use psychedelic drugs, then I urge them to do so with care. I am staunchly opposed to drug prohibition. The 'Just Say No' campaign is ineffective. Frankly, it is a waste of breath to tell someone 'don't take drugs' (I tell my son Huxley, daily, to 'tidy your room'. It does no good). Information is the essential feature people need to stay safe, and I will be pleased if this book can give people the necessary facts to minimize the potential harm of drug use. In later chapters, we will come back to the concept of harm minimization versus total prohibition and discuss these in the context of the War On Drugs. But for the time being the most important message is *Just Say Know to Drugs*.

Personally, as both a brain scientist and someone with a personal interest in the expansive capabilities of my own brain, I would feel it would be a disservice to my life's experience to disregard non-ordinary states of consciousness. Psychedelic drugs *can* be dangerous. Albert Hofmann — the discoverer of LSD and a proponent of its use throughout his very long life (he lived healthily to 102 years old) — was not shy of saying this[12]. These are immensely potent substances and they ought not be used lightly. But the actual rates of morbidity and mortality from psychedelic use are very low indeed. With due care and attention they can be used safely and be life-enhancing. Don't take my word for it, listen to the testimonies of the hundreds of millions of people who would tell you the same thing — if only they could put into words the ineffable nature of their experience.

Embracing the Challenge

The high-dose psychedelic experience is difficult, even gut-wrenching at times (often literally when one comes to ayahuasca). It is necessarily so. But what, I ask, is wrong with a little hardship? Take the analogy of climbing a mountain or running a marathon. It would be foolhardy to attempt these pursuits without preparation and care. Indeed, many hours of practising, training and exercise are required to climb mountains properly. One must go into the activity with a positive mind-set, be surrounded by skilled guides, trusted friends and stable conditions. Even with adequate preparation, once the marathon or climb is underway it will be difficult. Sometimes it will be exhilarating and euphoric; at other times it will be painful and challenging. But once one has reached the end of the race or climbed the mountain and come safely down the other side, one is full of the joys of life, proud of one's momentous and life-changing accomplishment. Nobody says 'don't climb mountains or run marathons' simply because they are difficult. Rather we caution them to do it with care, and allow (or even legislate for, in cases of officially organised events) provision of useful tools and advice.

Critics of this analogy might question comparing the 'natural' experience of rock climbing or running, with the 'unnatural' and seemingly indulgent easy-going drug-taking antics of a LSD user. Well, firstly, who says psychedelic drugs are unnatural? And secondly, there is nothing *easy* about navigating an experience on 300 micrograms of LSD. Our Western world's ingrained narrative that there is something inherently wrong or immoral about non-ordinary states of consciousness must be challenged. Why is playing golf or watching opera any more natural than eating fresh mushrooms one has just picked off a rainy Welsh hillside?

But as Donovan said in 1967: 'Don't do it if you don't want to, I wouldn't do a thing like that, oh no!'[13]

The Drugs Themselves

Classifying the Psychedelic Drugs

There are several ways of classifying and organising the wide variety of substances available. The range of drugs I will cover in this section is not by any means exhaustive. Indeed, I will not be exploring in depth the ever-growing list

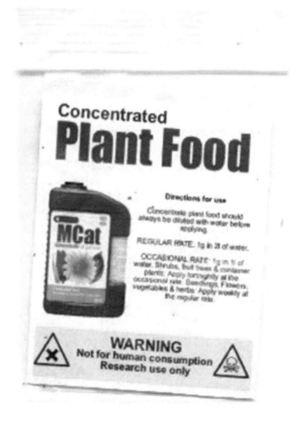

Picture 7: M-CAT. Originally sold literally as plant food. I bought some in 2007 when it was still legal and put it on my plants. The cacti loved it.

of *Research Chemicals* (RCs), new ones of which seem to appear for sale on the internet daily or, until recently, in Legal Highs in shops up and down the land, that is until the 2016 Psychoactive Substances Act pushed their sales into the black market. Through the darknet all drugs can be easily bought online. There is a growing subculture of self-confessed drug geeks, who swap their stories of internal voyages on an exponentially expanding forum of experiential drug blogs.[14] The RCs and all the political and pharmacological wrangling that go with them could constitute a volume of their own, so instead I will limit my lists to the more commonly known psychedelic drugs. Furthermore, most of the newly emerging RC drugs — some of which may certainly prove to be of clinical value in the future — are currently too much of an unknown quantity to be considered for research studies.

Most of the RCs, including the most well known in the UK, the cathinone mephedrone (M-CAT, 'plant food' or 'meow meow') have barely received even the most basic phase-one toxicology studies and in that respect, must be considered unsafe until more is known about their modes of action and effects on the human body. My advice is to steer clear of untested products. We have 60 years of reliable data on LSD, 25 years of toxicity data on MDMA and thousands of years knowledge of cannabis. One should be wary of something cooked up only last week in a test tube.

The Legal High that has caused the most problems in recent years is, ironically, not one that mimics stimulant or psychedelic drugs, but rather the group of synthetic cannabinoids, often referred to by brand names such as 'Spice'. Spice and its like are increasingly causing problems. Spice casualties are appearing in substance misuse services and particularly prisons. The fact that legal 'cannabis' (it is actually not at all like cannabis in either its effects or toxicity profiles) is causing so much trouble is, to me, the clearest example of the stupidity of the War On Drugs. Young people, scared of the illegality of cannabis, are choosing instead to dose themselves with highly potent Spice and thus are often experiencing psychoses and physical health problems that are rarely associated with natural cannabis. This is a situation in urgent need of reform — and one that will not be solved by simply banning the synthetic cannabinoids.

We must not demonise the skilled and diligent chemists who can teach us a lot about the possibilities for continued psychoactive cookery. For the most comprehensive guide to just about every psychedelic chemical conceivable, I direct readers to the late chemist Dr Alexander 'Sasha' Shulgin's two books *Pihkal* (*Phenethylamines I Have Known and Loved*)[15] and *Tihkal* (*Tryptamines I Have Known and Loved*)[16]. These treasure-troves of psychedelic cuisine describe the psychoactive effects and the chemical construction of hundreds of substances from the very common to the purely conceptual. In his books, which are co-authored by his wife, Ann Shulgin, alongside his recipes Sasha also tells some beautifully written stories about the last 50 years of psychedelic history. He has been dubbed 'the grandfather of MDMA' and was a much-loved figure in the psychedelic world. I will return to Sasha and his story later in this book.

Sticking, therefore, to the more common psychedelic substances, they can be organised according to their chemical structure or to their effects.

The 'Classical' Psychedelics

LSD, Psilocybin, Dimethyltryptamine (DMT) and Mescaline.

The Entactogens or Empathogens

MDMA, MDA, 2-CB, 2C-I, 2C-T-7 etc.

The NMDA-antagonist Dissociatives

Ketamine, Methoxetamine, PCP, DXM and Nitrous Oxide.

The Kappa-Opioid Agonist Dissociatives

Ibogaine and *Salvia divinorum*.

We could also classify the same drugs into groups depending on their chemical structure. Most of the common psychedelics fall into one of two distinct groups. There are those whose chemical structure is based around the tryptamine molecule, and those that are based around phenethylamine.

Tryptamines (or those psychedelic drugs closely related to it):
LSD, Psilocybin, DMT, Ibogaine, 5-MEO-DMT and Bufotenin.

Phenethylamines:
MDMA, Mescaline, MDA, 2C-B, 2C-I, 2C-T-4, 2C-T-7 etc.

Close relatives of both tryptamine and phenethylamine are found in their natural states in our brains, which have lead some scholars to suggest the presence of endogenous psychedelic chemicals might account for non-drug induced mystical experiences. For example, the common and immensely important neurotransmitter 5-hydroxytryptamine (also called serotonin or 5-HT) is a base tryptamine molecule plus an extra oxygen molecule in the fifth position of the benzene ring. And the immensely potent psychedelic substance dimethyltryptamine (DMT) is simply the same tryptamine structure but with two extra carbons atoms instead of the oxygen. Both are extremely close to tryptamine structurally, but the effects on the brain between the two substances could not be more dramatic.

Pineal Insufficiencies and Psychedelic Spirituality Pseudoscience?

There exist many theories that endogenous psychedelic drugs — particularly DMT — are released at times of intense, non-drug-induced religious, mystical or near death experiences. This is a fascinating possibility and makes sense intuitively. Some people within the psychedelic community postulate that the pineal gland is the site in the human brain where natural DMT is produced and released. This theory was made popular by Rick Strassman's work on DMT, whose year 2000 book *The Spirit Molecule* has been widely embraced[17]. My own take on this theory is that the pineal gland — whilst often idolised as a 'mysterious spirit gland' is, in fact, not the least bit mysterious. We have good scientific understanding of how the pineal gland works. It regulates wakefulness in response to light via the synthesis and secretion of the hormone melatonin.

I was delighted to find I share similar opinions about the pineal gland with the renowned psychedelic chemist David E. Nichols. During a long car journey together we reflected that the pineal gland is simply too small, with an insufficient throughput of serotonin, to produce sufficient amounts of DMT required (in the 7–30mg range) necessary for a psychedelic effect. This makes the little pineal a most unlikely site for production of

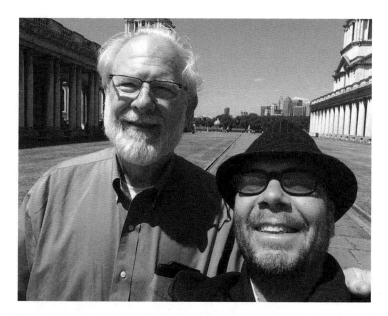

Picture 8: The chemist David E. Nichols. Side-chain sorcerer and molecular manipulator of mystical materials. Greenwich, London, Summer 2015.

endogenous DMT. If an endogenous psychedelic *were* being produced in the pineal from serotonin it would have to be far more potent than DMT; more like LSD, which works at the microgram dosage. Now, LSD is also a tryptamine psychedelic and could, theoretically, be synthesised from serotonin (via many other complex chemical processes), but there are no known mechanisms that have been elucidated to suggest this is happening or even *can* happen within the pineal gland.

However, there are other areas of the body — the gut and the lungs for instance — that contain far higher concentrations of serotonin, and are therefore better placed than the pineal to synthesize sufficient quantities of DMT. One scientist who is pursuing the lungs as a potential site for DMT synthesis is Ede Frecska, a psychiatrist at the University of Debrecen in Hungary. He is one of many whom believe endogenous DMT plays an important physiological role in protecting the brain against oxidative stress (e.g. hypoxia, lack of oxygen). Frecska and others hypothesise that DMT has the potential to extend the survival of the brain in clinical death. Frecska's goal is to have DMT ampoules for intravenous use on the crash trolleys of emergency vehicles, intensive care units and operating rooms, in order that it can be used to save the brain from unnecessarily severe damage, or indeed death, during hypoxic crises[18].

Nevertheless, the idea of the pineal gland as the spiritual centre of the human soul persists for many in the psychedelic community. Certainly, the lungs and gut lack the romantic qualities assigned to the pineal gland, which is seen by many as spiritual simply because it happens to fall anatomically within the same place in the brain where certain religions have assigned a 'chakra' point. (Something had to fall in that spot, assigned many thousands of years ago and well before we had any reasonable understanding of neuroanatomy. It could easily have been some other insignificant gland mediating, for example, bladder emptying). But many people like the fact that the pineal's position, deep within the brain in the midline, can be romantically regarded as a source of energy-rich vibrations. This 'pineal debate', whilst interesting as a cultural meme, is, I believe, a good example of psychedelic enthusiastic pseudoscience — of which there is plenty in this field.

Some Common Psychedelic Substances in More Detail

1. LSD

Of the group we call the classical psychedelics, undoubtedly the daddy, or mother perhaps, is lysergic acid diethylamide (LSD-25). Whether a fan of psychedelics or not, one must respect LSD for so many reasons: the way it was discovered, the incredible effect it has had on culture in the last 60 years, or simply its pharmacology.

Pharmacology of LSD

The compound has a plasma half-life of around five hours, and the experience lasts for between six and twelve hours, with some 'afterglow' effects often felt for several days. Comparing the short half-life against the lengthy subjective effects suggests LSD may trigger a central psychological reaction that self-perpetuates long after the chemical itself has degraded.

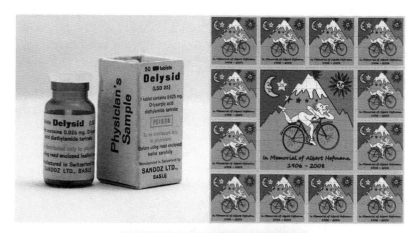

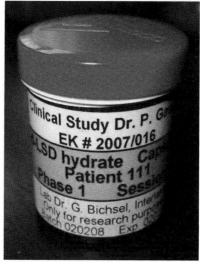

Picture 9: LSD: In its original, illicit and renaissance forms.

As described, the felt experience is highly dependent on set and setting. A user may take a given dose in a certain setting and feel virtually nothing, then take the same dose under different conditions and have an immensely strong experience. Multiple non-pharmacological factors contribute to the overall psychedelic experience.

The main psychedelic effects of LSD relate primarily to its role as a partial agonist at 5-HT2A receptors in the layer IV pyramidal cells of the cerebral cortex[19]. The exact mode of action — how this effect causes the extraordinary mental experiences that occur — is increasingly understood with contemporary studies, about which we will hear more later.

Aldous Huxley, in his description of the effects of mescaline and LSD, talked of the so-called 'reducing valve hypothesis', which he borrowed from the French philosopher, Henri Bergson, who proposed the concept of the brain as a 'reducing valve' in 1919[20]. Huxley suggested that psychedelics work by inhibiting the brain's natural role of filtering out a large proportion of the actual perceptual stimuli from the environment.[21] In other words, whilst our brains strive to intentionally present only a small fraction of the external material to our normal consciousness, psychedelics inhibit this process. As Huxley put it in *The Doors of Perception*:

> *The function of the brain and nervous system is to protect us from being over-whelmed and confused by this mass of largely useless and irrelevant knowledge, by shutting out most of what we should otherwise perceive or remember at any moment, and leaving only that very small and special selection which is likely to be practically useful.*

Huxley suggested that under the influence of mescaline or LSD this mechanism is switched off and we are treated to an overwhelming cacophony of sights, sounds and feelings — all of which are 'out there', but which we do not normally get the chance to experience.

Huxley was not a neuroscientist. Nevertheless, contemporary studies show that in some respects he was not far off the mark. Recent research on LSD and psilocybin by Robin Carhart-Harris at Imperial College London has demonstrated that the classical psychedelics do indeed 'turn off a valve' — but in a markedly different way than that proposed by Huxley[22]. Carhart-Harris' functional MRI scans of healthy controls injected with psilocybin demonstrate a *reduction* in cerebral blood flow, reduced glucose and oxygen consumption and an overall *decrease* in functional brain activity. This suggests that, rather than psychedelics 'expanding' our minds with an increased experience of external perceptions, the brain is put into a 'starvation state'. In this condition, it may be that, without the internal reducing valve, the external flood of perceptual information is allowed into our conscious awareness unchecked, thus presenting a kaleidoscopic display of 'what is really out there'. Or it may be that when the brain is shut down under psychedelics, we *lack* sufficient external information coming in, so instead are treated to a kaleidoscopic display of *internal* imagery, with all our top-down memories of the past no longer held back and free to fill our awareness. One way or the other, we certainly experience life as 'if the doors of perception were cleansed'.

The latter suggestion — that psychedelics block out the external world and leave us at the mercy of our internal world — feels more intuitively correct. One assumes the brain requires more, not less energy to process external material. Our brains use energy to keep the real world out. So psychedelics don't actually 'expand our minds' to the outside world. On the contrary, they temporarily *shrink* our ability to absorb information from the external world. This is not something that many psychedelic enthusiasts want to hear. Trippers typically like to believe that the dynamic movements of the breathing rocks and trees provides validation of a universal, living energy force alive in the external world and only glimpsed with the sacramental LSD. Unfortunately, contemporary research suggests this is not the case. The energy is inside.

However, this issue need not reduce our appreciation of the psychedelic state! On the contrary, as tools for psychotherapy, the concept that psychedelics can *shrink us* into our internal worlds is a good thing. On the other hand, given that I was one of the guinea pigs for Robin's research with LSD and psilocybin, and therefore some of the circulated fMRI images are of my shut-down brain, perhaps it is just me who has the shrunken mind.

Dosage and Usage of LSD in Popular Culture

LSD is the most potent drug on the planet bar none. This colourless, odourless, tasteless substance influences humans at doses below 20 micrograms; twenty millionths of a gram. An imperceptible grain of LSD on the head of a pin can alter one's consciousness for 12 hours. Some conspiracy theorists say that a few well-placed kilograms in the water supply could incapacitate a whole city. However, this is a psychedelic urban myth. It simply would not work in a city's water supply, as (quite apart from the actual quantities required to create a strong enough solution) the chlorine in the water would neutralize the LSD instantly[23].

In the 1960s, high doses of LSD were legendary. These were taken in a liquid form, dropped onto a sugar cube or blotting paper. Initially it had only been available from the Swiss company Sandoz, where it had been discovered and manufactured for medicinal use. But by 1966, Sandoz LSD was difficult to obtain, and underground chemists moved in to meet the high demand. Owsley Stanley III, the famous San Francisco chemist who produced millions of LSD pills for the burgeoning hippie culture, was proud to say he never dropped the bar below 200 micrograms. Whilst touring with The Grateful Dead in 1965 he met Tim Scully and production got serious. Between them Scully and Stanley put out one and a half million tablets of Purple Haze in 1966 and then White Lightning LSD tablets in 1967, which were carefully measured to be no less than 270 micrograms each[24].

In 1969 Scully teamed up with Nick Sand, a member of the global LSD manufacturing and distribution set-up, The Brotherhood of Eternal Love. This collaboration led to production of the famous Orange Sunshine LSD. Later, in the 1970s in the UK, the alleged doses of the millions of LSD tabs made in London and in an isolated Welsh cottage, famously busted by Operation Julie, were at least 200 micrograms each.[25]

Most of the LSD producers of the 1960s and 1970s were not in business for the money. Stanley, Scully, Sand, those behind the Operation Julie productions, and many manufacturers and distributors since, have often given away at least half of their LSD for free. They see their vocation as one of spreading around the world the message about this substance, which they hope will bring peace and harmony to millions of people. LSD has always been relatively cheap (an LSD hit in the UK was 50p until Operation Julie pushed it up to a pound). In 2013 I had the great pleasure of hosting Mr. Leaf Feilding, one of the key distributors in the Operation Julie days, to speak at our *Breaking Convention* gathering in London. His gentle and holistic approach to healing through psychedelics was appreciated by those who came to hear his talk.

Today in the UK, the typical dose of a single hit of LSD is between 25 and 50 micrograms — although most people may believe they are receiving doses in the 50 to 100 microgram range. The most common delivery medium of the drug now is the 'blotter', in which LSD has been absorbed onto a perforated sheet of paper that is divided into hundreds of single doses. The sheets are traditionally printed with colourful designs and (in their non-drug soaked form) become extremely collectable, especially when signed by psychedelic luminaries past and present[26]. Because of its infrequent, non-addictive pattern of use, selling LSD has never provided much in the way of financial value for dealers. Indeed, for many who distribute the drug it is often sold on at cost price within a tight community of selected users.

Risks and Safety of LSD

LSD is a very powerful drug. The inexperienced user may be terrified by the acutely unpleasant experience of a bad trip. But the risk of this happening can be minimized if the drug is taken with due care and attention.

For people with pre-existing mental illness, especially those with a personal or family history of schizophrenia, LSD could trigger a psychosis, which can be lengthy and lead to hospitalization. However, as any psychiatrist will testify, for people with such psychotic fragilities, it is the more potent dopamine agonists such as amphetamine, cocaine or even high-dose cannabis, that tend to trigger psychosis most frequently.

From a physiological point of view, LSD is virtually inert. With hundreds of millions of people taking it worldwide consistently for the last 60 years, there have been no confirmed deaths from the physical effects of LSD. Herculean overdoses have been reported when people have accidentally taken hits more than 5,000 times the normal dose, for example when mistakenly snorting a line of white powder assumed to be cocaine that turns out to be pure LSD crystals. Even under these circumstances physical reactions causing death have not been reported.

Of course, accidents have occurred to people whilst feeling disorientated on LSD. Stories about people believing they can fly and jumping off buildings are commonly told but difficult to confirm. However, in respect of the large international prevalence of LSD use it carries remarkably few risks. One is advised, nevertheless, when taking LSD to avoid great heights, traffic or complex spirals and instead simply wander nonchalantly around fields or sit (or lie) still, as close to the ground as possible.

Animal experiments and epidemiological observations confirm that LSD is not addictive. Rats in cages do not repeatedly self-administer themselves with LSD if given the opportunity to do so[27]. (Having said that, as Bruce Alexander demonstrated so brilliantly with his famous Rat Park experiments in the late 1970s, no animals (including humans) choose to abuse drugs when their psychological and social conditions are good[28].)

Many people have taken LSD just a few times, usually in their late teens or early 20s. The majority will say it was a positive experience, but only a small percentage go on to be longer-term users. Indeed, a 'regular user' may take LSD only a few times a year or even less. For many, LSD is a fulfilling and positive experience, something to be shared with close friends and family on a special occasion. Not the sort of drug one uses habitually every Saturday night.

There are many misconceptions about the harms of LSD. In the late sixties, an erroneous rumour circulated (based on a single, uncorroborated poorly controlled scientific study) that LSD caused chromosomal damage[29]. It doesn't. There are many scare stories about acid causalities; such stories are difficult to confirm. In most cases, in my opinion, they correlate with cases of pre-existing mental illness.

I experienced a good illustration of the fears surrounding LSD when presenting at a conference in 2015 to the Royal College of Psychiatrists about the benefits of psychedelic medicine[30]. A concerned Emergency Medicine doctor in the audience stuck up his hand and expressed his displeasure at hearing me suggest that LSD was safe. He described what he considered a dangerous incident in which a young person came into the Accident and Emergency Department having taken *seventeen* tabs of acid. The young person had removed his clothes and was performing somersaults in the hospital corridors. I asked the doctor whether the young person required admission to hospital, "No", he said, "After several hours of monitoring he was allowed home under the supervision of his friends and he required no further follow-up." I then put it to the challenging doctor what might have been the scenario had someone attended his department having taken 17 grams of cocaine, 17 grams of heroin or, for that matter, 17 bottles of wine. The doctor acknowledged that likely such a person would have ended up in the Intensive Care Unit or could have easily died because of their overdose. "So," I said to the audience member, "here is a young person who took 17 times the recommended dose of a substance and the only pathology was that he was performing naked somersaults?". There exist many fears about the toxicity of LSD. These are the sorts of attitudes that those of us in psychedelic medicine are up against daily.

Legal Status of LSD

LSD is illegal all over the world. It is a Schedule One drug in the USA and a Class A drug in the UK. Possession of any amount of LSD is a criminal offence and carries the risk of a lengthy prison sentence. Being prosecuted for a drug offence is by far the most dangerous aspect of using LSD. Prosecution could ruin your life with a severity that entirely eclipses any potential risks to your physical or mental health caused by LSD use.

Potential Role in Medicine for LSD

LSD has a rich history of use as a substance to enhance psychotherapy for patients with a wide range of mental health problems, particularly including anxiety-based disorders and addictions. It also has uses with autism, spiritual emergencies such as existential crises and end-of-life anxiety experiences.[31] All of these issues will be covered in more detail later on the book.

2. Psilocybin

Psilocybin is a naturally occurring classical psychedelic drug that can be found in many species of mushroom, particularly those of the psilocybe variety. In the UK, the most popularly used 'magic' mushroom is *Psilocybe semilanceata* — also called the liberty cap — whose distinctive pointy-headed appearance has become synonymous with psychedelic culture. There are hundreds of varieties of magic mushrooms, including the popular *Psilocybe cyanescens, Psilocybe mexicana* and *Psilocybe azurescens*.

Pharmacology of Psilocybin

The active component in the mushroom, psilocybin, is readily converted to the active component psilocin in the body, which affects the brain in a similar manner to LSD, as a partial agonist at 5-HT2A receptors.

As with LSD, the effects of psilocybin are those of the typical classical hallucinogens. Some users will say they can easily recognise the difference between the LSD experience and that of psilocybin, whereas others, even experienced users, cannot tell them apart at certain dosages. Interestingly, yawning — a serotonin mediated response — is a recognised common feature of the mushroom experience that one does not get so readily with LSD. As with all psychedelic drugs, the set and setting have such a

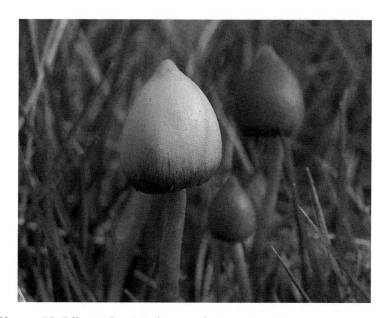

Picture 10: Liberty Cap Mushrooms from Wales: The magic mushroom has spawned generations of folklore tails, myths and legends — many of which are erroneous but have become ingrained into our social consciousness. It remains something of an enigma, with stalwart followers who often prefer its naturalness to what they consider to be the synthetic feel of LSD.

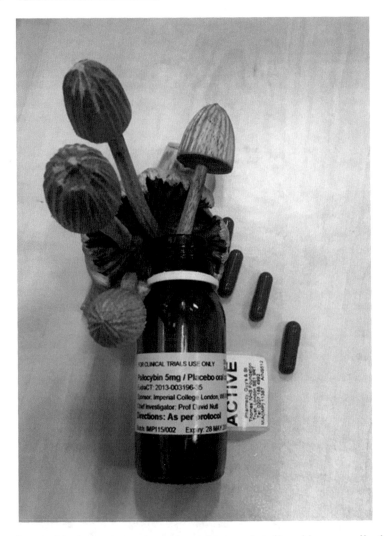

Picture 11: A renaissance version of research psilocybin, prescribed currently by the Beckley-Imperial Psychedelic Research team. Photo courtesy of Robin Carhart-Harris.

significant effect on the overall experience of the drug's intoxication that it is almost impossible to create equivalent testing conditions.

In general, psilocybin is shorter acting than LSD, its effects lasting between five to eight hours. Commonly it is described as 'slightly easier going', 'warmer' or 'more relaxed' than LSD. Again, however, there are many confounding factors as to why people may say this — perhaps influenced by people usually taking psilocybin mushrooms in a natural setting when they are freshly picked?

Dosage and Usage of Psilocybin

Magic mushrooms may be eaten raw and fresh, straight from the field. They are often dried, and can be brewed as a tea. As with LSD, psilocybin usage is generally not heavy or frequent for most users. Teenage usage is fairly common, especially in rural areas in the UK, where for two months of the year liberty cap mushrooms grow widely on many patches of short lush grass.

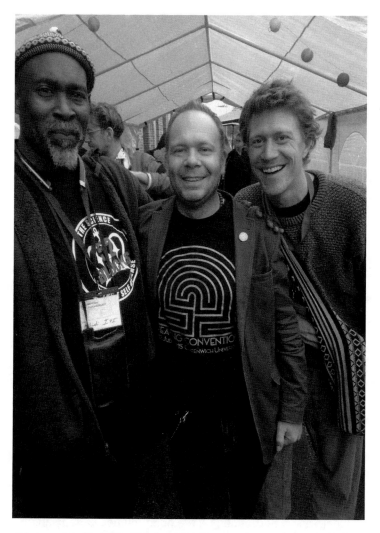

Picture 12: Dr Kilindi Iyi. At the Prague Beyond Psychedelics Conference in 2016, together with PsyPress UK publisher, Robert Dickins.

A typical dose of liberty caps, which are tiny things (the caps measuring just 10 to 15mm in diameter), would be between 10 to 100 dried mushrooms — these figures representing a very low to a very high dose. Of course, many serious 'psychonauts' would call for even higher doses. Notably, Terence McKenna often stated that the gold standard for a psilocybin-induced mystical experience was 5 grams of dried mushroom. This is echoed by contemporary writer and mushroom connoisseur, Dr Kilindi Iyi, who poetically describes his psilocybin internal shamanic journeys, 'alone in the darkness', accompanied by his plea that 'we need higher doses'. He is not shy of giving the following advice: 'If you feel worried and think "I may have taken too much," then that means you need to take more!'. This may sound reckless to some people. And one would have to be certain of one's psychological robustness to attempt Herculean doses.

Risks and Safety of Psilocybin

Like LSD, psilocybin is virtually inert physiologically, and recorded deaths from its toxicity are very rare. The lethal dose is over 1,000 times the typical intoxication dose, which equates to having to consume 17kg of fresh mushrooms to fatally overdose from psilocybin. This is unlikely to happen accidentally, unless the user has an unnaturally intense love of eating fungi.

One should bear in mind that, as with LSD and all psychedelic drugs, unpleasant psychological reactions and accidents may occur after consuming psilocybin. Paying attention to set and setting reduces the risks. Like LSD, a psilocybin trip *will* be a challenging experience at times.

Another potential problem with psilocybin mushrooms is that of picking and consuming the wrong type of mushrooms. There are a number of causalities every autumn in the UK from people who have accidentally eaten a poisonous mushroom that they wrongly identified as magic. Arming oneself with a colour photo guide to wild mushrooms and going with an experienced picker should protect against this. The wonderfully colourful book by Paul Stamets, *Psilocybin Mushrooms of the World*, is a good place to start[32].

Legal Status of Psilocybin

Psilocybin, the drug, is illegal. It is a Class A substance in the UK, and a Schedule One substance in the USA. Possession of psilocybin can lead to imprisonment and a destruction of life opportunities in a manner that far outstrips any of the health risks associated with using the drug.

It is against the law to grow or possess magic mushrooms, which therefore criminalises the entire farming population of South West England

and Wales. Apparently grazing mushrooms, directly from the ground, is currently legal.

Between 2003 and 2005 there was a loophole in the UK law in which it became legal to buy, sell and consume magic mushrooms as long as they were fresh. Nowadays, fresh or dried, magic mushrooms are illegal in the UK. Currently in Holland it is still legal to consume psilocybin in the form of truffles, which are the hardened mycelia (or sclerotia) of the *Psilocybe tampanensis*, *Psilocybe mexicana* and *Psilocybe Atlantis* mushrooms.

Potential Role of Psilocybin in Medicine and Neuroscience

Psilocybin is a remarkably versatile and useful medicine. It was studied extensively in trials in the 1950s and 1960s, and is now being researched internationally for potential development as a licensed medicine and as an agent to induce spiritual experience. Psilocybin has been preferred to LSD in several recent physiological, neuroimaging and clinical studies in the UK and USA. Partly because it is slightly shorter acting than LSD and therefore more clinically manageable, but mainly because proposing a study using LSD invites more media interest and unwanted ethical concerns than psilocybin.

The Heffter Research Institute concentrates primarily on psilocybin as its main research tool. Heffter projects at Johns Hopkins University, many overseen by Roland Griffiths, have been exploring psilocybin's capacity for inducing spiritual experiences with lasting positive personality changes[33].

In the UK Robin Carhart-Harris is currently leading an ongoing clinical study exploring the potential role for psilocybin-assisted psychotherapy in treating treatment resistant depression. The study arose from a chance finding in one of Carhart-Harris' earlier neuroimaging studies with the drug, in which it was discovered that psilocybin switches off a key area of the cerebral cortex which is usually overactive in cases of depression[34].

Furthermore, psilocybin has recently been used in a contemporary open-label pilot study by the US researcher Michael Bogenshutz to augment psychotherapy for people with alcohol dependence syndrome[35]. The subject of psychedelic therapy for people with addictions will be explored in greater detail later in this book.

3. *N,N*-Dimethyltryptamine (DMT)

Another classical psychedelic, DMT, is an extraordinary substance in that it occurs spontaneously throughout the animal and plant kingdom in a form that under normal circumstances (e.g. ingestion) has no effect on humans at all.

When smoked, it produces an intense but short-lived psychedelic experience, lasting just 15 to 25 minutes (though it may feel like several lifetimes). It rose to fame in the 1960s as 'the businessman's trip', capable of being enjoyed in one's lunch break. Today DMT use is on the increase, being one of the active ingredients in the South American brew ayahuasca. And as described earlier, its close resemblance to serotonin has led many researchers to suggest DMT is a good candidate for a human endogenous psychedelic.

Pharmacology of DMT

Like LSD and psilocybin, DMT's primary psychedelic effects are pro-duced at the 5-HT2A receptor in the cerebral cortex.

The effects of DMT are similar to the classical drugs LSD and psilo-cybin; including perceptual distortions, rapid fluctuations in thinking and, above all, an intense feeling of spirituality and connectivity with the uni-verse. When DMT is injected, or the crystals are smoked in a glass pipe, the drug effects occur rapidly. Users commonly experience a unique sense

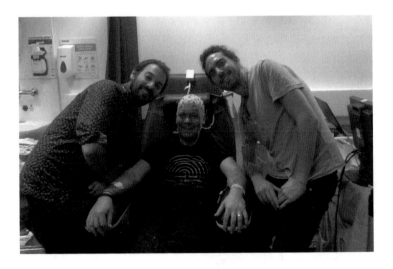

Picture 13: A healthy subject is injected with DMT whilst undergoing an EEG in November 2016. The team, led by Chris Timmerman, Luke Williams and Robin Carhart-Harris of the Beckley-Imperial College London group, are researching the neurobiology of this fascinating compound.

of otherworldliness with DMT and often describe seeing and interacting with 'entities', often reported as elfin-type aliens. However, it is possible that one person's trip report influences another. And there is now so much literature about meeting DMT entities that many users fully expect to (and therefore *do*) meet one of the little green (or, interestingly, more commonly blue) creatures when they take the drug.

Another area of science that has been historically connected with DMT is the phenomenon of the near-death experience (NDE). This is a massive topic, which we will not cover in detail in this book, other than to note that there are a lot of similarities between the psychedelic state and the NDE. Indeed, many scholars have proposed that during the throes of death the brain emits large quantities of endogenous DMT, to send us on our way, as it were. With over 15 million recorded occurrences, the NDE is a common psychological phenomenon but science has not yet come up with any substantial reproducible theories to explain how and why it occurs. It absolutely deserves further research. Unquestionably, the human brain is amazing and one's imagination is made of cosmic stuff.

Dosage and Usage of DMT

Until recently, pure DMT use has been relatively rare. It is not the sort of substance your average drug dealer is likely to come across and is certainly not a big money-spinner for a dealer. But with the growth of internet-based distribution networks for DMT or related analogues, such as 5-MEO-DMT, its popularity has grown immensely.

DMT is usually smoked, as it has no effect when eaten because it is broken down in the gut by the enzyme monoamine oxidase. It only becomes orally active when combined with a monoamine oxidase inhibitor (MAOI), as found in ayahuasca. The effects may then be equally intense, but with slower onset, and much longer lasting. We will come back to ayahuasca later in the book, which has seen a huge growth of interest in recent years both recreationally and in dozens of new scientific papers looking at the potential medical benefits of ayahuasca ceremonies.

Risks and Safety of DMT

As with other classical psychedelics, DMT produces relatively minimal physiological effects. Overdose is unlikely and no deaths have been recorded. However, as with the other classical psychedelics, the psychological reaction can be intense and unpleasant unless proper attention is paid to set and setting. Another risk factor for DMT occurs when its users take MAOI drugs without adequate understanding of their effects, which, as all psychiatrists know, can be potentially harmful.

Legal Status of DMT

Like other psychedelics, DMT is an illegal Class A and Schedule One drug. Possession risks imprisonment. The fact that it grows in abundance in every other blade of grass on the planet is a conveniently ignored legal peculiarity.

Potential Role in Medicine for DMT

As described earlier, our understanding of the role of endogenous DMT in mediating non-drug mystical experience needs further investigation. In 1995, Rick Strassman led the first psychedelic drug human study in modern times when he investigated the subjective psychological effects of DMT injected into a small group of healthy volunteers[36]. Strassman's study paved the way for the modern renaissance of psychedelic research. His postulations about the role of DMT as 'the sprit molecule' became immensely popular, with many enthusiasts believing the DMT state can teach us a great deal about the universe and the human condition. In his book Strassman rightly concludes that it is difficult to see a role for DMT as a therapeutic agent, as the intense short-lived experience (when smoked or injected) does not leave much room for therapeutic engagement. The therapeutic potential of ayahuasca, however, is a different matter and will be discussed later.

4. Mescaline

Mescaline is the last in the group we are calling the classical psychedelics. It is not very widely well-known or used in the UK, though is more popular

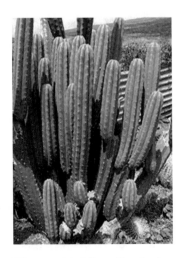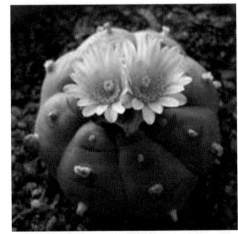

Picture 14: Mescaline is the principle active component in the San Pedro, Peyote and several other psychedelic cacti.

in the States. At the end of the 19th century it was the first psychedelic to be recognised in nature and then artificially synthesized.

It was mescaline that British psychiatrist Humphrey Osmond used when he dosed Aldous Huxley in the Hollywood hills in 1953[37].

Pharmacology of Mescaline

Like the other classical psychedelics mescaline exerts its main effects through its role as a partial agonist at 5-HT2A receptors in the cerebral cortex[38].

The effects include all the usual hallmarks of the classical psychedelic experience. Some users say there are less well-formed visual illusions or hallucinations compared to LSD, but more in the way of complex geometrical shapes and a greater sense of bodily or emotional changes, particularly those of a spiritual nature.

Dosage and Usage of Mescaline

While the commonest way of imbibing mescaline is through the ingestion of the cactus, it can also be synthesised and taken in an artificial form. In the UK, until the recent growth of internet access to psychedelic drugs, neither form had been especially popular, but now mescaline is increasingly available outside of specialist circles of psychedelic geeks.

The peyote cactus itself grows extremely slowly. It has a green, circular, non-spiny appearance — the 'button' that sits on the surface of the desert with a pointed root below the sand. Traditionally, the buttons are cut off from the surface with the roots left in situ, then dried and eaten. They are notoriously bitter.

The usual dose is between 100mg and 400mg (Huxley took 400mg), where one cactus button is equivalent to about 25mg. It is quite a feat, then, to eat enough buttons given their taste. The mescaline experience takes a long time to come on and is long lasting. Afterglow effects, in which one can be left wallowing in a state of pleasurable inner warmth and existential well-being, can persist for days.

Risks and Safety of Mescaline

Like the other classical drugs mescaline is physiologically relatively safe, even in high doses. But, as with other psychedelics, if mescaline is used without preparation the user may experience a transient state of panic. The existentialist philosopher, Jean-Paul Sartre is reported to have had an especially negative mescaline experience. Initial nausea is also commonly felt after taking mescaline. But then, as a famous psychedelic luminary once said: 'You have a tool to glimpse the secrets of the universe and you're worried you may throw up a little?'

Legal Status of Mescaline

Current prohibitive laws label mescaline a Class A (UK) and Schedule 1 (US) drug. To be caught with mescaline and be imprisoned could cause serious and lifelong catastrophic outcomes far beyond the physical or psychological harm induced by the substance.

However, there are some interesting exceptions regarding the legality of the peyote cactus. In the North American Church, it is legal for registered Native Americans to use peyote cactus as part of their religious ceremonies, as they have been doing for thousands of years. The colonization of Native American territories by Europeans all but eradicated their ways of life and replaced peyote with the modern intoxicant of choice, alcohol, leading to hundreds of millions of alcohol-related deaths compared to the zero deaths ever recorded from mescaline use. We shall return to this later.

Potential Role of Mescaline in Medicine

Unlike the other classical psychedelics, mescaline has received relatively scant clinical research attention. Its long duration of action makes it difficult to use clinically. Furthermore, in the US, where much of the contemporary psychedelic research has been taking place, the drug is relatively well known and there is an established racially motivated socio-political opposition to the peyote cult. One way or the other, the field is wide open for clinical mescaline research.

There has been one notable study by John Halpern at Harvard Medical School in 2005 that looked more particularly at the epidemiological aspects of peyote use amongst the Native American population.[39] It is noteworthy that rates of alcoholism are considerably lower among those Native Americans who use peyote, which suggests there is further scope for researching the role mescaline can play as a tool to combat addictions. This is certainly an area worthy of closer inspection.

5. 3,4-Methylenedioxymethamphetamine (MDMA)

MDMA is not one of the classical psychedelics. It was first described as an *empathogen* in 1983 by Ralph Metzner and David E. Nichols[40] and later rebranded again by Nichols[41] as an *entactogen*, meaning "touching within".

There is an awful lot to say about MDMA. Not only is it widely used recreationally in the form of Ecstasy, but it is also one of the psychedelic compounds rising to the forefront of research, proving to be most useful as a tool to enhance psychotherapy.

For example, if one were to invent a hypothetical drug for enhancing psychotherapy what qualities would it have? It would:

1. Be short-acting enough for a single session of therapy.
2. Have no significant dependency issues.
3. Be non-toxic at therapeutic doses.
4. Reduce feelings of depression that accompany post-trauma (PTSD) presentations.
5. Increase feelings of closeness between the patient and therapist.
6. Raise arousal to enhance motivation for therapy.
7. Paradoxically, increase relaxation and reduce the hyper-vigilance that accompanies PTSD.
8. Stimulate new ways of thinking to explore entrenched problems.

These are all the qualities of MDMA when used carefully in a clinical setting[42].

Receptors or Brain Region Involved	MDMA Effects	How effects relate to the treatment of PTSD		Neuro-biological Correlates
SEROTONIN	Reduces depression and anxiety	Provides patient with an experience of positive mood and reduced anxiety in increased engagement.		Release of pre-synaptic 5-hydroxytryptamine at 5-HT$_{1A}$ and 5-HT$_{1B}$ receptors.
	Stimulates alterations in the perceptions of meaning.	Opportunity to see old problems in a new light.		Increased activity at the 5-HT$_{2A}$ receptors
DOPAMINE AND NOR-EPINEPHRINE	Raises levels of arousal.	Stimulating effect increases motivation to engage in therapy	Optimum Level of Arousal	Release of dopamine and noradrenaline
ALPHA-2 ADRENO-CEPTORS	Increases relaxation.	Reduces hypervigilance associated with PTSD		Increased alpha 2-adrenoceptor activity.
HORMONAL EFFECTS	Improves fear extinction learning.	Allows reflection on traumatic memories during psychotherapy without being overwhelmed.		Release of noradrenaline and cortisol
	Increases emotional attachment and feelings of trust and empathy.	Improved relationship between patient and therapist. Capacity to reflect on traumatic memories.		Multiple factors, including release of oxytocin.
	More likely to use words relating to friendship, and intimacy	Generate discussion about wider aspects of the patient's social and emotional relationships.		
	Reduced social exclusion phenomena.	Opportunity to reflect upon patients' wider social functioning.		
REGIONAL BRAIN CHANGES	Improved detection of happy faces and reduced detection of negative faces.	Enhances levels of shared empathy and pro-social functioning.		Increased PFC activation and decreased amygdala fear response.
	Reduced subjective fear response on recall of negative memories.	Opportunity to reflect upon painful memories of trauma during psychotherapy.		Decreased cerebral blood flow in the right amygdala and hippocampus.

Picture 15: The subjective psychological effects of MDMA relate closely to 'the perfect psychotherapy session'[44].

Pharmacology of MDMA

The pharmacokinetics and pharmacodynamics of MDMA have been well studied in humans[43].

MDMA is a ring-substituted phenethylamine exerting its effects primarily through promoting raised levels of monoamine neurotransmitters in the brain, especially serotonin, but also dopamine and noradrenaline. Increased activity at $5\text{-}HT_{1A}$ and $5\text{-}HT_{1B}$ receptors reduces feelings of depression and anxiety, reduces the amygdala fear response and increases levels of self-confidence. Due to alpha 2-adrenoceptor mediated effects, MDMA makes an individual feel relaxed, which reduces hypervigilance. Furthermore, the effect of raised serotonin at $5\text{-}HT_{2A}$ receptors provides alterations in the perceptions of meanings and facilitates new ways of thinking about old experiences. MDMA has also been shown to facilitate the release of oxytocin — the hormone associated with early infantile bonding and increased levels of empathy and closeness. The combined dynamic interaction of increased serotonin, dopamine and noradrenaline in multiple brain regions modulating learning and memory, emotion, reward, attention and sympathetic/parasympathetic activity contribute to MDMA's subjective psychological effects. Based on doses ranging 100–125mg, the peak plasma concentration and subjective effects of MDMA are reached after 2–3 hours and the elimination half-life is between 7–9 hours.

As a psychotropic drug, MDMA provides a remarkably consistent pleasurable effect. It is shorter acting than LSD (2–5 hours' duration), produces less perceptual alterations and is difficult not to enjoy. Apart from perhaps the opiates, few other psychotropic drugs have this ability. However, there is some anecdotal evidence that the intensity of the user's initial experiences with MDMA diminishes quantitatively with prolonged use.

Dosage and Usage of MDMA

MDMA, in the form of Ecstasy, is the most popular recreational drug in the UK after cannabis. Ecstasy is usually taken as a tablet; often with a distinctive embossed design so users can compare batches. A lot has changed since we danced on Doves in the fields surrounding the M25 in England. Ecstasy tablets (often referred to as E's, X, pills, gurners, disco biscuits, little fellas, smarties, beans, eckies, rollers, etc.) are given popular brand names. Modern tableting methods means pills are no longer confined to simple white circular formulae, but now come in all shapes and sizes. I won't try to name them all; to do so will just show my age and not get anywhere near what the kids are calling them nowadays. They can be anything; whatever tickles the fancy of the producer and fits with the zeitgeist of the time, such

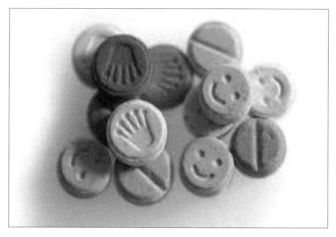

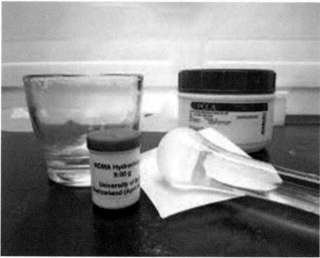

Picture 16: MDMA. In its illicit and renaissance forms.

as Mercedes, Euros, Homer Simpsons, Heinekens, Mitsubishis, Ferraris, Volkswagens, Red Devils, Blue Nikes, 007s, Playboys, OAPs, Vodafones, Swastikas, Barcelonas, Dominoes, Batmans, Supermans, Rolexes, Pokémons, Red Stop Signs, Buddhas, Butterflies, X-Files, White Diamonds, Yin Yangs, Armanis, etc. etc.

The dose per tablet varies. Ten years ago, the average dose of MDMA in a street tablet bought as Ecstasy was just 70mg, according to a study by Liverpool University's Dr. Jon Cole[45]. As well as, or instead of, MDMA, an Ecstasy tablet can contain ketamine, caffeine, BZP, heroin, brick dust, dog de-worming tablets, methamphetamine, mephedrone, opiates, fish tank oxygenation powder or anything else that can be pressed into a tablet and stamped with a Superman logo (hence my distinction between the words Ecstasy and MDMA when describing what one might imagine to be identical chemical compounds). In recent years — since the influence of Silk Road, Shiny Flakes and the darknet in general — Ecstasy tablets have become increasingly stronger; with some more than 300mg MDMA per pill.

Many recreational users also use crystal or powdered MDMA, which can be swallowed or snorted. Ecstasy, which has been an integral part of the dance music scene for over 40 years, is often taken together with other drugs — particularly cannabis and alcohol — but also frequently with amphetamines and cocaine. The sheer popularity of Ecstasy makes clinical research with MDMA a challenge for those researching the drug as a tool for clinical medicine. Of course, the doses, patterns of use and, subsequently, the risks associated with recreational Ecstasy use do not equate at all well with the proposed clinical uses of MDMA. Unfortunately, the popular media and even some parts of the scientific community cannot separate clinical MDMA from its historical association with Ecstasy. This obstacle needs to be tackled if we are to see the development of clinical MDMA in medicine[46].

Risks and Safety of MDMA

This is necessarily a long subsection, as there are a lot of important misconceptions about the relative risks or safety of MDMA and it is vital these are addressed accurately regarding contemporary research.

Using MDMA *does* carry a higher risk of physical harm than one sees with the classical psychedelics — no one will deny this. There have, after all, been no recorded deaths *due to physical toxicity* with the drugs LSD, psilocybin and DMT. But there *are* a notable small number of deaths each year attributed to MDMA or Ecstasy (and it is important we make the distinction between these two entities)[47]. The numbers themselves remain extremely low given the massive uncontrolled use of the drug — for the last 25 years, some 750,000 doses have been taken *every weekend* in the UK and the recorded *annual* death rate in the UK has been steady at around 20–40[48]. It may be that some users have a genetic predisposition to the potential harmful physical and psychological effects of MDMA, which then interact with certain environmental factors. More work is required to explore this phenomenon. A study in 2003 looked at UK coroners' reports of deaths attributed in part to Ecstasy between 1997 and 2000 and found 81 such deaths[49]. But only 7% of those 81 deaths involved MDMA alone. That is six deaths in three years, after some 120 million ecstasy tablets were consumed by over a million people. Of course, for the families and friends of those few young people that so tragically die because of ecstasy use, such statistics mean little. But as far as data goes, there is no denying that overall MDMA is a remarkably, staggeringly, safe compound; even when used in a non-controlled recreational setting.

There are two major ways in which recreational ecstasy users can suffer acute toxicity. The first is through hyperthermia, which may occur through prolonged physical exertion in a hot environment, combined with dehydration due to not consuming enough water. High temperature has also been demonstrated to further exacerbate the risk of longer-term neurotoxicity[50].

The second cause of acute toxicity is Ecstasy-induced hyponatremia, in which vulnerable individuals with a genetic predisposition experience an impairment of the kidney's normal water homeostasis mechanism[51]. This can be further exacerbated by excessive water consumption, which can occur, ironically, because users may be over-vigilant about the risk of dehydration.

In summary, then, when Ecstasy is taken in uncontrolled circumstances, by naïve individuals, in extreme heat and with vigorous exercise, there may be problems associated with either drinking *too much* or *too little* water.

Up until recently there was much debate about MDMA causing lasting neurotoxicity; often with a particularly political flavour[52,53]. Whilst some studies have suggested transient neuro-cognitive deficits associated with heavy, prolonged ecstasy use, others have reported a lack of such deficits, or only transient changes that revert back to normal after cessation of use[54]. Consequently, the vast majority of researchers today accept that at the typical doses used for low to moderate recreational use — and certainly at the low and infrequent doses proposed for *clinical* use, when pure MDMA is administered in a controlled clinical setting — MDMA is not considered a dangerous drug[55].

In the past, scare stories have arisen from studies on selectively biased populations of recreational Ecstasy users (who frequently use other drugs including alcohol, and/or have pre-existing mental health problems), or on animal models that translate poorly to humans. These are irrelevant to proposals for MDMA psychotherapy. In one such animal study subjects were dosed equivalent to a human consuming a total of 12 ½ ecstasy tablets[56], 40 tablets in four days[57] and in another, which "concluded neurotoxicity", the animals received the human equivalent of 160 tablets in a week[58]. One study has become infamous for its scientific flaws. Commissioned by the US government, George Ricaurte at Johns Hopkins University allegedly demonstrated severe neurotoxicity in primates given MDMA at equivalent human doses[59]. The paper received wide media coverage. However, it was later discovered that the animals were not given MDMA at all, but rather the (far more toxic) drug methamphetamine. The paper was subsequently retracted but it was too late to prevent the spread of an erroneous message about toxicity.

The media attention paid to the assumed dangerousness of MDMA is out of all proportion. It is bad science for people to make conclusions about the risks of neurotoxicity in humans based on irrelevant research.

Legal Status of MDMA

In the 1980s, the rise of dance-music culture saw MDMA take a path not dissimilar to that of LSD; leaking from the medical community and becoming widely used by young people. Despite little evidence of any actual harms, increasing negative reports of its uncontrolled use outside of the clinical environment led to the American Drug Enforcement Agency (DEA) calling for the drug to be banned. Those clinicians who had been using the drug safely and effectively for ten years appealed against the DEA and requested that further clinical research take place. But the DEA used emergency measures to bypass the hearing and make the drug a Schedule One controlled substance in the USA in 1985. Now labelled (erroneously) as highly addictive and of no medical use, MDMA research ceased overnight.

In the UK, the 1971 Misuse of Drugs Act (which had already been altered in 1977 to include all ring-substituted amphetamines, including MDMA) was further amended in 1985 to refer specifically to Ecstasy, placing it in the Class A category.

Potential Role in Medicine of MDMA

Using MDMA as an agent for psychotherapy can be significantly attributed to the Californian psychotherapist Dr. Leo Zeff. During the 1960s, Zeff had worked with LSD psychotherapy until it was banned. On discovering MDMA in the early 1970s, he came out of retirement and subsequently introduced MDMA (then still legal) to over 4,000 patients, many of whom went on to become therapists themselves[60]. Then known as 'Adam', from the mid-1970s to the mid-1980s there was a growth of clinicians using MDMA around California.

A paper by psychiatrist George Greer described the subjective reports of 29 patients safely administered MDMA as part of individual, group and couples therapy in the early 1980s[61]. The overwhelming majority of subjects reported positive individual effects, improved wellbeing and the resolution of relationship problems after their therapy. In a further case series study, Greer outlined the methods and experimental techniques that facilitate a successful MDMA-assisted session and suggested further, controlled studies occur[62].

However, the almost total prohibition of MDMA clinical research since 1985 has prevented such studies until recently. But since 2010 there have been several completed and published clinical MDMA studies. Most research centres around MDMA as a tool for the treatment of post-traumatic stress disorder (PTSD). We will return to MDMA and Ecstasy's history, and contemporary MDMA research, in more detail in later chapters.

6. Ketamine

Ketamine comes in the class known as dissociative anaesthetics and it exerts its effects as a powerful NMDA-antagonist. (Note: we are talking here about NMDA, which stands for *N*-methyl-D-aspartate, *not* the drug MDMA!) Other NMDA-antagonist dissociative psychedelic drugs include dextromethorphan (DXM), phencyclidine (PCP, which is also known as 'angel dust') and, to some extent, nitrous oxide.

The ketamine experience is best described as… *peculiar*. Its origins and place in medical history and the public's consciousness is also weird. Known to many as 'that horse tranquiliser' used by veterinary surgeons, it is also a useful short-acting anaesthetic for children[63]. During my paediatric training I learned that a brief shot of intramuscular ketamine is extremely effective when relocating a dislocated shoulder of a howling child. And a lot safer and easier to use than the high doses of benzodiazepines or opiates one would need to get an equivalent functional effect.

The mechanism by which ketamine works as a paediatric anaesthetic (pictured left) is the same reason recreational users enjoy its unusual effects. It doesn't simply block pain receptors, as an opiate might (though

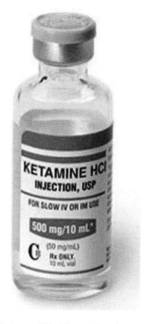

Picture 17: Ketamine is a synthetic drug, developed in 1962 and initially called CI-581, by the pharmaceutical company Parke-Davis.

it does do this to some extent). Rather it shifts attention away from the pain by producing a mental state of dissociation that *distracts* the user.

At low, sub-anaesthetic, doses, the effects are psychedelic. Users experience distortions of perceptions and time and an extreme sense of disconnectedness from the outside world, including otherworldly out-of-body experiences[64]. Spiritual experiences and hexagons are common.

It saw some medical and limited recreational use in the Vietnam War in the 1970s. There was some limited recreational use of the drug in the 1970s. The psychonaut John Lilly provided some beautiful stories about ketamine. His communications with dolphins, high altitude flight research, hours of high dose psychedelic sessions in floatation tanks with LSD, searching for extra-terrestrials with SETI and his methods for transcendence with ketamine are well worth checking out[65].

Ketamine became widely popular in the new (or 'nu') rave scene of the mid-2000s. Unfortunately, the horse tranquiliser adage and the image of a wasted raver slumped in the corner in a 'K-hole', distracts people from what an important substance ketamine is for clinical psychiatry and consciousness research. Like all the other substances discussed here, ketamine has its best days to come.

Mode of Action of Ketamine

As an antagonist at the NMDA receptors, ketamine inhibits calcium channel influx, which produces its analgesic effects[66]. This glutamate-mediated effect of ketamine makes it an interesting candidate for furthering our understanding of psychosis, which has been studied in recent years[67]. In 2011 I was lucky enough to be administered intravenous ketamine by colleague Dr. James Stone at the Institute of Psychiatry as part of his study developing ketamine as a treatment for depression[68]. Being let out into the streets of South London after that one, in a decidedly pleasant discombobulated state, was an unforgettable experience.

Dosage and Usage of ketamine

Medical ketamine is synthesised legally in large quantities worldwide, so there is no significant underground chemical synthesis of the drug. Most recreational ketamine is diverted from industrial production. Recreationally it is most often insufflated (sniffed) but may also be injected intravenously, intramuscularly or subcutaneously. Obviously, injecting produces a faster onset and shorter duration of action to when it is sniffed. Compared to many other psychedelics, at 2 to 4 hours, it is not a long-lasting experience.

Risks and Safety of ketamine

Remember, *any* drug can be dangerous and *any* drug can be used safely-depending on the circumstances (if this were not the case doctors would not prescribe chemotherapy to treat cancer and consumers would not drink coffee). Ketamine, used recreationally, certainly can cause problems for some users. It has higher addictive potential than other psychedelics[69] and there are also some worrying physical problems that arise with heavy sustained use.

The primary physical risk with sustained ketamine use is inflammation of the urinary tract; including reduced bladder volume, pain on urination, abdominal and pelvic pain and incontinence[70]. Symptoms often persist permanently even after stopping the drug. Furthermore, acutely, ketamine dosing involves a narrow therapeutic window. This means the desired psychedelic effects dose is close to the wasted, zoned-out, semi-collapsed, speechless 'K-hole' dose. This need not always cause casualties, however, because, as with cannabis, once one reaches such intense soporific effects one becomes unable to actively dose oneself any further and the brain recovers. But serious accidents can occur if one is injecting the drug. The terribly sad case of the American Marcia Moore is a particularly chilling account. An heiress to the Sheraton Hotel fortune, Marcia, like John Lilly, appreciated the aesthetic and spiritual properties of ketamine. She described her ketamine experiences in her book *Journeys into the Bright World*[71]. But one night in winter while partaking in a session of injecting herself with ketamine she went missing. Two years later, her skeleton was found crouched inside a hollowed-out tree in a forest near her house. The cause of death was never confirmed but it is hypothesised that she fell asleep and died of hypothermia. I find that image of a frozen skeleton sitting inside a tree extremely unnerving.

So, considered alongside the relatively safe psychedelic drugs LSD, MDMA and psilocybin, those images of addicted ravers lying in K-holes, incontinent with bladder problems — or, worse still, skeletons huddled in trees — gives ketamine a rather scary edge. Certainly, it is a drug worthy of care and attention.

Legal Status of ketamine

Because of its accepted medical uses, ketamine is Class C (or Schedule 3 in the States). This illustrates the peculiarities of the unfit-for-purpose classification schedule for controlled drugs. It has far greater toxicity than the other psychedelics drugs, but they all languish in Class A and Schedule 1. Oh, well. Ours is not to ponder nor question the wisdom of our sagacious governments who generously protect us with their drug laws.

In recent years, in response to ketamine's illegal status, the synthetic ketamine-like analogue, methoxetamine (3-MeO-2'-Oxo-PCE), has emerged as a popular Research Chemical. It has greater potency and duration of action than ketamine and was originally marketed as "bladder friendly". However, over time it has also been found to cause urinary tract inflammation and is therefore not necessarily a safer alternative[72].

Potential Role in Medicine of Ketamine

Ketamine is used extensively for minor surgery in emergency trauma, and as an agent to induce anaesthesia for major surgery. There is also growing interest regarding its use in psychiatry. We will come back to this in more detail in later chapters, describing some interesting studies exploring the role for ketamine as an antidepressant, used for treating depressive symptoms in people with bipolar disorder and in addiction therapies.

An off-label study, the 'Resistant Depression - Ketamine Infusion Treatment Evaluation' (RedKite), is currently underway in Oxford, run by the psychiatrist Dr Rupert McShane and colleagues. Rupert is investigating ketamine in the management of treatment resistant depression. This phenomenon could herald a radical new way of treating depression. Perhaps in the future, rather than use daily SSRI drugs, patients will adopt this 'dialysis' model, whereby a monthly infused dose of ketamine keeps their depressive symptoms at bay[73].

Also in the UK, a study started in 2016 by my colleague Dr Celia Morgan will explore the role for ketamine as a treatment for alcohol dependency syndrome. We will return to ketamine in greater detail in the section on psychedelic therapies for addictions.

In summary, there is far, far more to ketamine than simply 'that horse tranquilizer'.

7. Some Other Phenethylamines

It is worth briefly mentioning some of the less commonly used additions to the list of psychoactive phenethylamine compounds, which have emerged out of Alexander Shulgin's laboratory in the last forty years. These were documented, together with recipes of how to make them, in the book *PIH-KAL*[74]. A number of these compounds have proved useful in underground or unlicensed psychotherapy, but there are no published studies of their use 'legitimately', in clinical studies, to test them as adjuncts to psychotherapy. This does not mean that they may not prove to be useful clinical tools in years to come.

Drugs in the '2C-series' include 2C-B, 2C-T-7, 2C-T-2 and 2C-I. The one that has proved to be particularly useful for psychotherapy is 2C-B, often when combined with MDMA, because of its relatively short half-life and ease of use clinically. In the 1990s, the 2C-series became increasingly used recreationally, outside of the therapeutic context.

Mode of Action of 2C-B

2C-B does not have potent effects at the 5-HT2A receptor like the classical hallucinogens, nor does it cause a massive release of serotonin like MDMA. Rather it may have its principle effects at the 5-HT2C receptor[75].

Dosage and Usage of 2C-B

When 2C-B is used recreationally it is often taken mistakenly. Many clubbers do not know one pill from another, and may buy a 2C-B tablet expecting — and wanting — Ecstasy/MDMA. The dose range is different from MDMA, being between 15 and 25mg.

The effects of 2C-B are somewhat similar to MDMA, but with more visual phenomena such as illusions, patterns and halos. And 2C-B also characteristically produces distinct somatic sensorial changes, such as velvety textures and feelings of warmth. Mentally, one feels an increased sense of awareness, energy and stimulation and appreciation of music may be heightened. Many users say the come down from 2C-B is less harsh than that from MDMA.

Risks and Safety of 2C-B

As massive widespread use is not common, toxicity in the general population is rare. However 2C-B and the other 2C series have received relatively little in the way of toxicology studies and there have been some reports of deaths from its use[76].

Legal Status of 2C-B

As with most newly synthesised compounds, initially 2C-B was not illegal. It could be bought legally in head shops, especially in Amsterdam, under the name '*Nexus*', often marketed as an aphrodisiac, until banned in 1994. 2C-B and the other 2C series drugs are now illegal in most countries, classified as schedule One (USA) or Class A (UK).

Potential Role in Medicine for the 2C-series Drugs

Myron Stolaroff, in his books *Thanatos to Eros*,[77] and *The Secret Chief* (the book he wrote about Leo Zeff)[78] describes the therapeutic use of several of the 2C-series drugs, particularly 2C-B. Taken as part of a course of psychedelic psychotherapy using many different drugs, the 2C-series can be beneficial tools for psycho-spiritual development, both individually and as part of a group.

The German psychiatrist Friederike Fischer also describes her use of 2C-B alongside MDMA and LSD during her underground psychedelic practice in the 1990s. Only those patients who were sufficiently orientated with the mental spaces created by MDMA and LSD would then be given 2C-B, which she described as useful for its 'unforgiving insistence', to shift psychological resistence[79].

I am not aware of any contemporary planned clinical trials with 2C-B, though Stolaroff and others' experiences using the tools to assist stuck

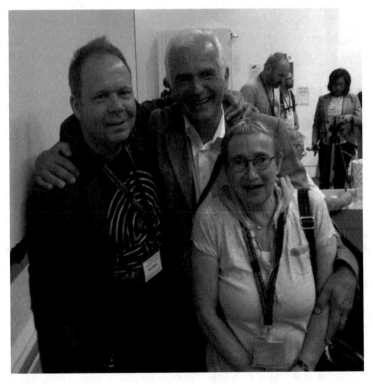

Picture 18: Psychiatrist, psychotherapist and pioneering guide Dr Friederike Fischer, with her co-therapist husband Konrad Meckel. At Breaking Convention, London, 2015.

patients through multiple situations of personal and interpersonal crises provide powerful anecdotal evidence that they could play a role in the future of psychiatry.

A Brief Mention of 2C-T-7, 2C-I and 2C-T-2

2C-T-7 has a greater mode of action at the 5-HT_{2A} receptor than 2C-B and is longer acting[63]. According to Stolaroff 2C-T-7 has the capacity to reveal deep levels of personal awareness. But it is certainly not as popular recreationally, as it has several unwanted side effects, including sexual dysfunction, muscular tension and cardiac symptoms in susceptible individuals[80]. More study is required before its safety and efficacy as a clinical tool could be assured.

2C-I has psychedelic and entactogenic qualities at higher doses. 2C-T-2 has similar effects to 2C-T-7 and provides a powerful psychedelic experience[81].

In summary, there are a host of established and new psychedelic compounds. As with all psychotropic drugs, they share similar core effects though with marked differences. We have been so distracted by their recreational use that we have only begun to scratch the surface of the potential healing effects of these substances. In the next chapter, we take a trip to a time before such drugs were well-known and demonised by society.

CHAPTER 3

Early Pioneers of the First and Second Psychedelic Eras

In chapter four we will visit some mushroom chewing cave-dwellers and also a sandal-wearing long-haired shaman from Galilee, but first we go back to review some important moments on the timeline of psychedelia.

Historically, there have been three great eras of psychedelic culture[1]. The first is centred on the dawn of the 20th century; the second, and generally the most well-known, incorporates the 'flower-power' era of the 1960s; and the third, well, that's the one we are rather excitingly in right now.

The First Psychedelic Era: 1880 to 1930

There was a stirring of interest in psychedelics between 1880 and the 1920s, mostly centred on the drug mescaline. Hashish was also popular at

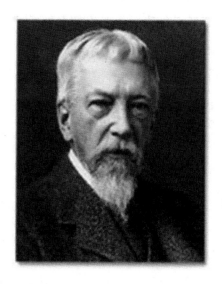

Picture 19:

The neurologist S. Weir Mitchell, whose various studies included the effects of weather on painful amputation stumps, the physiology of the cerebellum and a close examination of the cremasteric reflex, which every medical student should know.

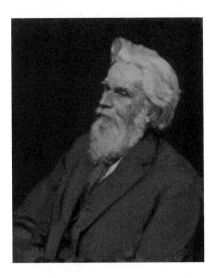

Picture 20:

Havelock Ellis. His broad interest in anthropology, archaeology, architecture, botany, ethics, ethnology, geology, history, literature, music, mythology, painting, philosophy, physics, and sculpture set him up perfectly as a psychedelic scientist.

the time, as was opium, which is not a psychedelic but its dream-like qualities were certainly responsible for many writers' creative meanderings.

People have known about mescaline, the active component in the peyote cactus, for a long time. But credit for the first formal scientific report on mescaline goes to the American neurologist and novelist S. Weir Mitchell. In 1896 Mitchell described the cactus in a paper for the *British Medical Journal* called '*The Effects of Anhelonium Lewinii (the Mescal Button)*'[2]. Like many others in psychedelic history, Mitchell was a colourful character. Prior to his interest in psychoactive cacti he had published works on subjects as esoteric as '*Gunshot Wounds and Other Injuries of Nerves*' and '*Researches Upon the Venom of the* Rattlesnake'.

Mitchell's paper was followed a year later by two reports from the British physician and psychologist, Henry Havelock Ellis: '*The Phenomena of Mescal Intoxication*' and '*Mescal: A New Artificial Paradise*'[3].

Havelock Ellis was another scientist with a broad knowledge base of atypical subjects. He led a most unconventional personal life and wrote extensively on the science of sex; publishing what was arguably the first medical textbook on homosexuality. A chronic sufferer of impotence, and reportedly a virgin at the time of starting an open marriage in the 1930s with his lesbian wife, he was also reportedly aroused by urolagnia, which I will leave the reader to investigate.

Havelock Ellis and Weir Mitchell were keen proponents of the mescaline experience and their works inspired others to explore the sensory and spiritual delights of the psychedelic cactus. A more scientific analysis of peyote had occurred ten years earlier by the German pharmacologist Louis Lewin, after whom the cactus was named[4]. Lewin was one of the first scientists to recognise the links between the pharmacology of different plants

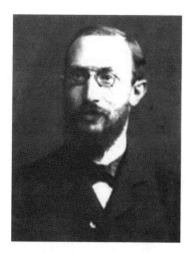

Picture 21:

Louis Lewin. His 1924 book *Phantastica* began the era of modern ethnobotany, combining pharmacology and toxicology to describe how plants produce their psychoactive effects.

and their mental effects, and attempted a classification of various psychoactive drugs based on their psychological effects, bringing new words into popular usage.

Louis Lewin Lewin's categories included the 'euphoriants', such as heroin; the 'inebriants,' such as alcohol; and the class of drugs he named 'phantastica', which later became the psychedelics. The words *euphoriant* and *inebriant* remain in popular usage today. And in 1947, when Werner Stoll, Albert Hofmann's contemporary, published the world's first report on the effects of LSD, Stoll referred to LSD as a *phantastica*[5]; there being no other word to describe it until later in the 1950s when the word *psychedelic* appears.

In 1897 another breakthrough occurred when German pharmacologist Arthur Carl Wilhelm Heffter, successfully isolated mescaline from the peyote cactus, which was the first time a naturally occurring psychedelic

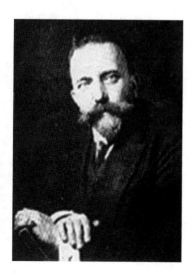

Picture 22:

Arthur Carl Wilhelm Heffter. Described on the Heffter Research Institute as "a brilliant and productive researcher and a warm human being loved by his colleagues."

72 THE PSYCHEDELIC RENAISSANCE

had been identified and extracted in this way[6]. Heffter's legacy continues to this day by his being the chosen name of a contemporary scientific group at the forefront of modern research into psychedelic drugs.

The Second Psychedelic Era: 1938 to 1976

The discovery of LSD in the 1940s, and the days of early psychedelic research in the 1950s and 1960s, are well documented, with numerous psychedelic folklore stories of Hofmann's magical bicycle ride through the countryside around Basel. Some of the UK-based contributions to psychedelic history are less well known, although they have been described superbly by my friend Andy Roberts in his outstanding book *Albion Dreaming*, which is highly recommended as a description of Britain's part in psychedelic history[7]. For those readers who have not already devoured every text available about the second psychedelic era, here is a brief potted review of those times.

Magnificent Realizations from Mouldy Rye

Albert Hofmann was a chemist working at Sandoz Laboratories in Switzerland. In the late 1930s, he was investigating a series of preparations based on the chemical lysergic acid, which is produced by the fungus ergot that grows on many different grasses and crops, but particularly on rye. For centuries, ergot (*Claviceps purpurea*) had been known to have psychotropic properties. It was recognised as having been responsible for outbreaks of St. Anthony's Fire in the Middle Ages, in which whole communities experienced peculiar epidemics of mass psychosis, hysteria and death after becoming poisoned by bread made from flour contaminated by the fungus. But Hofmann was interested in another known property of lysergic acid — its capacity to constrict blood vessels — and he was part of a team of pre-war chemists and psychopharmacologists developing possible vaso-constrictor drugs.

He diligently synthesised different combinations of chemicals based around the structure of lysergic acid and in 1938 produced the 25th in his series, lysergic acid diethylamide, which he called LSD-25; the 'S' abbreviation standing for 'saure', the German word for acid. Had the compound been discovered in an English-speaking country we may now be talking about LAD not LSD[8]. It is widely believed that this moment in 1938 was the first-time LSD had been brought into existence. However, by way of an interesting anecdote Leo Perutz, Austrian novelist and mathematician, published a story in 1933 about a scientist who discovers a psychotropic

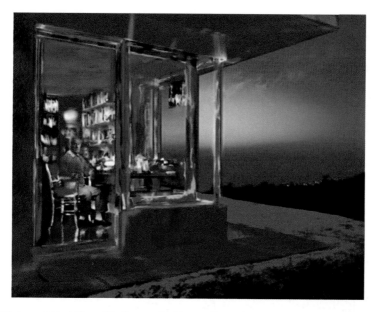

Picture 23: Albert Hofmann by Dean Chamberlain. This photograph appeared in the December 2006 edition of the *British Journal of Psychiatry* in celebration of Albert's 100th birthday. While the picture may look like a computer-enhanced image, it was made by shooting the subject in complete darkness with a several hours long exposure time. The artist then moved around the frame, exposing all the areas of the subject with a torch and a series of coloured gels. Used with kind permission of the artist.
Text by Dean Chamberlain.

drug based on wheat fungi which is used for mass spiritual transformation. This little-known fact certainly keeps psychedelic historians talking about wild conspiracy theories[9].

Having synthesised LSD in 1938, Hofmann subsequently shelved his new product before discovering its psychoactive properties. Then, fuelled by a strange presentiment that it may have further use, he returned to it again in 1943 and synthesised a fresh batch. It was during this process that Hofmann inadvertently imbibed a small quantity of the drug (possibly by absorption of the crystals through his fingertips or by inadvertently licking his fingers) and experienced a peculiar psychological episode character-ized by dizziness and hallucinations:

I became affected by a remarkable restlessness, combined with a slight dizzi-ness. At home I lay down and sank into a not unpleasant intoxicated-like condition, characterized by an extremely stimulated imagination. In a dream-like state, with eyes closed (I found the daylight to be unpleasantly glaring), I perceived an uninterrupted stream of fantastic pictures, extraordinary shapes with intense, kaleidoscopic play of colors. After some two hours this condition faded away.[10]

What happened next sealed the fate of the psychedelic culture and spawned a massive body of new research. It is a direct result of Hofmann's inquisitive personality that history turned out the way it did.

Hofmann the Creative Explorer

Many other scientists, having experienced what Albert Hofmann did that day with his accidental absorption, might have either ignored it, brushed it off, perhaps labelled the tube 'toxic' and never returned to it again. But for Hofmann, this was not enough. Always the exploratory scientist, with a creative imagination to boot, and a fascination for curious mental states, he decided to conduct a personal experiment.

A few days later, monitored by his colleagues he measured out what he thought was the tiniest possible amount of his LSD-25 — he chose 250 micrograms (a quarter of a tenth of a gram). The plan was to intentionally swallow this amount, which he did not expect to have any effect at such a small dose, and then slowly increase the dose by fractions of 25 micrograms until he felt something happening. For the record, 250 micrograms is a *whopping* dose of LSD — the average street dose today being between 75 and 100 micrograms.

What followed was another, even more intense experience, and that famous bicycle ride from his laboratory to his house. As he lay on his bed at home he was terrified and thought he was dying. His neighbour brought him a glass of milk and he saw her distorted image as that of a 'malevolent witch'. A doctor attended and reassured him that all his vital physical signs were normal and he was in no apparent physical danger. Then, as the hours passed and the intensity reduced a little, he was gradually able to enjoy the experience and drift languidly into hitherto unknown mental spaces of immense fascination and delight:

Little by little I could begin to enjoy the unprecedented colours and plays of shapes that persisted behind my closed eyes. Kaleidoscopic, fantastic images surged in on me, alternating, variegated, opening and then closing themselves in circles and spirals, exploding in coloured fountains, rearranging and hybridizing themselves in constant flux.

Again, at this point Hofmann could have shelved his LSD-25, passing the substance over to his toxicology colleagues and getting back to his day job

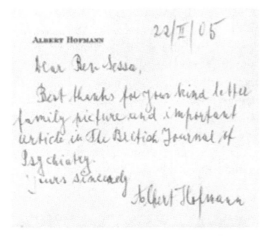

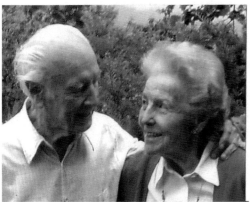

Pictures 24 and 25:
A postcard and photo from Albert Hofmann, on hearing the news of the publication of an editorial in the British Journal of Psychiatry; the first contemporary mention of psychedelic research in British mainstream medicine in modern times.

of synthesizing chemicals for circulatory problems. But he knew he was on to something. Here was a substance with immeasurable potential, powerfully active even in the most miniscule of doses (it is still recognised today as the most potent psychoactive substance known to science by an order of magnitude far beyond the next contender). But which field of science could possibly be interested in such a thing? The answer, clearly, was (and is) psychiatry.

Self-experimenting was the only viable method of believing the chemical's fantastic properties and he convinced his seniors to try the drug themselves. They were similarly impressed by its importance. There followed several years of phase one investigations of the drug by staff at the Sandoz laboratories, testing it on animals to evaluate its degree of toxicity and potential safety for human consumption. The Second World War delayed progress for a while until, eventually, in 1947 Hofmann's colleague Werner Stoll at the University of Zurich published the first academic description of the mental effects of LSD on humans[11].

The laboratory studies had concluded that despite the drug's intense mental effects, LSD appeared to be largely physiologically inert, causing little more than mild fluctuations of the pulse and blood pressure, and a dilation of the pupils. It had minimal effect on laboratory animals apart from causing some mild restlessness. Of course, had those rats and mice been able to talk we would doubtless have heard a very different story (but then, had they talked we might have wondered what we too had taken). In conclusion, LSD-25 was considered, rightly, to be physiologically non-toxic. Now deemed perfectly safe for human consumption, the plan was made for its distribution to psychiatrists worldwide under the brand name *Delysid.*

LSD Comes to Blighty for the First Time

Of course, no one can know for certain who first brought LSD into Britain. A possible candidate was either Dr Joel Elkes, a highly

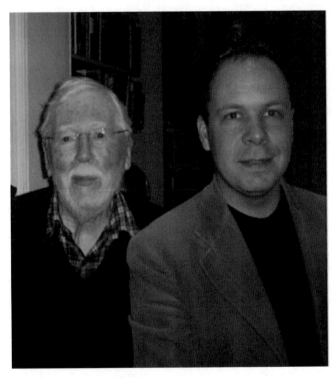

Picture 26: Dr. Ronald Sandison at his home in Ledbury, Herefordshire, in 2006.

influential doctor and psychopharmacologist working at the Birmingham University department of Experimental Psychology, or his Birmingham colleagues, William Meyer-Gross. However, the psychiatrist Dr Ronald Sandison, whilst maybe not the first person to bring LSD into the country, is arguably the British doctor who did the most to develop research with the drug in the earliest days of 1950s Britain. He described to me when I first met him in 2006 the academic climate in psychiatry at that time:

"It was immensely exciting. We were looking for a new world. It's hard now to recapture the excitement of those years. During the decade or so after the war we were talking about the new Elizabethan age; everything seemed possible[12]."

In 1952 Sandison, like almost everyone else outside of that single laboratory in Basel, had never heard of LSD. But he went on an international study tour of Switzerland that year and, while he was travelling around looking at different psychiatric institutions, he got the opportunity to visit the laboratories at Sandoz. Sandison was fascinated by Hofmann's research with LSD, and was surprised that none of the other members of his party showed much interest in the work of the Swiss chemist. He made a point of returning to Sandoz two months later, in November 1952. Hofmann was gladly giving out LSD to any respectable psychiatrist who thought they might be able to develop some useful research utilising the new compound. And so Sandison came away with 100 vials of *Delysid*.

Sandison immediately began using LSD as part of his psychotherapy program at Powick Hospital in Gloucestershire. Giving the drug to patients who had become stuck in traditional psychotherapy, Sandison soon collected a sizeable cases series for publication. In 1954 he published an early paper describing a large group of LSD-assisted psychotherapy patients, 'The Therapeutic Value of Lysergic Acid Diethylamide in Mental Illness', in the British publication, *The Journal of Mental Science*, the forerunner of the *British Journal of Psychiatry*[13]. In it he described how, using LSD, he was able to re-awaken a therapeutic response from 36 patients who had become stuck with treatment resistance. His managerial colleagues at Powick backed the research and in 1954, with financial support from Joel Elkes' team at the Birmingham Regional Hospital Board, Sandison built a special purpose LSD clinic — the world's first — attached to the outside of the main old hospital building by a corridor. 'Of course it has all been demolished now', said Sandison in 2007. 'They kept the main building, but the very fine ballroom was demolished and luxury flats were built on the site'.

Just an Average Day at Work

Prior to starting the LSD work, all of Sandison's patients had already been in traditional psychotherapy for varying periods of time; some for many years. There was no set rule but all of the patients had been failing to progress in normal psychotherapy.

There would be up to five patients for each LSD session. A volunteer driver would bring them to the clinic at nine in the morning and the patients and clinical staff would meet briefly. Then the patients would take their LSD dissolved in a glass of water. Generally, they would begin on a low dose, around 20mcg, which would be increased week on week until Sandison saw some progress. The average weekly maintenance dose was

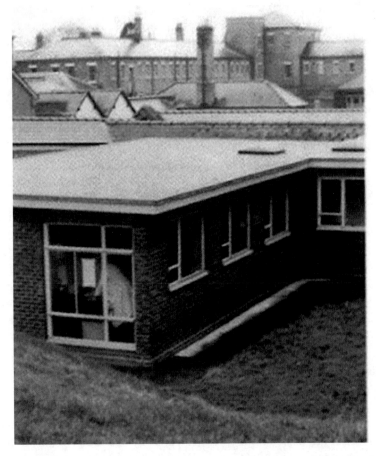

Picture 27: The world's first purpose built LSD unit at Powick Hospital in 1955. Up to five patients at a time received their medicine under the care of Ronnie Sandison.

150mcg. After taking the drug the patients would then retire to their rooms. There was a main corridor with the five individual session rooms extending off it. Here they would stay for the main part of the session.

During the next few hours, the nurses or medical registrars would go in and visit the patients as they lay on their beds. There was not someone with them always as many of the patients often preferred to be on their own. There was a record player available for them if they wanted to listen to music, and a blackboard for drawing on. Some patients brought teddy bears.

Then, at about 4pm, the patients got together for a 'wash up' group session to talk about the day's proceedings, before their drivers arrived and took them home. The LSD clinic staff had a very good working relationship with the drivers who played an important role. The patients got to

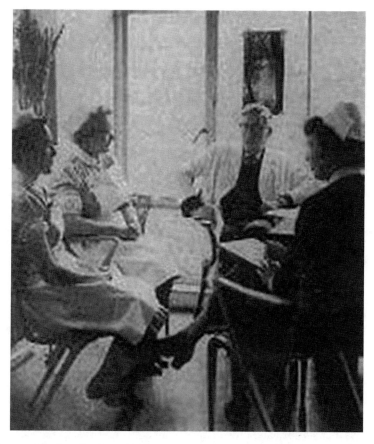

Picture 28: Sandison and his team of LSD nurses. Patients brought their power object teddies and drew their experiences on blackboards.

know their drivers well during their treatment because at the end of the day when they were still experiencing the effects of the LSD they would often chat to their driver on the way home. So the doctors and nurses endeavoured to make sure the patient got the same driver each time. Hence these volunteer car drivers became part of the therapeutic team.

Generally, patients had weekly sessions with LSD. Some had it twice a week. There was no set limit about how many sessions were offered, but generally if a patient had shown no response or progression after 20 sessions they might stop the treatment as by then it was assumed it probably wasn't going to work. Following Hofmann's later synthesis of psilocybin in 1957, which was then distributed by Sandoz as the product *Indocybin*, Sandison also tried using this with some of his patients. He recognized and appreciated that psilocybin had its place, as a shorter-acting and therefore slightly more clinically manageable alternative, but he generally found LSD to be more effective.

Will LSD be the Next Big Thing in Psychiatry?

The staff at Powick were a committed and involved team. The BBC made two films at the clinic: *The Magic Mushroom* in the 1950s and later *The Beyond Within*. The psychiatric profession, and the public, quickly began to take notice of this new experimental approach and a major LSD conference was held during part of the annual Conference of the American Psychiatric Association in 1955. Ronald Sandison was invited, and spoke about the work he had been doing at Powick. Aldous Huxley was also present, speaking about his own life-changing experience with mescaline two years earlier.

In 1959 Sandison introduced the term *psycholytic* ('mind-loosening') to describe the action of LSD, and in 1961 he organised a three-day symposium for the Medico-Psychological Association, the forerunner of the Royal College of Psychiatrists. Several eminent psychiatrists, psychoanalysts, writers and commentators spoke at that event, including Tom Main and Ernst Gombrich, and all were very well received. Also at the conference was the British Member of Parliament Christopher Mayhew, who, in 1960, had famously taken mescaline in front of a BBC film crew[14].

This was all happening in an era before the popular knowledge and misuse of LSD. Drug abuse on a large scale was an unrecognized phenomenon, and even within medicine there was no Committee of Safety in Medicines as there is now, and little in the way of ethical boards. Evidence-based medicine was not recognized as a concept, and clinicians were effectively left to get on with whatever treatment they felt was right for their patients.

LSD as a Psychotomimetic

Sandison and UK psychiatry led the world in the early 1950s by developing the earliest centre for large-scale psychotherapeutic use of LSD. But his was not the first paper to describe LSD being given to psychiatric patients. That occurred in 1949 and is credited to psychiatrists at the Boston Psychopathic Hospital (now the Massachusetts Mental Health Center) in the States. They believed LSD's main role was not as an adjunct to psychotherapy, but as a tool to mimic and model psychoses; a tool for doctors and other clinicians to take *themselves* in order to glimpse what it feels like to have schizophrenia. The remarkable psychological qualities of LSD, coupled with the fact that it was a known organic agent with a demonstrable (though at the time poorly understood) mode of action, excited many researchers that here was a way of understanding how schizophrenia works at the brain level.

Theories were put forward, many involving the possible role for adrenaline or noradrenaline (epinephrine or norepinephrine), which excited interested researchers at the Boston Psychopathic Hospital, not least because they supported the prevailing opinion of one of their contemporaries, Dr. Daniel H. Funkenstein, who had proposed a pituitary-driven physiological explanation for the modulation of mental states.

In 1950, in a study with far more in common with the European development of psycholytic psychotherapy, Anthony Busch and Warren Johnson of St. Louis, Missouri, USA, published the results of a small case series describing the effects of LSD when given at low doses (maximum 40mcg) to 29 patients, mainly with paranoid schizophrenia or mania[15]. They concluded that the drug appeared to safely allow for improved access to their otherwise inaccessible mental states, and proposed further studies to consider whether the drug had a role in enhancing psychotherapy.

Enter Dr. Humphrey Osmond

The suggestion that LSD could be used as a psychotomimetic, and that the psychedelic state could teach us something about the natural process of schizophrenia, prevailed in the USA and particularly caught the attention of Humphrey Osmond, a British psychiatrist based in Canada. Working at the Weyburn Mental Hospital in Saskatchewan with his friend and colleague, Dr John Smythies, he further proposed links between the mescaline state and schizophrenia. Smythies and Osmond published a small essay on these matters in 1952, 'A New Approach to Schizophrenia'[16], and introduced the Adrenochrone Hypothesis for schizophrenia, which suggests that adrenaline undergoes a degradation process in the brain and becomes a psychoactive compound, adrenochrone, which was known to have a low potency psychedelic effect and therefore could explain the symptoms of schizophrenia. Osmond went on to conduct several important psychedelic drug trials in Canada throughout the 1950s in collaboration with Abram Hoffer. He gained attention for his work utilising LSD therapy for patients with alcohol dependence.

Using LSD to Treat Alcohol Dependence

It is well known, both back then and today, that for a significant proportion of alcohol dependent patients when they 'hit rock bottom' and experience the terrifying effects of the Delirium Tremens (DTs) this leads to spontaneous sobriety. For around 10% of patients the DTs, a profound organic psychosis brought on when heavy dependent drinkers undergo a rapid withdrawal from alcohol, prompts an immediate and intense distaste of alcohol.

From their interest in mescaline, Osmond and his colleagues in the 1950s in Saskatchewan knew of the experimental compound LSD, which was being shipped around the world free of charge from Hofmann's laboratory to any psychiatrists who thought they might be able to do something useful with it. The product information for Delysid said on the bottle that it produced a physiologically safe organic psychosis.

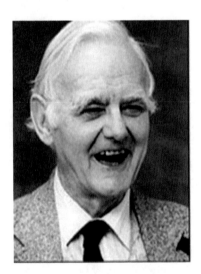

Picture 29: The British Psychiatrist in Canada, Dr Humphrey Osmond.

Osmond's theory was that, as the DTs is a severe and dangerous psychosis that can lead to sobriety, why don't we give our alcoholic patients this new drug LSD and see what happens? The hope was that the LSD would scare the willies out of the patients but with none of the physiological risks of the real DTs. It might just work. So, they gave their patients LSD. But much to their surprise it did not frighten them out of their wits in quite the way the researchers had imagined. On the contrary, many of the patients quite enjoyed the experience, and moreover, it did lead to abstinence from alcohol. Osmond and colleagues fine-tuned the process further, adding elements of supportive psychotherapy and, before long, could boast of abstinence rates of 50–90%, which far surpasses all other treatments for the condition before or since. So impressed was the Saskatchewan Bureau on Alcoholism that in 1962 it went as far as to report that 'such excellent results have been noted by the bureau staff in individual cases, usually with resistance to other forms of therapy, that LSD treatment, which was originally regarded by the bureau as experimental, became a standard form of treatment to be used where indicated'.

There have been notable critics of the Saskatchewan experiments, with some people stating that the team did not use adequate controls. And some researchers — particularly Ludwig in 1970 — set out to rubbish the experiments by repeating them but with no attention paid to set and setting. When patients became overwhelmed by the experience they were restrained and tied to the bed, which did frighten them. Unsurprisingly, Ludwig yielded poor results[17]. Nevertheless, the topic of using psychedelic drugs as treatments for addiction has remained hot ever since.

In 2012 the Norwegian couple Teri S. Krebs and Pål-Ørjan Johansen published an important meta-analysis paper reviewing six randomized trials of LSD-for-alcoholism from the 1950s and 1960s. They tackled the heterogeneity of the early studies; which had wide ranges of doses, varying control conditions and variable degrees of support and follow-up. Taken together, the early studies describe generally favourable results, with 59%

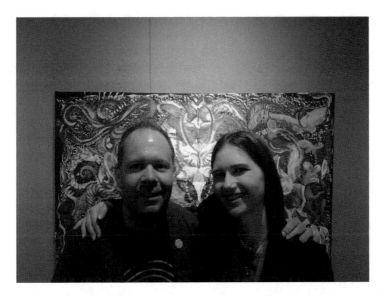

Picture 30: Celebrated psychedelic researcher, Teri Krebs, director of the Emma Sofia programme. In Prague, 2016

of the LSD-treated participants significantly improved compared to 38% of the controls. This demonstrates a strong case for revisiting classical psychedelics in the treatment of addictions[18].

There is a lot of sense in the idea that once a person has experienced a reaction as intense as a high-dose LSD session (Osmond was using mega doses), other drugs such as alcohol, cocaine and heroin seem rather paltry by comparison. This leads to cracks appearing in the hold of addition, which can then be further widened by focused psychotherapy. This was also the rationale behind Evgeny Krupitsky's work in 1990s Russia, using ketamine-assisted psychotherapy to treat addictions[19] — a topic we will cover later.

A notable further word in the Humphrey Osmond story is that of his relationship with Bill Wilson, who had formed Alcoholics Anonymous (AA) in the 1930s, and took LSD under Osmond's auspices in the 1950s. AA applies an essentially spiritual model of treatment through which to attain and maintain sobriety. In this context, Wilson could see the potential role LSD could play, saying:

> *It is a generally acknowledged fact in spiritual development that ego reduction makes the influx of God's grace possible. If, therefore, under LSD we can have a temporary reduction, so that we can better see what we are and where we are going — well, that might be of some help. The goal might become clearer. So I consider LSD to be of some value to some people, and practically no damage to anyone.[20]*

But, funnily enough, Wilson's support for LSD in the 1950s is rarely mentioned to the two million AA members today, nor does it figure in the organisation's famous Twelve Steps method. However, watch this space to see how the field of addictions — an area of psychiatry fraught with ineffective treatments and high remittance rates — might be transformed by the development of new research into psychedelic drugs.

Enter Aldous Huxley

The final mention of Osmond is to report on his famous meeting with Aldous Huxley, perhaps one of the most famous and noteworthy historical episodes of all, as it not only led to the writing of the one of the most celebrated popular texts on the subject, but also generated the very word that appears in this book's title.

Aldous Huxley was already in his 60s when he wrote to Humphrey Osmond in 1953, having been intrigued by one of the British psychiatrist's papers on the effects of mescaline. Huxley was a lifelong writer and lover of all things mystical. He was known internationally for his highly intellectual novels and essays, which covered history, philosophy, all aspects of the arts, human lives and relationships. He had explored in detail the religions of the East and was fascinated by the subject of mystics and altered states of consciousness, but had never actually experienced these first hand.

By the 1950s, Huxley was living in Hollywood, where the sunlight suited his poor eyesight better than his native Oxford, and he invited Osmond over to chat, but with an ulterior motive.

He expressed a keen desire to take mescaline.

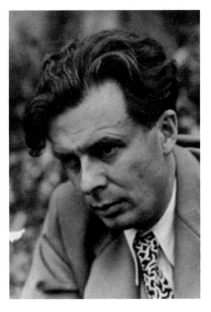

Picture 31: The academic literary mystic, Aldous Huxley.

On a bright morning on May 4, 1953, Osmond nervously handed Huxley a glass of water in which was famously dissolved 'four tenths of a gram of mescaline'. Huxley was excited about the event, having effectively waited his whole life to glimpse the realms about which he had been writing for decades. Osmond remarked later just how anxious he had been about the situation, concerned that he would be forever remembered in history as 'the man who drove Aldous Huxley mad'. He need not have worried. Huxley loved the mescaline experience, and went on to write one of the most widely read texts on the subject, *The Doors of Perception*[21], which takes its name from William Blake's observation that:

> If the doors of perception were cleansed Everything will appear to man as it is, infinite.

Sharing British roots, both men were academics living abroad and both keen writers. The relationship between Huxley and Osmond grew, and a series of letters passed between them in which they discussed all aspects of this curious group of chemical compounds, the hallucinogens. Among other things, they pondered what these drugs should be called. Neither was comfortable with the emerging suggestion of 'psychotomimetic', as they felt the effects of these drugs went far beyond that of simply mimicking psychosis — after all, there were all the aspects of the undeniable spiritual experience that needed to be accounted for in a name.

Huxley suggested *phanerothyme*, which means 'to make the soul visible' and wrote to Osmond illustrating his proposed name with a brief poem:

To make this trivial world sublime Take half a gramme of phanerothyme.

This suggestion led to Osmond's now famous reply, thus concluding the issue and creating an entire culture:

To fathom hell or soar angelic Just take a pinch of psychedelic[22].

Thus, the term *psychedelic*, which means literally 'mind manifesting' was born, and Osmond first used it publicly at a meeting of the New York Academy of Sciences in 1957.

A Brief Mention of Al Hubbard

Huxley spent the last ten years of his life deeply ensconced in the — at that time — small and exclusive psychedelic culture. In 1955 he tried LSD that was given to him by Al Hubbard — a mysterious and shady character from LSD history[23]. An entrepreneurial shape-shifter, Hubbard is reported to have worked both within and outside official government departments, been a scientific director of the Uranium Corporation of Vancouver, and owned his own fleet of aircraft, a 100-foot yacht, and a Canadian island. He also travelled around the world propagating LSD along the way.

Huxley the Conservative

Aldous Huxley wrote several other works relating to his experiences with psychedelic drugs and his last novel, *Island* (which was the antithesis of *Brave New World*, his most famous book written years earlier in 1932), tackles the issue of the role psychedelic drugs could play as part of coming to terms with death in a utopian world[24]. Given the popularity of *The Doors of Perception*, Huxley can be credited as one of the first people to effect a crossover of these drugs from the exclusive world of the scientists into popular culture. This is ironic, as Huxley himself held rather conservative views about how psychedelics ought to be used. He did not believe these drugs should be taken by the masses (as was the role for *soma* in *Brave New World*), but that they should, rather, remain within the realms of intellectuals, writers and artists like himself. In fact, he was a very reluctant figurehead of the emerging psychedelic movement, who had crowned him as their leader in the wake of his little essay on his mescaline experience.

Huxley died of laryngeal cancer on November 22nd 1963, the same day as President Kennedy was assassinated — most likely a fortuitous event as far as Huxley would have been concerned, as it nicely overshadowed his own departure. On his deathbed, he instructed his wife, Laura, to inject him with 100mcg of intra-muscular LSD[25]. This she did. And whilst the other occupants of the house watched in horror as the news of Kennedy's assignation came on the television, Huxley slipped peacefully into the white light of infinity, cradled by Laura, soaring on the molecule he had discovered so late in his life. A molecule that so perfectly celebrated the state of mystical bliss and enlightenment he had been searching for with all his marvellously erudite books about the human experience of living and dying.

Stanislav Grof and the Perinatal Matrices

In continental Europe, psychedelic research was taking off. Stanislav Grof began sitting in on LSD psychotherapy sessions as an observer in 1954 when he was a medical student. He had his first personal LSD experience after graduating from Charles University School of Medicine in Prague, Czechoslovakia in 1956. This first psychedelic experience occurred as part of an experimental study in which he was required to undergo an EEG measurement at the same time as being asked to lie beneath a powerful strobe light whose flashes were calibrated to tune in to his corresponding brain waves. The experience was life changing and resulted in a career studying non-ordinary states of consciousness[26].

Grof moved to the States in 1967 to work at John Hopkins University, later holding a position at the Maryland Psychiatric Research Centre, and serving as scholar-in-residence at the Esalen Institute in Big Sur, California. Through a lifetime of work with psychedelic drug and non-drug induced non-ordinary states of consciousness, Grof has developed a systemised theory describing how early pre-natal and birth experiences can be re-experienced when in non-ordinary states of consciousness. He described a detailed cartography or map of the inner space of consciousness and used these methods clinically with his patients to help them recognise how their very early infantile and foetal experiences continue to influence their lives.

This form of psychotherapy differed considerably from Sandison's psycholytic method, which used low to medium doses of LSD in repeated sessions. In contrast, Grof has often proposed using a single — or infrequent, such as monthly — high-dose session (up to 500 micrograms of LSD) followed by subsequent non-drug sessions in which the patient explored and integrated the massive outpouring of psychological material that occurred in the drug session.

Grof has carried out pioneering clinical work on the use of non-ordinary states of consciousness in the therapeutic management of easing anxiety associated with the experience of dying. Together with Joan Halifax he published his work with patients suffering mainly with cancer at the Maryland Psychiatric Research Center. Then, when LSD was banned in the late sixties and most research fizzled out, Grof, in collaboration with his wife Christina, developed a unique technique of breathing, involving hyperventilation, to induce the experience of a non-ordinary state of consciousness. His Holotropic Breathwork© method endures as a popular form of healing today, and is used by many people around the world[27]. Since 1994, Grof has been professor of psychology at the California Institute of Integral Studies in San Francisco. He remains one of the leading figures in contemporary transpersonal psychotherapy and psychedelic research.

Harvard University and Timothy Leary

No history of the roots of psychedelic research would be complete without the Timothy Leary story. This chapter is no exception, although much of Leary's story, because it strays from the subject of developments in the clinical aspects of LSD, best belongs in chapter five, Hippie Heydays.

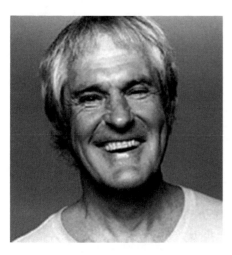

Picture 32: The much-maligned, erudite and visionary anti-establishment trickster, psychologist Dr Timothy Leary, whose message by today's standards was relatively benign.

Leary, of course, would be proud to be remembered for straying away from the 'mainstream game', as he called it[28].

Leary was a successful research psychologist by the time he got to Harvard in 1959, having previously written a well-received academic paper on the measurement of personality characteristics. He was interested in how the human personality could be dissected into its constituent parts according to a fairly rigid set of rules that govern personality traits. His design even gained the name of the Leary Circumplex or Leary Circle in which he described, 'a two-dimensional representation of personality organized around two major axes'[29]. His system found patterns in human personality traits and focused on how the interpersonal process could be used to diagnose mental disorders. However, his life was to take a sudden change in direction, when, in August 1960, on a visit to Cuernavaca in Mexico, he was given the opportunity to try the local *Psilocybe mexicana* mushrooms.

A self-confessed hard-drinking Irishman, who, prior to Harvard, had been enrolled as a cadet at West Point Military Academy (before resigning following a court martial for a bout of drinking), Leary's experience of altered states of consciousness up to that point had not strayed beyond that of alcohol. On leaving the army, he studied psychology and then gained his PhD at the University of California, Berkeley in 1950. But it was that day in 1960, by the pool in Mexico, that was to change his life forever.

Leary Discovers the Divine Mushroom

Leary had decided to travel to Mexico inspired by a *Life* Magazine article by the amateur mycologist Gordon Wasson. After the experience, he was so convinced of the transformative powers of the magic mushroom to positively alter an individual's personality and life course that, on his return to Harvard, he decided to dedicate his research to this newly discovered focus of enquiry, namely, the psychedelic drugs. After the mushroom trip Leary commented:

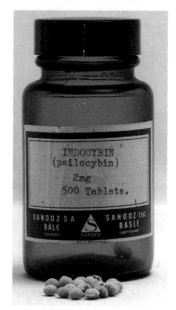

I learned more about my brain and its possibilities in the five hours after taking these mushrooms than I had in the preceding fifteen years of studying and doing research in psychology.

He set up the Harvard Psilocybin Project with colleague Richard Alpert using a supply of synthetic psilocybin provided by Sandoz. Leary and Alpert (who later became Ram Dass) set about running experiments in which they gave psilocybin to 36 inmates at the local Concord Prison[30]. Combining the drug with guided psychotherapy, the experimenters hoped to demonstrate that psilocybin therapy could lower criminal

Picture 33: *Indocybin,* the infamous little yellow pills from Sandoz that prompted Ginsberg to pick up the phone to JFK.

recidivism rates, which they claimed to have reduced from 60% to 20% in their experimental group (these figures were challenged when MAPS founder Rick Doblin reviewed the study data much later)[31].

Leary Graduates to LSD

In 1962 Leary graduated from psilocybin to LSD when dosed by British researcher Michael Hollingshead[32]. Another flamboyant figure from LSD folklore, Hollingshead is not only credited with introducing Leary to acid, but is also allegedly responsible for giving the drug to, among others, Paul McCartney, John Lennon, George Harrison, Charles Mingus, Maynard Ferguson, William S. Burroughs, Roman Polanski, Allen Ginsberg, Donovan, Keith Richards, and the philosopher and immensely popular figure of comparative religion, Alan Watts — who applied the insights from their psychedelic experiences to their various trades.

When Hollingshead turned up at Timothy Leary's place at Harvard in 1961, having been directed towards Leary by Aldous Huxley, he had with him a now legendary supply of LSD in a mayonnaise jar, mixed into a sugary paste. Although he had just one gram of the then still legal drug, this was enough for five thousand 200 microgram hits. Famous for saying, 'Acid was a bundle of solutions looking for a problem', Hollingshead lived in Leary's house, taught at Harvard and participated in the Concord Prison Experiment.

Leary and Alpert soon expanded their project and set up an organisation called The International Federation for Internal Freedom (IFIF), and gave their psychedelics to a wide variety of people, including artists and writers. The scientific controls around the experiments gradually loosened and they encouraged the trippers to simply experience whatever arose, then describe how it was. Their voyagers included Arthur Koestler, Neal Cassady and Jack Kerouac, amongst others, who dutifully recorded their impressions.

During the summer recesses from Harvard, Leary and Alpert set up The Zihuatanejo Project, which was an idea based on Huxley's utopian novel *Island*. Paying members of IFIF gathered at the beachfront Catalina Hotel in Zihuatanejo in Guerrero, Mexico, where with Leary, Richard Alpert and another Harvard researcher, Ralph Metzner, they took part in group LSD sessions. But soon the Mexican authorities became suspicious of the crazy Americans' all night sessions of love and music on the beach, and when the media started to report their 'LSD Paradise' Leary and colleagues were ejected from Mexico and returned to the USA on a specially charted jet. Leary returned to Harvard only to find he had been fired.

The official reason for the loss of his job was given as absenteeism, that he had been in Mexico when he was meant to be teaching classes. But rumours were circulating with the Harvard authorities that he had given drugs to undergraduate students outside of his project. The truth is the authorities had been getting increasingly uncomfortable about the amount of attention Leary and his crew were attracting on campus. For his part, Leary was making no efforts to play down the anti-authority viewpoints that spontaneously emerged in the context of his repeated high-dose psychedelic drug use[33].

Timothy Leary's proselytizing of psychedelics did not end there, of course, and his influence on the developing 1960s countercultures in America and beyond became legendary — a story we will pick up later in the book.

God in a Bottle

Before his departure from Harvard, Leary played his part in a very important research study, The Marsh Chapel Experiment, which has since gone down in history[34]. Also called 'the Good Friday Experiment', it was the PhD project of Walter N. Pahnke, a student in theology at Harvard Divinity School. Leary was supervising Pahnke as part of the Harvard Psilocybin Project at the time. Pahnke was investigating whether psilocybin could induce a spiritual-type experience in religiously predisposed subjects. The study stands out in psychedelic history partly because of the elaborate surroundings (it was conducted on Good Friday, 1962, at Boston University's Marsh Chapel), partly because of Leary's connection, and partly because it was one of the most beautifully designed double-blind placebo controlled psychedelic studies of its day — one of the very few from that that period, in fact, with such a high degree of scientific robustness; most other psychedelic studies of the time produced mere anecdotal data by comparison. Rick Doblin of MAPS reviewed this crucial moment in psychedelic research history many years later, in 1991, when he revisited the original participants of the Good Friday Experiment. They described how the insights and spiritual awareness gained that day have stayed with them throughout their lives as Christian ministers[35].

But another reason why the Marsh Chapel experiment became so talked about was because it sparked a controversial debate, one which still rages today, about the extent to which a drug can reliably mimic or, indeed, *induce*, a genuine spiritual experience.

To study whether the drug had actually *created* a mystical experience, Pahnke used a structured set of criteria designed by W. T. Stace, which were agreed to accurately represent such an experience. Stace developed the scale for evaluation by conducting a review of multiple written examples of the characteristics of the (non-drug) mystical experience, identifying nine core criteria that were shared and essential to characterise a true mystical experience. These, which were translated by Bill Richards and Pahnke to directly describe the psychedelic experience, are listed in the last chapter of this book.

In his experiment, Pahnke gave half the group (ten subjects) an active placebo, nicotinic acid, which produces a mild tingling stimulation to fool the subjects into thinking they may have had the active drug. The other ten people received a 30mg dose of psilocybin — a large dose by any standards. However, despite the efforts to blind the experiment in this way, it became obvious within half an hour who had had which drug: members of the psilocybin group were lounging around the pews of the church in awe at the booming voice of the minister delivering the sermon; the other group members were feeling somewhat short-changed. The participants, all of whom already had a strong Christian faith and were studying theology as part of a path towards becoming ministers, were later required to complete a battery of tests that measured the quality of their experience. The outcome was a success, with results very positively in favour of psilocybin inducing a mystical or spiritual experience. Nine out of ten of the psilocybin group fulfilled the criteria for having had a fully-fledged spiritual experience, compared to just one of the placebo group. Pahnke thus concluded:

> The results of our experiment would indicate that psilocybin is an important tool for the study of the mystical (transcendence, ecstasy, cosmic) state of consciousness. . . . This is a realm of human experience that is reproducible under suitable conditions and should not be rejected as outside the realm of serious scientific study. . . . Our data suggests that when a person existentially encounters basic values such as the meaning of his life (past, present, and future), deep and meaningful interpersonal relationships, and insight into the possibility of personal behavior change, can be therapeutic if approached and worked with in a sensitive and adequate way.

God in a Bottle? Not Everyone's Cup of Tea

Pahnke's work and the ideas that sprang from it stimulated a lot of debate, not least from the likes of the ex-intelligence officer and Catholic academic R.C. Zaehner, who at the time was the Oxford University Spalding Professor of Eastern Religions and Ethics. Zaehner was not a fan of psychedelics, having previously experienced a bad trip with mescaline, and he went out of his way to rubbish the insights many people at the time (including Huxley) were attributing to psychedelic drugs[36]. Zaehner's conservative views contrasted significantly with the more esoteric reports coming from those who championed the psychedelic experience. He claimed that any mystical state other than those that are theistic or attached to an organised religion, must be inherently amoral.

Zaehner was certainly not alone in wishing to rubbish the value of the psychedelic state and distance it from other 'more natural and proper' routes to godliness. In a pamphlet released in 1966 called *God in a Pill?*, Meher Baba, an Indian guru popular in the West at the time, was keen to discredit LSD's ability to induce a genuine spiritual state, claiming psychedelics were harmful for the user[37].

However, this did little to curb the enthusiasm of the psychedelic researchers. Many other experiments besides Pahnke's investigated the potential role of psychedelics as agents to induce spiritual experiences. In their 1966 book *The Varieties of Psychedelic Experience*, Masters and Houston wrote that after ingesting LSD, 96% of subjects had 'religious imagery'[38]. Similarly, in 1964 a study by Downing and Wygant found that 60% felt 'a greater trust in God'[39]. A further study by Walter Clark, published in 1974, claimed that, after taking LSD, 100% of his subjects felt a subjective experience of "being in the presence of God"[40].

Pahnke's influential study continues to inspire today. It was the subject of another famous study in modern times when, in 2006, Roland Griffiths' team at Johns Hopkins University recreated many aspects of the Marsh Chapel Experiment — a subject about which we will learn more of in a later chapter on contemporary psychedelic research.

Things Start to Change and Doctors Get Nervous

Sandison's approach to LSD was different to those of researchers in America. In the UK, there was little support for the hypothesis that LSD could be a psychotomimetic. The nature and quality of the experience was not considered to be at all like schizophrenia, mainly because of the thorny issue of insight. On LSD, you know you've taken a drug and you can be assured that in the space of a few hours the experience will have subsided and you'll be back to normal. This is a radically different situation from someone who has a fixed delusional belief that will not go away. Consequently, few psychiatrists in Britain thought LSD helped them to understand schizophrenia. Sandison never liked the term *psychotomimetic*, which is why he coined the term *psycholytic*. And unlike Leary's approach in the States, self-experimentation in the UK was less prevalent amongst health professionals in the 1950s. Sandison himself took LSD only once:

"It was an enlightening and valuable experience. Some people showed more of an interest in self-experimentation, but not me. I mean, how far does one go with self-experimentation in psychiatry? Does one have ECT?[41]*"*

Personally, I and other contemporary researchers today, believe self-experimentation is an essential part of being a psychedelic therapist. The clinician must have knowledge and understanding of the mental spaces through which she is steering her patient. This will be discussed in more detail later in the book.

By the late 1950s, there were some serious problems emerging; not from the medical uses of the drug, but from the military. The role played in the development of psychedelic culture by government military agencies in America and Europe is undeniable and well documented. At the time, the CIA had a low-profile project, which is now well known, called MK-ULTRA. The CIA project included activities such as agents slipping high doses of LSD to unsuspecting members of the public, and then studying them through two-way mirrors as they interacted with stooges, to see whether LSD could be developed as a truth drug for military purposes. Many horror stories have subsequently emerged that demonstrate that the sanctioned government agencies carrying out this kind of work used methods and produced casualties that far outstrip any of the complaints of unethical practice that could be rallied against the medical profession at the time.

But another, greater phenomenon threatening to undermine medical research was the rising popularity of recreational LSD use. By 1964 the mass use of psychedelics within mainstream culture was only just beginning, but Sandison was becoming worn out. He had already been running his LSD clinic for over twelve years and wanted a rest. Conducting LSD sessions was a time-consuming and draining experience. Also, by the early sixties Powick Hospital was beginning to change. It was moving towards a centre for community psychiatry, and the hospital directors were increasingly pushing it in that direction. There was also the emerging dominance of new neuroleptic (antipsychotic) drugs to treat mental illness, which placed less emphasis on outpatient psychotherapy sessions. For Ronnie it was time to move on.

It is estimated that by 1964 over four million people in the USA had used LSD outside of medical treatment centres. Causalities (which were few and far between when the drug was used under medical supervision) began to appear. Sandison was asked to advise as an expert witness to a high-profile murder trial in 1964 involving a man called Robert Lipman who apparently murdered a sex worker while under the influence of LSD. There was a lot of negative media surrounding the event, and more and more horror stories about the drug were emerging in the press. Many were erroneous, but this negative publicity undoubtedly scared off many fine doctors from entering this field.

A Good Thing Turned Sour, But Outcomes Remain Good

By the mid-sixties, there was a general feeling among most psychiatrists that they didn't want anything to do with LSD. Patients, too, were reluctant to undergo the therapy if they had heard negative reports. It all became very complicated. Of course, there were increasing ethical considerations and bodies forming to control and regulate the profession. In the UK, The Committee for Safety of Medicines was formed in 1966, which introduced new regulatory procedures.

Nevertheless, by this stage there were already many other psychiatrists in the UK other than Sandison who had developed their own LSD psychotherapy services, all of which maintained good results when the drug was used under careful medical supervision. There were treatment facilities at Roffey Park, Surrey; Guys Hospital, London; Netley Hospital, Southampton; and Bromley Psychiatric Clinic. After Sandison's large-scale Powick LSD Clinic the next most prolific provider was The Marlborough Day Hospital in London, which conducted over six thousand LSD sessions and fifty psilocybin sessions on more than five hundred patients during the early 1960s. It had very good results, with no suicides, no serious suicide attempts and only four psychoses throughout this period[42].

Indeed, the evidence base and success of the early use of LSD when used within the clinical environment was very good. Europe's use of psycholytic psychotherapy (using small to moderate doses on a regular basis with patients alongside traditional psychoanalytic psychotherapy) and the USA-based method, psychedelic psychotherapy (using a single high-dose session followed by non-drug sessions to explore and integrate the material that emerged in the drug session), were used to treat a wide range of anxiety disorders.

The 'peak experience' qualities of psychedelic therapy were useful for treating alcohol addiction. And the mystical and reflective qualities of the psychedelic experience were shown to be useful for relieving the pain and anxiety of end-stage cancer, as demonstrated by a series of very positive trials by the psychiatric Eric Kast at Chicago Medical School in 1964[43]. Kast demonstrated that even when LSD was given without any formal psychotherapy it produced dramatic and sustained analgesia that out-performed traditional opiate-based drugs. This phenomenon highlights an interesting mode of action of the classical psychedelic drugs that may be due to its effects on vasoconstriction, and we will return to this later on when we look at some contemporary research with classical psychedelics to treat cluster headaches.

Did Psychedelic Therapy Actually *Work* in the 1960s?

In the 1950s and 1960s, before LSD was banned, throughout the world tens of thousands of patients were treated with psychedelic or psycholytic therapy by the medical profession. When the use of LSD stayed within the medical context, before it became widely used publically, the adverse results were low and success rates were generally good[44]. Over 2,000 papers were published on LSD during that period, and psychedelic therapy was truly considered the next big thing in psychiatry. Widespread popular use of the drug outside of the medical environment had yet to happen (certainly in the UK, though in the USA even by the mid-sixties its use had begun to grow, especially on college campuses) and the treatments were legal and freely available to psychiatrists. None of the media scare stories about nightmarish casualties had appeared. Instead, those psychiatrists who were increasingly choosing this avenue of treatment for their patients were seeing results that were overwhelmingly positive, describing safe and effective therapeutic interventions.

Dr Nicholas Malleson, a member of the Royal College of Physicians and the Advisory Committee on Drug Dependence, carried out an important meta-analysis of psychedelic therapy in the UK at the end of the 1960s. He reviewed 20 years of psychedelic therapy in the UK, which included the pooled results of 4,303 patients over 50,000 psychedelic drug-assisted sessions (most which used LSD, though some studies were also included using psilocybin and mescaline). On reviewing this vast meta-analysis, Malleson found there had been only *two* completed suicides and only 37 patients who had demonstrated a prolonged psychotic reaction lasting over 48 hours[45]. Despite these isolated tragedies, these results are very positive, especially when one remembers that at this time, LSD therapy would generally have only been recommended for the most treatment-resistant chronic cases — for those patients who had failed to progress with other more mainstream treatments of the time, as was the case for most experimental and innovative treatments, both then and now in medicine.

By today's standards, to give an example for comparison, if one looked at a random group of over 4,000 severe psychiatric patients over

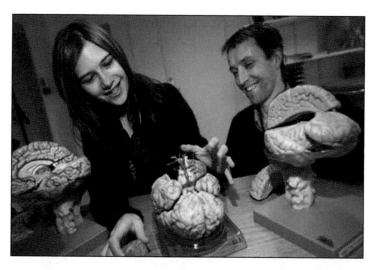

Picture 34: Teri Krebs and Pal Johansen. Two Norwegians whose work, which involved temporarily removing the brains of their subjects and examining them on the lab surface before reinstalling them into their subjects, has done so much to further the field of psychedelic research.

time one would see a great many more than just two completed suicides. This observation further strengthens the agreed opinion at the time that LSD therapy was both effective and safe when used in the context of the clinical environment, under appropriate medical supervision by carefully trained professionals using structured and controlled therapeutic paradigms.

Indeed, in 2013 a highly influential paper by that dynamic Norwegian duo, Teri Krebs and Pal Johansen, describes a large sample of participants whose use of recreational psychedelics have not only caused them no harm but appear to have had an additional *positive* effect on their mental health above that of people without psychedelic experience[46]. This paper has provoked a welcomed positive reaction from the public, suggesting what many in the healing profession have believed for some time; that far been from being a demon to be feared, used wisely psychedelics could be beneficial for people.

Back in 1969 Malleson had already come to the same conclusion in his review of psychedelic drugs applied in the clinical environment thus adding:

> *Treatment with LSD is not without acute adverse reactions, but given adequate psychiatric supervision and proper conditions for its administration, the incidence of such reactions is not great.*

As the sixties wore on, it was not only larger hospitals that were developing LSD services, but also many small and private organisations who were not subjected to anything like the sorts of controls around clinical practice that one sees today. And in those private practices clustered around Harley Street and Wimpole Street in London there was one such doctor who became an enthusiastic advocate of psychedelic drug therapy. It was the Scottish psychiatrist Ronald David Laing.

The Anti-Psychiatry Psychiatrist with a Passion for LSD

Dr R. D. Laing saw LSD as an essential tool to assist professionals in experiencing the inner world of the psychotic or neurotic patient and as a valuable therapeutic device for loosening the ego defences of highly strung patients.

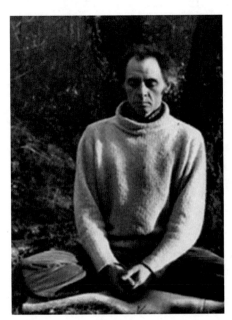

Laing spearheaded the anti-psychiatry movement, which influenced many of us deeply — including myself[48]. Looking back now, with almost two decades of clinical psychiatry behind me, I see many aspects of the anti-psychiatry movement of the 1960s that bear little resemblance to our present system. Back in the sixties, there were still many institutions that had failed to move on since the days of those dreadful 19th century asylums. Practices such as psycho-surgery and ECT without anaesthesia were mainstream treatments, and many patients were still confined in hospitals because of their 'moral weaknesses'. For example, homosexuality was considered a 'treatable mental disorder' until as late as the 1970s. Even Timothy Leary himself, who one might have

Picture 35: R. D. Laing first took LSD in 1960 and was so smitten that, when asked what advice he would give for those wishing to become a psychoanalyst, he answered: *'Number One, read the works of Freud. Number two, undergo a personal analysis and number three, take LSD.*[47]

assumed to be more broad-minded on the issue, was not shy of talking about how LSD could 'cure' homosexuals by 'turning them on to women'[49]. So Laing had a lot to complain about, and what he did 50 years ago was essential and right for the time.

The profession needed to have its cobwebs shaken off. In 1965, he founded Kingsley Hall in East London, an experiment in psychiatric communal living, in which the boundaries between patients and doctors — who lived side by side — were blurred. Psychedelic drugs were an integral part of the community. Traditional concepts of diagnosis and treatment were absent. The guiding principle was that 'to break down is to break through'. A resident of Kingsley hall in 1968, Paul Zeal, now a psychotherapist in Taunton, told me how group LSD sessions helped the residents to learn that 'rules were for discovering'. He described Laing as a containing presence who was respected by all, even when dissent was actively encouraged as an important tool for self-discovery[50]. Laing rose to celebrity status because of his work, and had many famous patients from the London glitterati for LSD sessions that he conducted in their homes, including Sean Connery, where his standard fee was a bottle of fine Scotch whisky and a limousine home.

However, psychiatry today is considerably different than it was back in the sixties. The system now is not in any way perfect, and there is always room for a good anti-authority stance in any institution, but today we have well established structures of external regulatory control, powerful and empowered patient groups, clear lines of accountability, ethics committees and all the other joys of clinical governance and health and safety that are found in the modern world. But from my own clinical experience, the reason much of Laing now seems dated is in his concept that psychosis is nothing more than unrecognised creativity, a position that seems somewhat romantic and unrealistic. The idea that we should 'free the schizophrenics' by flinging open the doors of our hospitals and giving them an easel and canvas to express themselves (with the hope that they will teach us something about the world) just does not cohere with so much of the personal experience of people with severe mental illness. Most people with schizophrenia and mania are *not* closet artists, any more than most artists have psychosis.

Having said that, a recent study by Simon Kyaga et al. from Sweden, on 300,000 patients with psychosis *did* see a link between creativity and severe mental disorder, which could be a good thing, I suppose, depending on how one looks at it[51]. This is certainly a field worthy of more research, which could be informed by the psychedelic experience. In a later chapter, we concentrate on the close relationship between psychedelics and creativity.

Prohibition and Ecstasy

Before we finish this chapter, there are two more important pieces of history from the second great psychedelic era that need to be addressed: the change in the legal status of LSD, and the emergence of Ecstasy.

Despite the protestations of those therapists who were using it safely and effectively with their patients, by 1966 tens of millions of people had used the drug outside of the medical environment. Rather than listen to the views of many academic and spiritual leaders at the time, who proposed a system of control that would allow for the safe use of the drug, the authorities made LSD illegal. Suffice to say, this legislation did nothing to curb LSD's recreational use — which continued to grow, alongside the illegal use of every other drug — but the move was very effective at halting practically all medical research. The doctors, unlike the unscrupulous hippies who had no qualms about taking a banned drug, simply couldn't associate themselves with such a red-hot product. Consequently, medical licences to use LSD experimentally became harder to get and many interested psychiatrists moved on to other projects, namely, those new antipsychotics that the burgeoning pharmaceutical industry were now pushing with vigour. Psychedelic research ground to a halt, not because it wasn't safe or effective, but simply because of socio-political reasons, which, in my view, is terribly bad science and deprived a lot of patients who may have benefitted from its use.

But the banning of LSD opened a new development, one that may promise to *really* be the next big thing in psychiatry: MDMA. However, before we get onto that topic, we are going to explore whether psychedelic drugs could be responsible for the very emergence of human consciousness in the first place. To do this, we are going back about one million years to some psychedelic cave-dwelling folk.

CHAPTER 4

The Prehistory and Ancient History of Hallucinogens

Contemplation of Navels

Today, it seems, the concept of spirituality — especially that version of it we term religion — exists on a separate plane from that of science. Some people, whether religious fundamentalists, or scientific materialists and atheists, will say they subscribe to either one approach or the other. For many others these subjects are grey, or perhaps more colourful, areas. Whereas spirituality is supported by faith and immediate inner experience, science uses a system of experimentation and testable evidence to support its claims. For the most part, science is comprehensible and verifiable and those things we do not yet comprehend, such as the exact nature of the universe at its moment of conception, remain nothing more than a transient gap in our knowledge, which we hope those clever chaps at the Large Hadron Collider at CERN in Geneva are soon to determine. The world disclosed by science suggests that everything is ordered and efficient, as we move inexorably towards a complete understanding of all there is to know.

I like the way Stephen Hawking put it:

> *'We are each free to believe what we want and it is my view that the simplest explanation is there is no God. No one created the universe and no one directs our fate. This leads me to a profound realization. There is probably no heaven, and no afterlife either. We have this one life to appreciate the grand design of the universe, and for that, I am extremely grateful.'*[1]

For the record, I am a deeply unspiritual, irreligious and scientifically agnostic person. I believe there is little empirical evidence for consciousness existing outside the brain. My understanding of consciousness is therefore best explained by the epiphenomenalist point of view, namely, that consciousness is a consequence of our highly complex brains, producing the illusion of this phenomenon we call consciousness and that without a human brain there to appreciate it, no such thing would exist.

I would also propose that the very concept of spirituality — as a non-material phenomenon — is, for me, another example of humanity's arrogance and anthrocentric approach to nature. Not only do we, when we fall for the delusion of non-material spirituality, fool ourselves into believing our own brain-synthesized delusion, we even have the superciliousness to project this onto the environment around us; making illusory statements about how the plants, rocks and animals possess souls and are part of a global non-material spirituality. In my opinion the trees are most likely standing there laughing at us, saying, "Do me a favour, humans. Just because you fell for your own delusion there's no need to make out I'm part of it too. I'm just a tree and proud of it. Materialism is good enough for me. You can keep your gods, thank you!".

While I realize this view separates me from many in the psychedelic community, for me Occam's Razor (the principle that one should choose the simplest, most obvious explanation) supports my understanding of consciousness. On the other hand, the experience of God — if there is such a thing — can, I believe, be known through the psychedelically-induced peak experience. And in the meantime, science — if there is such a thing (which might then mean there is no need for God) — can tell us everything there is to know about the universe. However, I appreciate this viewpoint I hold is ambivalent — paradoxically, I have a love of both spirituality and science, and so I remain agnostic.

The trouble with our current level of understanding is that it leaves little room for mystery and myth within the modern scientific worldview, and there is little to justify revelling in ignorance or lazing around pontificating about the important things in life, a practice traditionally indulged in by myth and religion; which I feel is somewhat sad. Making up stories and inventing untruths, such as 'there may be a dragon over that hill' or 'don't go in the forest because therein live trolls that will eat you' are considered childish or superstitious nonsense and dismissed by modern religious and scientific adults alike. And yet as we know, children can teach us a lot about how to live fulfilled and joyful lives.

There was a time — not so very long ago in the grand scheme of things — when these myths and mysteries did occupy our thoughts. They were not merely stories and time-wasting fantasies; they were seen as true, revealing something real about existence. Until modern science emerged in the 16th century we needed these facts — dreamt up by wise and knowledgeable elders — to protect us, to explain the unpredictability in our environment, to fill the gaps in our knowledge about the irrepressible forces of nature that controlled the hapless lives of fragile communities. Myth, understood as primitive explanations of the workings of nature, was effectively the science of the day. But this is only one view of myth. Myths also reveal something that science misses; spirituality, connection to land, environment, the past; moral instruction perhaps, illumination to guide us through different life stages. In the ancient world, there was no dichotomy between science and spirituality; they were one and the same thing, because these categories were not distinguished. No one felt the need to invent spirituality. It didn't arise out of some intellectual need for a greater depth in our lives.

It was only once our discovery of the objective scientific method developed in the 16th and 17th centuries that it overtook religion and spirituality, and created the separation. Cartesian philosophy was also foundational to this direction in thought. But why and how did spirituality arise in the first place? In the next section, I will attempt to tackle this question from my limited perspective as a medical scientist and armchair enthusiast.

Sitting Around and Coming Up with God

A good question to consider first is this: Is it an intrinsic part of our experience to look beyond the superficial aspects of life and strive for something more? To do so, to make that metaphysical leap of faith from a purely intellectual standpoint would, from a modern scientific perspective, seem to be such a wild and fanciful thing to do that it is almost inconceivable that it happened. Even the most intelligent and worldly-wise humans of their day, gathered together in a cave around a crackling fire, are unlikely to have 'invented' gods and goddesses. Such ideas can't possibly have arisen from an intellectual or logical beginning. Personifications of natural phenomena arise in our first attempts at origin stories, hanging on to this day as giants or similar brutish forces, but elevating them to the rarefied status of deity needs an extra boost.

Many people are very fond of the works of Terence McKenna. His ideas are certainly sufficiently 'out there' enough that one is forced to react, either for or against. Arising from his exploration of the internal and external landscape disclosed by high-dose psilocybin, he makes speculations delivered in a trademark American drawl. His ideas range from the most astute scientific points to the most ridiculous, fanciful dreams and he himself does not always make efforts to distinguish which is which. He prefers the reader or listener to sort the wheat from the chaff and make their own mind up. In 2016 I wrote to the popular UK physicist Professor Brian Cox, who had recently created a book and TV programme on the human species, to ask his opinion on McKenna's proposition of the role of psychedelics in the evolutionary development of consciousness. In doing so I found McKenna — and

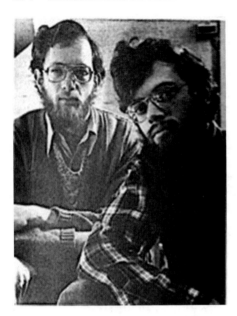

Picture 36: Dennis and Terence McKenna. Pruning the dendritic jungle of popular cosmic narratives with their systematic cultural and scientific secateurs.

myself! — quickly rubbished by Cox's supporters on Facebook. It seems McKenna (pictured left, with his brother, Dennis McKenna) is certainly not everybody's cup of yage tea.

McKenna quixotically proposes that psychedelic plants and fungi played a central role, if not *the* central role, in the development of humans as sentient, spiritual, socially complex animals, which led in turn to our increased survival rates, the evolution of intelligence and the development into what we are today[2].

In describing this below, I have expanded McKenna's ideas a little by throwing in some observations about autism and language that I have made through my own clinical practice and knowledge about the effects of psychedelic drugs.

Portal for the Immortal

The reason Terence McKenna's mythology resonates so well with his readers is that it appeals to many scientists as well as spiritual believers. What he proposes — to loosely paraphrase — is that the essential catalyst that sparked the development of spirituality in early humans was a psychedelic mushroom. This suggestion attributes that miraculous leap of faith not to a group of philosophers using the powers of their intellectual functioning to invent God, but rather to the organic outgrowth of a spontaneous mental effect. We have already established that the psychedelic experience frequently causes intense sensations of cosmic oneness. Many experiments, both from the 1960s and more recently, have demonstrated that previously atheistic people, when given a psychedelic drug or undergoing a non-drug peak experience (induced by other techniques such as asceticism, fasting, breathing, rites of passage), may describe their experience as spiritual. So it is highly plausible that it was a non-ordinary state of consciousness that first opened these ancient human's eyes to the possibility of a spiritual dimension.

Of course, it starts getting complicated when one asks whether or not psychedelic drugs simply act like lenses that allow us to see a god that was always there, or whether they simply mangle our brains and make us think there is a god when there isn't. Regardless of one's answer to that question, as a neuroscientist I am more interested in the simple and well-established fact that when we put psychedelic drugs into our brains, at the very simplest interpretation, it *feels* as if a god is out (or in!) there. And furthermore, striving to understand what might be taking place here could teach us an awful lot about the actions of psychedelic drugs and the mechanism of brain function. We'd also probably learn a thing or two about God at the same time.

Back to the Cave People

McKenna backs up his proposition that mushrooms played a major part in the development of human consciousness with the evidence that something peculiar happened in our development. After making stone tools for millions of years with little deviation, no art, and no biological evidence for spoken language (regarding brain structure and larynx position), the animals which gave rise to *Homo sapiens* and related species changed rapidly.

So, if we follow the essence of Terence's tale, what happened during that brief million years? An awful lot it seems. *Homo sapiens* is a far more advanced model than *erectus*, with some great new added features including opposing thumbs, bipedalism, binocular vision and a throwing arm. But above and beyond these useful skills, by the end of this period we had developed language and spirituality. In the blink of a hairy eye, we had advanced beyond mere primitive animals into a race of sentient, artistic, spirit-worshipping humans, with increasingly sophisticated social communities, complex relational ideas and all kinds of stories for our young about the creation of the world, the deeds of gods and goddesses, and cosmic oneness of which we are a part. As phrased in *2001: A Space Odyssey*, we had well and truly stepped through the portal for the immortal.

Mushrooms Gave Us Thought, and Thinking Gave Us Language

With the advances in our ability to manipulate our environment, we evolved from simple cave-dwelling hunter-gatherers towards complex farmers and keepers of animals. Following Terence's storyline, early people lived around cattle and other large herbivores, and where there are cattle there are cow pats and where there are cow pats there are... wait for it... mushrooms! These early humans would have been in the habit of eating everything they see around them, which would include the strange blue-staining toadstools growing out of the cow pats. What happened next was nothing short of the opening of their eyes — or, rather, as Carhart-Harris at Imperial University has established with his recent psilocybin and LSD neuroimaging experiments, a closing of the eyes and an opening to the depths of the inner world of mind. These mushrooms, we can speculate, forced our cave-ritual-people to go within, while spontaneously inducing feelings of oceanic boundlessness and unity. The ancient humans, their sensibilities heightened by the mushrooms, had no choice but to ask themselves some very novel questions: *What is going on? Is this it, or are we part of something bigger? Are those really just clouds up there or is there some grander scheme at work?*

It was but a short jump from there to the development of cave art, culture and stories. Furthermore, McKenna goes on to argue that, at low doses, psilocybin increases visual acuity, which gave the mushroom-eating hunters an advantage over those who hadn't eaten the mushroom, and led to further selection for mushroom eating. But even more important is that we developed language.

The subject of language development is vast and far beyond the scope of this book, but one popular and interesting theory, proposed by Steven Jay Gould, is that language initially developed not as a means of communication with others, but rather to hold a personal dialogue with ourselves[3]. To understand the complexity of our expanding, increasingly sophisticated external world — and, perhaps the new world of spirituality revealed to us by mushroom experiences — we needed to be able to have a personal dialogue to make sense of our stream of consciousness, to help us to *think,* to understand different concepts and hold internal representations of objects. In other words, when we looked down and saw a piece of fruit we were holding in our hand and then we lifted that fruit into our mouths we began to recognise that this series of events could be strung together into a meaningful sequence, or sentence: desire-fruit-hand-lift-mouth-eat. According to this view, it was only at a later point in evolution that these internal *thoughts* became externalized speech and communication: 'I want to get some fruit and put it in my mouth.'

V. S. Ramachandran expands on Gould's concept in *The Tell-Tale Brain*[4] when addressing the subject of neurological evolutionary theory, though he fails to consider the role psychedelics might have played in the development of humankind[5]. He describes how the human ability of

Theory of Mind (ToM) — the capacity to appreciate that other people have minds — allows one to see other people's point of view and, by extension, reflect upon *one's own* internal mental state. Such a unique skill, which appears to set us apart from other species of animals, has allowed us to advance beyond the slow pace of genetic evolution to develop more rapidly reproducible tools for transmitting information such as teaching. Freed from genetics as our only means of progress, we have since left all other species behind. And there are clear links between ToM, psychedelics and autism. Indeed, Dr. Alicia Danforth, a psychedelic researcher in the USA, and others at MAPS, are currently undertaking a study to explore whether drugs such as LSD and psilocybin, that produce recognised expansions of one's boundaries beyond those of one's own fixed ego, or drugs such as MDMA that have known empathic-boosting effects, may have clinical value in the treatment of social anxiety associated with autism[6].

As a psychiatrist who has worked extensively with children with autism, I would echo that it feels intuitively right that the extraordinary mental states produced by these drugs could have therapeutic uses with autism. Autism is often about being trapped within one's own shrunken, asocial universe. A drug experience that opens the individual to feel instinctively part of a greater whole could be a valuable tool. A few studies were done in the 1960s giving severely autistic children high doses of LSD, with some noteworthy results[7,8,9]. Children who were previously shut off from the outside world or mute became animated and verbal, and laughed and engaged with their carers for a few hours, before returning back to their internal worlds when the drugs wore off. Such studies, which by modern standards provide little more than anecdotal evidence, are certainly worth revisiting with contemporary scientific methods. But can one even begin to imagine the ethical issues in proposing such a research study on children today? If Alicia Danforth — who we gratefully welcomed as a speaker at *Breaking Convention* in 2015 — is successful in her study with adults with autism, I may one day take steps to propose something similar for children, who more than anyone deserve a way out.

The Mushroom Cycle

So, imagine the scenario: Once the cave-people have gathered their cattle around them, munched the toadstools, increased their visual acuity, and improved their hunting ability, they can now also develop a method for sophisticated internal dialogue with themselves. They can fathom out what the universe is all about, now they have glimpsed the cosmic wonder given to them by the mushroom experience and this expanded internal conversation may also be used as an external communication tool. And it seems that those who eat the mushrooms, in low doses, also show an increased interest in sexual activity, which further boosts their numbers. Higher doses of the mushrooms — which, we can speculate, they began to go out of their way to look for rather than just eat accidentally — were contributing to their development of language by providing them with even more novel ideas to think, and then talk, about. ToM begins to appear. They have an understanding about themselves, that they exist, and that one day they won't. They can talk to other people about their thoughts, wants and desires because once they start sharing their internal thoughts it turns out that others have minds too. Bigger brains, more food, more sex, more ideas lead to more sophisticated communal groups. A sense of shared identity bonds multiple individuals ever more strongly into a tribe. Language and ideas spread by example.

If the cave-people begin to notice that the mushrooms — which by now may have risen to a position of high status in the community — only grow at certain times of the year, then cyclical and seasonal life starts becoming even more significant. It becomes a communal ceremonial event to consume the mushrooms. This would fit in well with their increasing knowledge about the year's seasons. Then, imagine that high doses begin. For a few months of the year, a few people, those with the appropriate genetic predisposition for channelling and communicating the mushroom's message, become held aloft as tribal leaders, soothsayers, holy people.

It is notable that, thanks to the work of Roland Griffiths at Johns Hopkins University, we are now getting excitingly close to knowing in advance which of us have an increased genetic predisposition to experiencing spiritual thoughts on psilocybin and which of us don't. Now that the cave people are thinking in an increasingly cyclical and spiritual manner they can reflect upon past generations, and this naturally leads to the development of myths, legends and stories. Cause and effect becomes the name of the game. The seasons change like they do because of the forces that we glimpse when we eat the special fruit — we know this to be true as we have seen and felt it. *There is something out there.* It's not just about chasing mammoths around. There is a god. The mushroom is the god. Terence McKenna is quite a guy.

A final word, for now, from McKenna, which ties in nicely with the cyclical nature of psychedelic mushrooms (and also appeals to my love of brewing cider). McKenna and others have postulated that these ancient people preserved their psychedelic mushrooms by storing them in honey. In this way, the early humans could make their magic fruit last all year, so their precious opportunities to worship their ecstatic gods were not confined only to the winter months. Storing mushrooms in honey is a fine way

of preserving them and one technique (among others) that some hallucinogenic fungi enthusiasts still employ today. The trouble is that if one leaves
honey uneaten for too long it tends to ferment. McKenna speculates (there
is little empirical evidence for this, incidentally) that storing mushrooms in
honey accounts for the gradual loss of these ancient mushroom cultures
and a development of an alcohol culture. He suggests that from time to
time there might be years when the mushroom crop was low and few caps
were gathered and stored. Then, when the communal psychedelic ceremonies came around, the revellers, we can imagine, would be consuming far
more in the way of fermented honey than that of magic mushrooms. So, if
this theory holds up, they didn't trip and speak to their gods like they
intended, but rather had a right royal knees up. Laughs, sex and drunken
fights were enjoyed instead of spiritual awakenings. The likely result, sad
though it may seem, was that the people began to gradually *prefer* the easy
drunkenness to the more challenging psychedelic experience. Over generations, by this account, the mushrooms were lost altogether, except for a few
chosen members of the community who continued the sacred tradition: the
shamans. Meanwhile, alcohol became the community's drug of choice and
more sophisticated methods of preparing fermented (non-psychedelic)
fruits were developed.

So, according to McKenna's speculation, not only do we owe spirituality, consciousness, cognitive development and language to the mushrooms but they themselves were also responsible for the rise of their very
nemesis, alcohol. I guess, if it is to be believed, we could all drink mead to
that.

The Birth of Religion

If one follows McKenna's speculative argument through, one might conclude that the influence of psychedelic plants and fungi over human psycho-spiritual development gave rise to the birth of modern humans. There
are cultures, for example the Mazatec Indians in Central America, where
psychedelic plants and fungi became the heart and soul of social and religious life for the community. For the Mazatec, the mushroom was revered
as a sacramental tool.

The notion that religion develops as a direct consequence of the
organic influence of psychedelic chemicals feels intuitively correct to
many followers of McKenna; even those who doubt his particulars might
have some sympathy for the general idea that '*Homo psychedelica*' might
play a part in our cultural evolution. Just as other major evolutionary steps
took place through the accidental influence of some organic or physical

intervention — such as lightning striking a tree leading to the discovery of fire, or iron rich rocks falling into fires giving rise to the discovery of metal — the inadvertent, *non-intellectual* influence of accidental mushroom consumption growing into religion through the spontaneous catalytic inducement of spiritual thoughts resonates with many people.

No one knows how, when, where or why religion, and the accompanying ritual practices, began. We rely on archaeological evidence to give us clues about how the earliest humans approached spirituality. But there is general acceptance from the scientific community that when ancient humans begin to bury their dead this represents an emergence of sentient intelligence and ceremony — something one does not see with any other animals except the elephant, who famously buries its dead and even returns to the graves of long deceased relatives as an apparent form of pilgrimage[10]. It is perhaps worth mentioning in passing that elephants are often very keen to indulge in states of intoxication.

The emergence of complex burial rituals among early humans amounts to the beginning of symbolic representation of non-material beliefs. And some of the earliest rock art, that of the Middle Palaeolithic period, up to 300,000 years ago, involves geometric shapes carved into pieces of bone which may suggest that the artist was experiencing an altered state of consciousness, whether drug induced or arising spontaneously. Certainly, by the Upper Palaeolithic period (40,000 years ago), anthropomorphic images and those representing half-human and half-animal images appear, as in the many splendid paintings of this period unearthed in deep caves in Lascaux, France, that suggest these early humans were the first people to believe in many gods whose very image was fused with that of nature. With this development, we enter the territory of shamanism.

Shamanism

This is another vast subject and one that underpins so much of what is understood about the origins of religion and the role played by psychedelic drugs. The fact that shamanism is still practiced today throughout the world by non-Western societies gives us clues that shamanistic practices go back a very long way. For those readers interested in shamans, look for Mircea Eliade, who is generally accepted to be the 'father of the study of modern shamanism', with his 1951 book *Shamanism: Archaic Techniques of Ecstasy*[11]. A notable critic of Eliade, and the supposed link between modern day shamanistic practices and those of the Palaeolithic humans, however, is the anthropologist Alice Kehoe, who criticises Eliade partly because he was a religious historian and not an anthropologist, and also for not backing up his claims of direct links between Palaeolithic religious practices and modern shamanism with appropriate field study data[12].

Scholars agree, however, that the essential feature of shamanistic belief is that it is a method of communication between the human and the spiritual world. And there is often an implied healing or medicinal purpose to the methods and practice. Shamans themselves were — and still are — considered skilled herbalists, botanists, anatomists and physicians, not to mention their role as psychiatrists and priests; as well as engaging in combat (on the outer and inner planes) as defenders, hunters and warriors. They can be seen as messengers, carrying knowledge and information from one dimension of reality to the other, transcending time in both directions to provide for the health of their community.

An essential component of their practice is that of the use of altered states of consciousness. This may be done using a number of different techniques. The healing or medical component is inherent in the technique, and the shaman — doctor, priest, psychiatrist — is often assumed to live *primarily* in the spirit or animal world, which is accessed by others through altering their state of consciousness in a ceremony directed by the shaman. For shamans, who *live* in the spirit world, the ceremonies can sometimes represent their opportunity to take a foray into the normal waking consciousness of everyday people[13].

Consciousness is altered using trance-like drumming, dancing, chanting, and songs sung by the shaman which have personal and group significance for the prospective spiritual travellers. Usually the experience takes place at night, and involves many members of the tribe, which makes it cohesive and empowering for the community, not just for an individual.

Sacred plants are powerful tools for altering consciousness. In this context, they are referred to as entheogens, which translates roughly from the Greek as 'that which creates the God from within'. There is robust anthropological evidence for plenty of psychoactive plants and fungi being used in a shamanistic context for at least 5,000 years — basically since written records began. The links back to pre-historic religion may be more tenuous because, without any written records, no one can be sure what took place before 5,000 years ago. But it seems unlikely that entheogenic use only started at the same time as records began. One way or the other, formal organised religions are very recent; while the vast majority of the human spiritual lifetime has been lived for hundreds of thousands of years prior to the emergence of organized religions. If we can accept there is evidence for the role of psychedelic drugs in modern religions, it is a fair assumption to imagine that psychedelic drugs had an *even greater* role in spiritual practices during pre-historical times.

Put plainly, despite the relatively very recent influence of Christianity's attempt to eradicate psychedelic spirituality — whether at the hands of the conquistadors or the Republicans — it really has never gone away and entheogenic spirituality still plays a vital part in today's multi-faith secular society[14].

Many Religions Can Trace Their Roots to Psychedelic Drugs

Although contemporary organised religions have clearly contributed much to modern life and culture, including communal living — indeed, such a lifestyle might have served an evolutionary purpose itself — their autocratic structures are a considerable departure from the individualised experiential aspects of the psychedelic experience. When, on imbibing a fungus, one believes with all one's heart that the universe is good and that possessions, hierarchies and ego boundaries are meaningless, it is difficult to subscribe to the autocratic dogma of most organized religions. But the roots of the roles psychedelics have played in our spiritual development are not lost altogether, and can be traced back with good evidence to several examples of recent human history. Some of these are discussed below.

Soma

This was a psychedelic drink taken in a ritual manner by the early Indo-Iranians, the descendants of the Proto-Indo-Europeans known as the Andronovo culture[15]. Helped by their invention of the chariot, they spread throughout Asia from the area stretching from Hungary to Mongolia around 5,000 years ago. *Soma* is first mentioned in the Sanskrit texts that form the basis of the Hindu and Zoroastrian traditions. Of the 1,200 texts of the Hindu Rig Vedas, over 100 describe the mystery substance *soma*, which, when consumed, allowed for direct communication with the gods. The Rig Veda describes *soma* simply as 'God for Gods', suggesting it carried the highest accolade of all. There are lots of clues hidden in the Rig Vedas that suggest the substance was psychedelic. Many passages describe the visions and magic to be gained by drinking *soma*, the manner in which it transports one to be with the gods and become immortal.

Like a stag, come here to drink!
Drink Soma as much as you like.
Pissing it out day by day, O generous one,
You have assumed your most mighty force.
(The Rig-Veda 4.10)

We have drunk Soma and become immortal;
We have attained the light, the Gods discovered.
Now what may foeman's malice do to harm us?
What, O Immortal, mortal man's deception?
(The Rig-Veda)

No one knows for certain what the exact ingredients of *soma* were, but there are many substances pressing their claims. Some scholars suggest it is ephedra, others, notably R. Gordon Wasson, suggest it was the hallucinogenic mushroom *Amanita muscaria* (fly agaric) which, when urinated, retains its psychedelic qualities, pointing to the Rig Vedas mention of 'pissing'. The *Psilocybe cubensis* mushroom, cannabis, and opium, have also all been considered as potential candidates for key ingredients of *soma* at one time or another. The jury remains out as to exactly what soma was.

Eleusinian Rites

In ancient Greece, there was a 2,000-year-long practice of worshipping the goddesses Demeter and Persephone, called the Eleusinian Mystery Rites[16]. The ceremony occurred annually and was part of a major festival, but the rites themselves were shrouded in secrecy — at pain of death — so very little in the way of written information is known about what took place. The known details suggest that the ceremony began with a procession, followed by a day of fasting and then the initiates drank a special brew made with barley called the *kykeon*, before entering a great hall called the

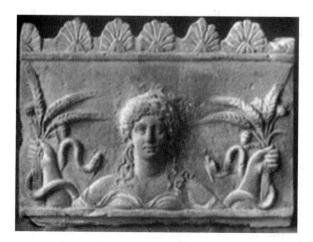

Picture 37: The goddess Demeter with her gifts for humanity: barley and poppies.

Telestrion, which held a thousand participants. Here, revealed unto them, were mysterious visions, including knowledge about how to attain life after death. There then followed a great party with feasting and entertainments, including a bull sacrifice.

There are, as with the Vedic *soma*, several potential pharmacological candidates to explain the apparent psychedelic effects of the *kykeon*. Suggestions have included opium, various types of psilocybin mushrooms and the *Amanita muscaria* mushroom again (this mushroom, with its classically magic appearance: bright red with white spots, crops up everywhere in psychedelic folklore). But most attention recently has been turned upon the known fact that 'barley' was used to make the *kykeon*. This may have been dallis grass *(Paspalum dilatatum)*, which is known to readily become impregnated with *Claviceps paspali,* a form of ergot, which contains high concentration of ergotamine, a precursor for lysergic acid on the synthesis pathway for LSD.

The author Carl Ruck presented an excellent paper on the subject at the 2006 conference in Basel to celebrate Albert Hofmann's 100th birthday. We subsequently invited Carl to speak at our 2015 *Breaking Convention* meeting, where he postulated it is possible to recreate the conditions of the preparation of the *kykeon*[17]. Mixing together barley water and mint (readily available ingredients to the ancient Greeks), impregnated with ash to provide the appropriate alkalinity to power partial hydrolysis, the *kykeon* could potentially become a powerful brew. Whatever it contained, the result suggests it is perfectly possible that a psychedelic experience was at the heart of ancient Greek culture. The Eleusinian Rites were held in very high regard, and respected for a long time by the Greeks, with a great deal of attention paid to inducing a non-ordinary state of consciousness.

During the secret ceremony, the initiates — who reportedly included Plato and Cicero — described their experience of 'seeing and communicating with the Goddess herself': 'Trembling, vertigo, cold sweat, and then a sight, a sense of awe and wonder at a brilliance that caused a profound silence'[18]. It seems, then, as if there were something incredibly profound going on for such a ceremony to endure for such a long period. And, as mentioned, this example of psychedelics at the heart of an ancient human culture may owe much to a considerably earlier use of the drugs in a shamanistic setting.

Psychedelic Drugs at the Heart of Christianity

Going into a church today one is bombarded with devices and tricks to evoke a spiritual mood and to honour God. Such devices also have the effect of mildly altering one's state of consciousness: the ethereal music, the coloured dim light coming through stained-glass windows, billowing incense, the assumed awe-inspiring mind-set is further induced by hushed voices and an obligatory reverence. All these features are merely quantitatively, not qualitatively, different from the psychedelic experience.

Yet, prevalent views underpinning Christianity are those of chastity and sobriety, a rejection of intoxication with any substance other than alcohol as requirement on the pathway to God. Only shamans and witches adulterate their bodies with the devil's poisons. It seems there is little room for psychedelic mushrooms in the Christian way of life.

But, as with Hinduism, perhaps Christianity has hallucinogenic roots? We have already noted that, by a very long way, the majority of human contact with the life of the spirit occurred as part of pre-historic, unwritten

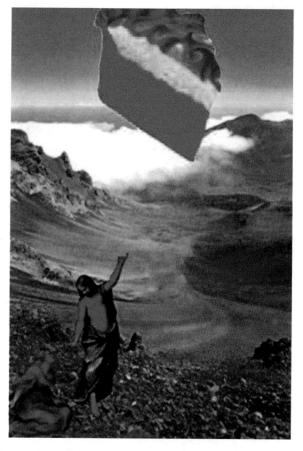

Picture 38: Pie in the Sky (1994) Photograph collage, by Clark Heinrich.
Used with kind permission of the artist.

religions in which shamanistic rituals were the form of worship, directly linking humans to the natural world of plants and animals around them. And we know that psychoactive plants and fungi provide the perfect psychological cauldron, as it were, in which to experience such a connection with nature and the universe.

Perhaps Jesus was a shaman? A long-haired sandal-wearing magic medicine-man with an intimate knowledge of the herbal and fungal botany of the day; an influential mystic whose stories have been distorted with equal measures of pious veneration and immoral bastardisation by those who wished to suppress shamanic culture?

Historically, there is certainly a good chance that psychedelic plants and fungi, had they been available to Jesus, would not have been subject to the same restrictions — legal, societal and moral — that we associate them with today. Elaborate mushroom cults at the heart of Christianity have been proposed by several scholars and (unsurprisingly) rejected by the church. Of note is the theologian John Marco Allegro's 1970 book *The Sacred Mushroom and the Cross*, which, whilst contentious, is well worth a read[19]. The Bible itself is full of psychedelic imagery, despite attempts to eradicate this in the many versions that have tried to tell the Old Testament and New Testament stories in retrospective recall. Further contemporary constructive deconstructions of established ideas — particularly those that have emerged from the bible — can be found in the writings of the Reverend Danny Nemu, with his two books *Science Revealed*[20] and *Neuro-Apocalypse*[21]. It seems nothing is sacred these days.

Thank God.

For an excellent account of the influence of magic mushrooms — particularly *Amanita muscaria* — on the development of Christianity, I direct the reader to the seminal text by writer, artist and photography, Clark Heinrich, *Magic Mushrooms in Religion and Alchemy* (2002)[22], which is an improved second edition of his earlier *Strange Fruit* (1995). And Rick Strassman's new book, *DMT and the Soul of Prophecy*, provides a further reflection on the Old Testament, with a slant towards the DMT experience[23]. Assuming the gospel accounts are factually accurate, exactly what, we might wonder, was the forbidden fruit that opened Adam's and Eve's eyes to see the world as it truly appears? Some have suggested it was the *Psilocybe cubensis* mushroom that grows in that part of the world, often at the base of trees.

And were there psychedelic mushrooms growing in the Sinai desert when Jesus went to where the angels were waiting for him, and was overwhelmed by a kaleidoscopic display of colour? One may also wonder whether those shepherds were eating the fungal fruits of the meadows that night on the hill above Bethlehem when the shaman himself was born.

Another beautifully psychedelic description from the Old Testament is that of manna, which, when fed to the Israelites by Moses made them look toward the wilderness and behold the glory of Yahweh in a cloud. The early morning gathering of manna is described in the book of Exodus thus:

Then said the LORD unto Moses, Behold, I will rain bread from heaven for you; and the people shall go out and gather a certain rate every day, that I may prove them, whether they will walk in my law or not.

And when the dew that lay was gone behold, upon the face of the wilderness there lay a small round thing, as small as the hoar frost on the ground. **(Exodus 16:14, King James Bible)**

All the usual suspects of the field have given their support to the theory that manna is a psychedelic mushroom. Dan Merkur, in his book *The Mystery of Manna: The Psychedelic Sacrament of the Bible*, seems to have found enough personal evidence to substantiate his claim, but as it stands there is not a lot of support from many other notable figures of learned theology[24]. I must say, however, for anyone who has ever ventured out over the autumn fields of South West England at the crack of dawn looking for liberty caps amidst dripping fog, they will contest that this description of 'small round things' in the dew does not sound unlike a mushroom hunt. The Rev. Nemu, in his above mentioned *Neuro-Apocalypse*, suggests ergot secretion; for which he gives a persuasive argument.

Modern Spirituality in Europe: The Middle Ages and Witches

The Greeks were psychedelic users, and it was the ancient Romans that saw off the shaman Jesus. The Romans were themselves firm believers in hosts of gods and pagan deities, and were well-known to be rather partial to opium, cannabis and datura.

By the 4th century CE, the Romans had, of course, chosen Christianity as their primary religion and, in doing so, thereby ushered in the development of the modern world as we know it. As we head into the Middle Ages in Europe we see Christianity running roughshod over everything in its path, sweeping away any remaining vestiges of belief in the ancient religions.

On the surface, the links between witchcraft, mental illness and psychedelics are, to the untrained eye, obvious. Ask any child for their classic images of a witch and one will be bombarded with the full regalia of psychedelic and shamanistic imagery: She lives alone in the wood, has an intimate knowledge of nature and collects herbs, roots, flowers and toadstools to make her magic spells, which she brews up as a bubbling potion in a cauldron that give her special powers such as the ability to fly on a broomstick, the ability to change her shape and to cast spells on others. However, this fairy-tale image of the old crone nature-loving witch is totally modern era; hints appearing in Shakespeare's blatant propaganda for the paranoid James I at the earliest. We need to look beyond such erroneous stereotypes to get a clearer picture.

Psychoactive Plants Available to Europeans in the Middle Ages

While there is no historical evidence for the use of powerful psychedelic drugs such as psilocybin by Europeans in the Middle Ages, what follows is a summary of some of the plants that we know *were* used.

Deadly nightshade (belladonna), has been long known as a poison. All parts of the plant contain high concentrations of the drug atropine, which causes a powerful anticholinergic reaction of blurred vision, dilated pupils and tachycardia. Used by ancient people as a toxin, it can be lethal and still causes death for a significant number of people every year who mistakenly eat its berries. But when mixed with other ingredients and applied as a tincture, it also has a rich history as a medicine. However, as well as the deadly physical symptoms it causes on the way to death, the Belladonna intoxication also produces a dreamy state of delirium and powerful hallucinations.

Closely related to belladonna is the **datura** plant, a very powerful substance associated by some with medieval European witchcraft as a 'flying ointment'. Other names include jimson weed, devil's apple and thorn apple. It is a woody-stalked, leafy herb, growing up to two metres high, which produces spiny seedpods and large trumpet-shaped flowers. Datura contains several tropane alkaloids, including scopolamine, hyoscyamine, and atropine. The seeds and flowers are more potent than the leaves and roots. Taken orally the effects include confusion, disorientation and hallucinations, which can last for days. It is difficult to find a non-toxic psychedelic dose and there are few positive descriptions of human consumption. It is still used today by Native American Navajo and Havasupai, and in India and Africa by shamans. Indeed, when I was in Northern India I met a traveller in the ashram where I was staying who warned me off the local 'moon flowers', telling me that after eating datura she spent three weeks entwined in her mosquito net, believing it to be a magically possessed wedding dress. Suffice to say, on that occasion I stuck to meditation.

Another favourite plant for European magic men and women was the **mandrake root**. Apart from being a fabulously psychedelic song by Deep Purple in 1968[25] (more in the way of psychedelic music later!), it is also a fascinating plant, whose roots contain high concentrations of hallucino-genic alkaloids. It is also rather cool because of the roots' twisted crazy humanoid shapes that resemble a little person. Legend has it that the roots scream when pulled from the ground and there are heaps of legends and stories associated with this plant. It is well worth searching for at your local vegetable market. Just don't ever look one in the eye.

Another is **henbane**. This rather beautiful flower has been associated with datura, deadly nightshade and mandrake because it was historically combined with the others to produce anaesthesia. Henbane contains plant alkaloids like belladonna and, alongside producing hallucinations and delirium, can also be deadly.

Witches, Witchcraft, Ergotism and Witch-hunts

The concept of witchcraft, which is broad and includes many variations all over the world, incorporates some fundamental common defining features. The main feature is the magical (I would say psychedelic) nature of the witches' practices, but another is that witches are commonly maligned and oppressed. Witch-hunts were frequent and span a long period of history in Europe between the 14th and 18th centuries. They were a systematic demonization of anyone differing from accepted church doctrine, including pagan religions, by a dominant and often paranoid Christian church.

But witch-hunts were much more than religious persecution. They also represent sexism, stigma against mental illness and a clear attack by the (drunken) sober herd on the oddball minority. In some cases, the so-called witches might have been intentionally practicing forms of shamanism that incorporated the use of entheogens. In other cases, it could be that individuals, and indeed whole communities, were inadvertently victims of mass psychedelic poisoning. Ergotism has been postulated as the cause of the famous Salem witch trials that occurred in 1652 in Salem, Massachusetts, in which a group of young girls fell into a terrifying state of paranoid delusion, confusion and hallucinations accompanied by vomiting and convulsions. They survived and were subsequently accused of being witches. There ensued a mass hysteria fuelled by the fundamental Christian beliefs that underpinned the community, and the girls were eventually put on trial and executed. But it didn't stop there. By the time the mass hysteria was over, a further 20 locals had also been accused of witchcraft and met the death penalty. It was an American writer, Linda Caporael, who proposed in 1976 that ergot poisoning might have been the cause of this phenomenon[26].

Also, called St. Anthony's Fire, ergotism occurs when the ergot fungus grows on several different damp crops, especially dark rye, where its black nodules are less easily noticed. It was not just confined to the Middle Ages and cases may still occur. Indeed, there was a famous case as recently as 1951 when an entire French village was poisoned by bread made from flour poisoned with ergot. Some scholars have claimed that the 1951 outbreak was not ergotism, but rather a clandestine project by the CIA to test LSD as a weapon of war[27]. However, closer examination by critics of this theory (including Hofmann himself when asked to investigate) have highlighted some significant reasons — largely those relating to the pharmacological impossibility of disseminating the drug on such a scale — why this is a highly unlikely proposition[28].

Stigmatisation of Mental Illness

While ergot poisoning may explain some reports of witchcraft in mistake for madness, in other cases witches may have simply been old men and women who were mentally unwell. Mentally ill people, often maligned and rejected, often drift towards loneliness and isolation. At best ignored, at worst they are persecuted and, in the case of witches, hunted down and victimized simply because of their difference. Thomas Szasz likened witch-hunts to stigma against mental illness. His book *The Myth of Mental Illness*[29], Michel Foucault's *Madness and Civilization*[30] and Erving Goffman's *Asylums*[31], which were highly influential for me during my medical education, are all important texts for anyone wishing to become a psychiatrist, rightly attacking the fundamental flaws and pitfalls that anyone so arrogant as to declare themselves knowledgeable about *other people's* mental states may face in their coming careers.

Hunting Down and Persecuting Psychedelic Users Has Not Gone Away

Today's 'War on Drugs', as it applies to contemporary judicious users of psychedelics, is our version of the historical witch-hunts. In many countries people are imprisoned and even executed for their drug use. In 2016 the murderous president of the Philippines, Rodrigo Duterte, waged war on drug users, slaughtering thousands of innocent people in the name of stamping his twisted morality upon his subjects. Prosecuting victimless psychedelic users is a stark example of an alcohol-supping, pharmacology-driven 'masculine' dominance over the peaceful 'feminine' Earth movement. The

War on Drugs has as much scientific validity as the historic persecution of witches. Punishments are metered out arbitrarily according to the whims and fancies of local authorities. Media driven mob rule takes control. Being seen to be 'tough on drugs' by vilifying the local pot and acid seller is a sure way of catching an easy headline and Middle England votes.

In the UK today's drug laws have deteriorated into dangerous chaos. The pot-selling 'witch' may get lucky and simply be sent home by the police with as much as an ounce of cannabis in her pocket. A tolerant police officer, who cannot be bothered to fill in the paperwork, might turn a blind eye to a fellow smoker and send him on his way with a nudge and a wink without even confiscating his stash. In stark contrast, whole squads of detectives can descend on a person's house, kicking his door in at 4am, and haul him off to a custodial sentence for the merest crumb of hash down the back of the sofa — especially if he is wanted for some other heinous crime, such as having been identified on video taking part in a direct action anti-establishment protest. Of course, there are many issues to the fore here, but the links between the way drug laws can be applied and the arbitrary nature of the historic witch-hunts are not lost on many people.

Further comparisons include the way drug users today are so often medicalised and pathologised; described as 'mad'. Their ways are different from the norm, which is the same as saying not-as-good-as-the-norm. They are held up and humiliated to make the healthy non-users look good, and described by a political and medical model that rejects and, at best, pities the drug user. But the situation today is even more complicated and inter-esting than that of the past. Back then those accused of witchcraft were in a minority; they represented the last vestiges of folk traditions being weeded out by propagators of a monocultural Christianity. Whereas now, it is the majority (within certain age groups) who use drugs. Among today's youth, there are more who have used illegal drugs like cannabis and Ecstasy than there are who have not. The recent closure of the legendary London night club *Fabric* is a good example of reactionary persecution[32]. Surely they cannot *all* be witches.

With the recent developments of the Psychoactive Substances Act (2016) we are now more than ever in danger of a truly occult situation in which the hidden majority are victimized by a political system they voted in but are too scared to vote out. Talk about Emperor's New Clothes!

Spaghetti Monsters and Pot Head Pixies

As we shall see in the next chapter, there remain many ways to appreciate gods and goddesses. It is a brave person who dares suggest one way is better

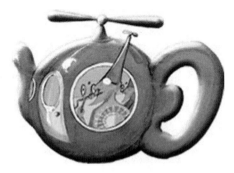

Picture 39: Break off and eat the corner of your mind. Gong's Pot Head Pixies arriving in their tea pot taxis to deliver the message of cognitive liberty and freedom of expression.

than any other — which means, of course, there are billions of brave people in the world. Whether they were discovered recently (in the last ten thousand years) or earlier, it could be argued that each religious belief system is an equally valid tool with which to experience the spiritual realm — no matter how fanciful it seems. Clearly it is easy to intellectually challenge religious beliefs. In 2005 a man called Bobby Henderson was so incensed that Creationism might be taught in Amercan schools that he came up with the idea of the Flying Spaghetti Monster; a god with a wonderful story about its creation, existence and continued presence in our lives[33]. Henderson proposed that his 'Pastafarianism' had equal rights to be taught in schools alongside Creationism and evolutionary theory, if school boards were so crazy as to accept Intelligent Design in the first place.

Another equally spectacular story is that of the Gong Mythology, with its detailed and colourful descriptions of Pot Head Pixies (pictured below, in their flying teapot), as influenced by a psychedelic band with their hallucinogenic imaginations working in overdrive[34]. 2015 and 2016 saw the sad loss of Gong's deeply inspirational leader-guru Daevid Allen[35] and space-whisperer Gilli Smyth[36], both of whom are now looking down on us from Planet Gong, smiling benevolently and enjoying a nice pot of tea.

Given these brilliant interpretations of our fragile minds' incessant need to dress up the complex yet horribly simple understandings of our existential meaning, psychedelic spirituality ends up standing out as a perfectly valid — if not crystal clear — explanation of What It's All About.

The Varieties of Religious and Psychedelic Experiences

The psychologist and pragmatist William James (pictured below) wrote *The Varieties of Religious Experience* in 1902[37]. His simple, no-nonsense description of the wonderful colourful versions of spiritual experience to be found throughout the world captures both the imagination and logical persuasion of anyone who reads it.

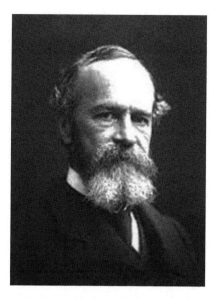

Picture 40: "Our normal waking consciousness, rational consciousness as we call it, is but one special type of consciousness, whilst all about it, parted from it by the filmiest of screens, there lie potential forms of consciousness entirely different. We may go through life without suspecting their existence; but apply the requisite stimulus, and at a touch they are there in all their completeness, definite types of mentality which probably somewhere have their field of application and adaptation. No account of the universe in its totality can be final which leaves these other forms of consciousness quite discarded. How to regard them is the question, for they are so discontinuous with ordinary consciousness."

—**William James**, *The Varieties of Religious Experience*, 1902

Masters and Houston subsequently borrowed the title of that book for their own, brilliant *The Varieties of Psychedelic Experience*, which approaches the apparently chaotic display of psychedelic experiences with a similarly erudite and exacting science[38]. Both books are a great read and the latter is, in my opinion, perhaps the best introductory text to psychedelic drugs available — compiled, as it is, with the greatest precision and charm from hundreds of psychedelic therapy sessions in the early 1960s.

Above all, these texts show us that there are many ways to be, and to worship, the Unknown. Not only are all these ways of worship as valid as one another, but they are also, very often, relatively reproducible. Similar mental states — and indeed spiritual experiences — seem to crop up again and again regardless of historical and geographical boundaries. The presumption, as far as I can see, is that there is an innate human psychological capacity for what we categorise as spiritual feelings and thought — and since our brains are pretty much the same as they have been for at least the last 100,000 years, this would make sense. What we need is a Church of the Temporal Lobes.

Wrestling Bliss Off the Church

Language has provided us with some beautiful words used by various religions to describe both the spiritual and the inseparable psychedelic experience: *satori, unio mystica,* the *Tao, nirvana, fana.* Many words, such as *illuminating, transforming, bliss,* and *cosmic oneness* have been hijacked by religions. One must head to the nearest church, mosque or synagogue to use these words safely. There is little place for them in a scientific or traditional academic environment. If one dares utter the words *transformation, illumination* or *bliss* in front of a psychiatrist, for instance, one risks being carted off to hospital, diagnosed with psychosis and treated to the finest wares of the pharmacological industry.

But, in my opinion, these words are not *religious.* They are everyday human psychological terms describing valid mental states. I believe we as psychiatrists need to wrestle these words away from the church, and bring them into the clinic as valid mental states. Just as we use medical terms to describe the mental states of anger, lust, fear, love and agitation, so too can we use words like bliss and enlightenment. The concept of the spiritual emergency is long overdue in psychiatry, and psychedelics are the best placed tools to remind us of the validity of these mental spaces. For if we confine ourselves only to the normal waking state, we risk missing a whole level of understanding about the brain, and humanity's place in the universe. Psychedelics may be an essential tool in helping us understand this level of meaning in our lives and the lives of our patients.

Conclusion and Confusion in Collusion with the Delusion

So why are these fascinating drugs so misunderstood? Is it because they are associated with drug abuse? Or is it because of the erroneous belief that there are significant physical dangers involved with using them? Perhaps it is because the War on Drugs campaign has been so successful at labelling all illegal drugs as useless and not worth investigating. Or is it simply because some people are scared of the transpersonal realm itself?

In many non-Western cultures, psychedelics are used as viable tools to access the spiritual world. Whereas most of those Westerners who claim to lead 'religious lives', never actually personally experience a truly transforming or enlightening moment. There are similarities between the psychedelic experience and the experience of religious or mystical transcendence. This has been so hotly debated in the 1960s and beyond that in this modern age of neuroimaging it has become an almost moot point. It seems, in the wake of sexual abuse atrocities carried out in the name of religion by greed and power-hungry individuals who have taken advantage of their positions as 'holy men', that humanity is wising-up to the delusion of 'official' spirituality and seeking, in my opinion, a far more rational approach to why humans have found the need to invent religion. Richard Dawkins' excellently controversial book *The God Delusion* (2006) describes such atrocities with startling effect[39].

However, although as a self-confessed materialist I personally reject the idea of consciousness existing outside the human brain (and therefore also reject the empirical reality of non-material spirituality), I nevertheless believe that we *need* the delusion of non-material phenomena. It is a delusion that serves an important evolutionary function (or why else would it have survived?). Perhaps to experience the fullness of our material lives in our friable physical bodies in its beautiful entirety we *must* fall for our delusion. For many people their belief in spirituality forms an important bedrock of their experience of human consciousness. That, of course, leaves me in a difficult position from a phenomenological point of view. Because if know I need to believe my own delusion in order for it to have a positive effect on my well-being, then, by definition, it ceases to be a delusion. Oh dear, it seems I have talked myself out of, then back into, a dualistic hole.

The way I get my head around this paradox, as a neuroscientist, is to tell myself that it *does not matter* to me whether the spiritual experience is genuinely non-material or not. The point is it *feels* as if it is. Or might be. And that forces us to ask some interesting questions about how the brain works. Particularly, can exploring these mental states be useful for understanding the nature of consciousness and, crucially, can they have therapeutic value in psychiatry? We will be investigating these questions in the chapters to come. But first we are taking off our shoes and putting flowers in our hair for a trip back to the sixties.

CHAPTER 5

Hippie Heydays, Ravers and the Birth of Ecstasy

'Meet the Hippies'

Where did the hippies come from and where did they all go? The simple answers to these questions are that they have always been there and they haven't gone anywhere. There was merely a brief psychedelic flowering of recognition of their existence in the late 1960s and early 1970s, deftly sandwiched between the grim post-war years and the screaming rejection of all things corduroy with the birth of punk.

The first 'Summer of Love' took place in 1967 in the United States and is probably best encapsulated by the 'Human Be In' gathering held in Golden Gate Park, just off the Haight-Ashbury district of San Francisco. That timeless moment of white lightning drenched epoch-shattering glory is generally considered to be the symbolic point at which the hippie counterculture and psychedelia reached their peak in the United States. (And by *White Lightning* I don't mean the popular cider consumed by English teenagers, but rather the Owsley acid created especially for the occasion and scattered freely into the loved-up crowd).

But for those in the know, who had been using psychedelics for at least six years before 1967, by then the party was well and truly over. And, of course, by the time we reach Woodstock in 1969 — coming as it did after the bloodshed and riots of 1968 — the 'come-down' was in full swing. As Danny said in *Withnail and I,* referring to the last months of the sixties:

'The dream is over. They're selling hippie wigs in Woolworths, man.'[1]

In the UK, however, our best hippie years were yet to come; they happened in the early 1970s, with the development of the tremendous Free Festival movement, the Peace Convoy, the traveller lifestyle and the Stonehenge festivals, which kept those flared loons flapping right through into the punk era and encouraged an entire team of undercover police officers to lie around in hedges with long-range binoculars surveying a remote cottage in Wales occupied by goat-loving chemists.

Who's Going to Take All the Credit — or the Blame?

No single person can take the credit for the movement of these psychedelic drugs away from the psychiatric clinic and into the mainstream consciousness. Rather, there were several simultaneously occurring threads operating independently, together with the groundswell of social changes linked to the end of World War Two. Some of these contributory factors will be discussed in this chapter. Or then again perhaps it was simply the alignment of the planets, the Age of Aquarius, or whatever other bit of narrative dogma one chooses to follow. One way or another, once Hofmann's cat had been let out of Pandora's box it was only a matter of time before the world turned on.

The Beat Generation

At the end of the Second World War, there were a lot of disillusioned men and women, young and old — some who had fought, some who had experienced the horror of war through their parents — who then met head-on the growing circus of post-war 1950s America in which shopping and entertainment were peddled to the masses as the perfect antidotes to the intrusive memories of recent violent conflict. The Beats were at the forefront of the beautifully slovenly protest to this homogenized bastardisation of aesthetics. A decade before the hippies did their thing, these bearded visionaries trudged barefoot through the streets of New York, San Francisco, Paris and Tangiers, hitched and rode boxcars writing poetry, and listened to jazz, taking whatever consciousness-altering utopiant they could lay their hands on.

Allen Ginsberg first took LSD in 1959 at Stanford's Mental Research Institute, as part of an experimental programme run by the revolutionary anthropologist Gregory Bateson. Good friends with the psychedelic crusader Al Hubbard, Bateson had been involved in developing Systems Theory, but is better known to most psychiatrists as the brains behind the double-bind hypothesis of schizophrenia; a theory exploring abnormal parenting styles as a cause for schizophrenia[2]. Ginsberg was deeply enamoured by the astonishing higher trance state of consciousness provided by his LSD experience, in which 'everything seemed to be permanent and transcendent and identical with the origin of the universe', and afterwards he famously wrote his poem 'Lysergic Acid'[3].

Later, in 1960, while on a trip from New York visiting Tim Leary, Ginsberg was offered some of Leary's Sandoz psilocybin pills which the psychologist had at home as part of his mushrooming psychology project. Ginsberg enjoyed another intense psychedelic experience and reportedly stripped naked, cavorted outside in the snow, and tried to use Leary's phone to call Kennedy and tell him how psilocybin could be used to unite the world's political leaders. As we shall see, perhaps JFK took some notice[4].

The Beats subject matter, for Corso, Kerouac, Ginsberg, Burroughs and Ferlinghetti, was the streets and the real people they encountered on their travels across America and beyond. They wrote as they thought, fuelled by Benzedrine and cannabis, with a stream of consciousness, a flowing of words that cared less about structural form and more about meaning and feeling. Their approach was an antithesis of the ludicrous addiction of the consumerist hell sprouting up and being mindlessly absorbed by the growing generation of middle-class Americans proud to settle into their TV-driven quest for ever higher standards of living. It was the Beats that provided the backdrop for the psychedelic revolution. They were the ones who drove the bus that the stoned kids were on. They rapped like embarrassing, but very *cool,* parents while a new generation of teenagers prepared themselves for a massive social revolution. But it was a revolution in need of a magic potion.

There appears to be a clear paper trail in which Humphrey Osmond in Canada (who started out with mescaline in the 1950s) tweaked Aldous Huxley's imagination, leading to *The Doors of Perception.* But it seems a different independent thread took R. Gordon Wasson into Mexico, which lead to his mushroom excursions and that highly influential *Life* magazine article, which subsequently stimulated Tim Leary's fancy and sent him, too, to Mexico. One way or another the stuff got out there.

The decision by Sandoz to try to recuperate research-and-development costs by titillating psychiatry with Delysid, available free of charge to anyone who asked politely, did a lot for worldwide distribution of Albert's potion. And the CIA certainly played its part by setting up MK-ULTRA, which frightened, disgusted and enthralled scientists, military people and unsuspecting members of the public in equal measures, while also very effectively disseminating LSD into the wider population. Some would say, that the US military did more to bring on the psychedelic revolution than Tim Leary. There are lots of conspiracy theories around this issue, but some of the best books on the topic of how LSD leaked from the laboratory to the college campuses and became a worldwide phenomenon are *Acid Dreams*[5] by Lee and Shalin, *Storming Heaven*[6] by Jay Stevens, and *The Brotherhood of Eternal Love*[7] by Stewart Tendler and David May.

One Flew East, One Flew West and One Took LSD and Bought a School Bus

Scientific experiments on members of the public are a great way for the Men in Suits to let the public know they have got something good in their medicine cabinet. In 1959, Ken Kesey, an aspiring writer needing the cash, agreed to take part in a series of tests on new drugs as part of the CIA's MK-ULTRA program at the Menlo Park State Psychiatric Hospital where he was working at the time as a night porter. Week after week he was given a collection of different jabs and tabs and told to lie around and then report his findings. It certainly beat the usual drab surroundings —especially when the white-coated experimenters gave him a little pill they called 'LSD-25'.

Kesey had access to the medicine cabinet, smuggled out the experimental LSD and began having soirees in the La Honda area of California where he lived. In the early sixties the time was right, as he said later, 'to push the boundaries, to go down deeper in the oceans and up higher in the skies'. The space race was in full swing, he was an artist on the edge of the Beat Generation and people everywhere were being encouraged to climb their way out of the PTSD-induced experience of the war, and to expand their cultural, societal and personal horizons. Besides, it was great fun.

Fun, riotous fun, was a central part of the subsequent Merry Pranksters group that emerged, forming around Kesey like a high, grinning cat. Kesey was growing in stature as an artist, alongside the creative imaginations stimulated by the LSD he and his friends were using. It was while under

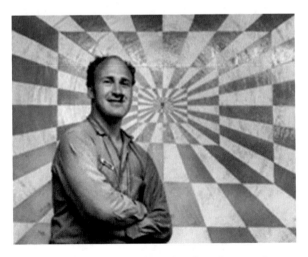

Picture 41: Ken Kesesy. The cool dad leading the way into psychedelia for a generation of early 1960s proto-hippie kids.

the influence of LSD in 1959 that he wrote large sections of his book *One Flew Over the Cuckoo's Nest*, which was soon to become a massive best-seller and catapult him into the literary history books[8]. The story centres upon a broom-pushing psychiatric patient, the giant Native American, 'Chief', and describes the impassive agony of life in the mental institute, endlessly sweeping the spotless corridors. There are sections in Kesey's famous book (which never actually refers to LSD, yet is an undoubted psychedelic classic) in which there is a 'white cloud', described as 'the combine', the insidious controlling force that keeps all the hapless patients institutionalised. The cloud descends over everyone, blunts their minds and blurs the edges of acceptable familiarity, moulding the inhabitants of the hospital into a conglomerated mass of brainless automatons. This is a far cry from the joyous experience of taking a psychedelic drug in sun-drenched hippie meadows that was to come later in the decade. Instead, it is a reliable description of what happens when no attention is paid to the set and setting, and the internal worlds are left to run with abandon in the frightening environment of an authoritarian mental institution.

On the back of the success of his book, Kesey and his tribe of Merry Pranksters took off in 1964 on a legendary road trip, in an old Harvester school bus painted in fabulous psychedelic regalia, driven by Neal Cassady; the larger-than-life Beat extraordinaire, friend of Jack Kerouac and the

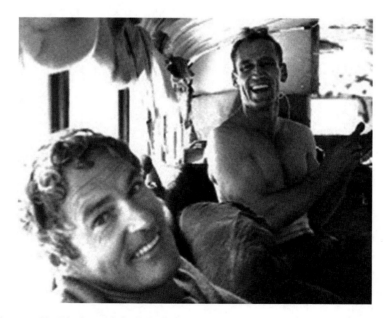

Picture 42: The speed-fueled sledge hammerer, Neal Cassady. On the bus with Timothy Leary.

inspiration for the wonderful character Dean Moriarty in Kerouac's *On the Road*[9]. Cassady, high on amphetamine, came with the perfect credentials to carry the tripping crew at breakneck speeds through the unsuspecting innocent towns of middle America. The Pranksters mission was to cause havoc, to push boundaries and excite and shock people. It worked. Later these adventures were immortalized in Tom Wolfe's *The Electric Kool Aid Acid Test*[10]— an absolute must-read for a wonderful description of this period of American history; recently re-issued in 2016 in a special edition of signed copies.

The Californian Proto-Hippies Get a Place of Their Own

In 1962, on the impossibly beautiful coast in Big Sur, California, Michael Murphy and Dick Price brought the Esalen Institute into existence. Its stunning 120-acre site provided a perfect platform for the discussion and dissemination of humanistic and transpersonal ideas, as it still does today. All manner of Western and Eastern philosophical thinking, from yoga to ecology and massage, have been explored over the years; with residents staying amidst the serene landscape perched on the cliffs above the crashing waves of the Pacific Coast south of San Francisco. Since its inauguration, the likes of Aldous Huxley, Stanislav Grof, Allen Ginsberg, Carlos Castaneda, Gregory Bateson, Deepak Chopra, Albert Hofmann, Richard Alpert, Rupert Sheldrake, Terence McKenna, John C. Lilly, Ken Kesey, Abraham Maslow, Fritz Perls, Carl Rogers, Alan Watts, Andrew Weil, Robert Anton Wilson and Joseph Campbell have all held workshops and talks at the institute; and Gary Snyder, Michael McClure, Lawrence Ferlinghetti, Allen Ginsberg, Kenneth Rexroth, and Robert Bly have held poetry readings there too. Naturally, such a place became a central stop for many on the psychedelic intellectual journey of the sixties and since, including many popular music stars[11].

Literally, Psychedelically Mind-expanding Words

In the early 1960s, not only was the use of LSD as a recreational drug growing, but there was also a blossoming appreciation of the multicultural aspects of natural psychedelic drugs. People became interested in peyote, magic mushrooms and ayahuasca, and all the colourful culture that surrounds these practices.

Shamanism became a popular subject and people swallowed the whole caboodle of holistic change, embracing a new paradigm of thinking, alternative medicine and ecology, just as they swallowed their acid. Literary works alluding to alternative lifestyles — from Alistair Crowley or the idealists of the 1920s Bloomsbury set — were embraced. LSD encouraged an escape from the city and a drift towards Mother Nature, an acceptance of seemingly archaic ideas about communal living and getting back to the land. Large sections of contemporary society had their eyes opened to the destruction of the environment, the modern green movement emerged, and previously decimated sections of the population — for example, the Native Americans — were embraced, and protests about their mistreatment by modern America grew.

Twentieth century shamans wrote about their experiences and new awakenings. Carlos Castaneda's 1968 book *The Teachings of Don Juan* described a personal journey into contemporary shamanism and remains a student classic today[12], although many have since rejected Castaneda's apparent shamanistic experiences as a fraud[13]. Throughout the sixties and since, there has been a seemingly endless stream of books about the politics, science and art of the psychedelic experience, not to mention many people's accounts of their personal experiences using a whole host of drugs; some of which are tremendously interesting and some, as one can imagine, are mind-numbingly dull. I suppose you had to be there.

Did JFK Drop LSD?

This question has been asked by a lot of people. The association between Kennedy and acid comes from a three-way friendship: Kennedy had a close relationship with the socialite painter Mary Eno Pinchot Meyer and she was also in a close relationship at the time with Tim Leary. Mary's friendship with the president was intimate, and, meanwhile, her regular visits to Leary in Harvard made sure that plenty of cannabis and LSD found its way into the White House during 1962 and 1963. Mary considered herself on a secret mission to propagate LSD to as many powerful members of the government as possible in order to spread the love and avoid nuclear war. In his memoirs from much later in life, Leary confessed that he felt Mary was at least partially successful in encouraging the president to take a few steps closer to nuclear disarmament because of the transformative influence of LSD. But we may never know the truth of what went on between Mary Eno Pinchot Meyer and Kennedy, as she was mysteriously murdered in 1964 — a year after Kennedy[14].

Unless one is open to conspiracy theories, it is probably best not to speculate what might have been going on. That said, there is nothing especially conspiratorial to imagine Kennedy took LSD. After all, he was an intelligent, switched-on and highly perceptive person. It is certainly conceivable, especially given the anecdotal circumstantial evidence, that he might have engaged with what was one of the most important social and philosophical pastimes of the day.

Leary Leaves Harvard and the Fun Begins

Earlier, we left Tim Leary's story as he was given his marching orders from Harvard. Interested to see how creative people behaved under the influence of the drug, he set about giving LSD to as many people as possible outside the clinical environment. Several important writers and musicians of the day were introduced to its unique mental milieus during this period.

In 1963, Leary eventually found his spiritual home in the form of a massive mansion set in over 100 acres of private countryside estate near the town of Millbrook, in New York State. Lent to him by the millionaire Hitchcock family, this became *the* place to go and be part of the newly developing psychedelic scene. It was from here that Tim Leary, having now shed what fragile ties he might still have held to Harvard and the conventional world of the establishment since taking his first mushroom trip, allowed himself and his willing followers to enter a beautiful, swirling maelstrom of colours and escapades that were new to them all. As Jefferson Airplane said, 'I'm doing things that haven't got a name yet'.

Leary's mental development was going deeper than anyone thought imaginable, heading into the territory of a fully formed religious movement. His *League for Spiritual Development* (nice acronym) was shaping into a loosely structured method of attaining spiritual enlightenment using LSD and other psychedelics. Perhaps because of, or despite, his grounding in clinical psychology, there was a great deal of method and purpose to Leary's work. In his spoken words and writings, despite how he might have been misrepresented by the media, then and now, Leary *always*, without exception, talked of the respect one must have for psychedelic drugs. He never promoted a gung-ho or frivolous approach. Leary was clear that caution and a judicious and reverent attitude were essential to their use. Although he was not as tightly restrictive as Huxley (who suggested that psychedelics ought not be available to the general public but only to appropriately highly-tuned academics and artists), Leary was a good distance from the Ken Kesey approach, whose prankster attitude was always, quite blatantly, to go too far and get as freaked out as possible. For Kesey, after all, life may have been interpreted as but a joke — and few experiences are better at pointing this out than a high-dose psychedelic session.

Suddenly LSD is Everywhere

Nevertheless, both Kesey's madness and Leary's controlled approach provoked total revulsion in the authorities, who were keen to hold on to their grip of consciousness-control. If people looked within too often, the authorities realized, consumers forgot to look in the shopping malls and sign up at the military academies, and that simply wasn't good for business or for the country. But there was little they could do. LSD was fast becoming the next big thing on the US college campuses. By 1965 over two million people in the States had taken LSD beyond the confines of the clinical or military test environment. This was never supposed to happen! Consciousness-expanding LSD use coupled very neatly with left-wing protests, anti-authority sentiments and, above all, the arts. And an awful lot of this crystallization of expanded thinking was concentrating increasingly on the populous West and East coasts of America.

New York was a melting pot for the growing underground movement, always frequented by the Beats, together with a healthy folk and art scene clustered around the coffee shops of Greenwich Village. San Francisco has always accepted the cultural waifs and strays of the planet. Since the 1940s, it had seen a drift of open-minded people congregating in the wooden housed hills over-looking its foggy bay, especially the Haight-Ashbury district. LSD was bound to flourish here.

The role of the Vietnam War — and the protests against it – in the development of the psychedelic scene is undeniable. What better antithesis could there be of the LSD experience than a brutal televised war that dragged teenagers kicking and screaming away from their books and music and dropped them into the dark jungle thousands of miles away from home? If it is an intrinsic and spontaneous characteristic of an LSD trip to feel the love, then people now had many more reasons to strive for it. Britain lacked such a war, which might explain in part the more nostalgic, gentle approach to psychedelia that we saw in the UK.

The Psychedelic Music Scene

The genre of music dedicated to psychedelia is very close to my heart[15]. There are lots of good books to read about Haight-Ashbury and the development of the psychedelic scene. One of my favourites, with lots of local information and stories of the bands from the area, is Charles Perry's *The Haight-Ashbury*[16]. There are a lot of potential contenders for 'the first psychedelic band' so I will not try and speculate who it might be. One might imagine it is a safe bet to suggest they came from around the Bay Area, but maybe not...

Around 1963, an unusual scene, centred on a strange cowboy-throw-back establishment, The Red Dog Saloon in Virginia City, Nevada, was developing. Growing numbers of artists and musicians were gathering there, dressing in vintage threads, carrying guns and getting loaded on peyote as part of an experimental tribal family established by Chandler A. Laughlin III. By 1965, this had become the place to hang out if you were a band interested in taking LSD and other substances. People came to get stoned, up close to nature, and in touch with the historical roots of Native America. Among other bands that played the Red Dog Saloon were Big Brother and the Holding Company, Jefferson Airplane, Quicksilver Messenger Service and The Charlatans — who, more than the others, are often credited as being the first *truly* psychedelic band.

By this time, if one were interested, one was no longer entirely reliant on the increasingly hard-to-find Swiss Sandoz LSD, but could opt for the widely available sacrament being produced locally in vast quantities by the chemist Owsley Stanley III, who was living in Berkeley in 1965, and flooding the San Francisco scene with his chemical product. It is arguable, then, that 1965 San Francisco was where hippies, and the public phase of non-medical psychedelia all began. Especially the music.

On his return to La Honda from his bus trip in 1964, Ken Kesey held frequent psychedelic parties in the woods at his house. These became the basis for the famous 'Acid Tests' during which he and the Pranksters colluded to create spectacular environments for people to try LSD in for the first time. Visitors knew what to expect. The sign at the end of the lane that lead to his cabin in the woods had been modified to read 'No Left Turn Unstoned'. At this time the drug was not yet illegal, and it was increasingly available for anyone interested in trying it. Many people were wishing to do so and they congregated for these parties firstly in their dozens, then in the hundreds. Before long the Acid Tests were taken on the road, with happenings rolled-out throughout California, played to packed halls of thousands of saucer-eyed revellers, put on by Kesey and the Pranksters with their Day-Glo painted craziness and improvised sounds. Using banks of audio equipment and cameras they wired the place for sound and projected back to people their own wails of ecstasy and confusion live as they happened — everything designed to twist the senses and expand the boundaries of reality.

And there was no better soundtrack for this experience than a weirdly familiar traditional country-roots-jazz-rock improvisational jam band like The Warlocks, a bunch of kids from San Francisco who played extended instrumental sets under the influence of swirling dials and patterned sounds emanating from the speaker stacks. They were later to become The Grateful Dead, and they had their first gig in 1965 at Ken Kesey's Acid Test in

San Jose, California. An excellent recent book, describing the intrinsic role of The Grateful Dead in the propagation of LSD culture from the 1960s to the present day, is Jesse Jarnow's *Heads*[17].

Read All About It

By 1966 the Haight-Ashbury hippie scene had its very own shop and newspaper. 'The Psychedelic Shop' on Haight Street, run by Ron and Jay Thelin, became the place to go for candles, papers, comics, posters, clothes and all the other necessary paraphernalia for those looking to get involved, or just hang around and ossify into the surroundings. The Thelin brothers subsequently put up cash to start the first underground newspaper, *The San Francisco Oracle*, which was edited by Allen Cohen and showcased the latest sounds and parties, and provided a place to read about the exploits of Ginsberg, Leary and the rest of the characters embodying/portraying alternative versions of American life. The paper was known for its colourful psychedelic artwork, directed by Michael Bowen. From here on, psychedelia expanded exponentially.

By way of a brief diversion before we launch into a spiel on psychedelic music, whether or not one believes psychedelics improve the production of music, most people would not deny that the experience of music listening is enhanced by psychedelics. It was only a matter of time before some clever soul got around to formally testing this well-known

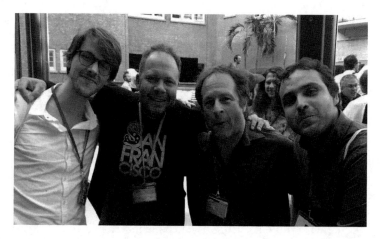

Picture 43: Mendel Kaelen, left, at the end of a busy day of presentations at the June 2016 Amsterdam conference, with Rick Doblin and Iker Puente. Now, where are those coffee shops?

phenomenon: That person was my colleague Mendel Kaelen, at Imperial College London. As part of the study team exploring the neural correlates of LSD (on, among others, my brain), Mendel subjected participants to a range of different music styles whilst under the influence. And, surprise surprise, he found that LSD enhanced aesthetic appreciation of sounds[18].

Hundreds of bands were developing their peculiar brand of esoteric sounds. In Berkeley, a 'right on' student activist jug band, Country Joe and the Fish, were brewing up their own versions of electric music for the mind and body, spawning a brilliant album that could well hold the prize for being the first record entirely conceived, written, produced and performed on LSD. As Joe McDonald said: 'In our quest to be the greatest psyche- delic band we must have taken more acid than all the rest put together!'

Psychedelic music was clearly designed both to emulate the sensa- tions of the acid experience and be enjoyed in a similar state of mind. This movement was converging on San Francisco and would lead eventually to the Bay Area's first major record-label signing for a psychedelic band, which was for Jefferson Airplane with their *Surrealistic Pillow* album in 1966. Psychedelic music had well and truly arrived, and it was very West Coast California. But the most influential musical force at the time — and soon to be leading the genre of psychedelic music itself — was coming from the other side of the pond.

It's All Too Much

The album *Rubber Soul* was The Beatles' cannabis LP and marked the per- manent loss of the mop-top clean image. Bob Dylan had introduced them to weed in 1964 and those introspective, soul-searching mellow acoustic songs on *Rubber Soul* had pot all over them. By the time *Revolver* came out in July 1966, they were increasingly experimenting with LSD (at least John, George and Ringo were — they had begun taking the sacrament shortly before the more cautious Paul). When the album ended with the splendidly psychedelic *Tomorrow Never Knows*, it was as if mainstream psychedelic music was here to stay. With its lyrics taken from Tim Leary's version of *The Tibetan Book of the Dead*, *The Psychedelic Experience*, the opening line 'Turn off your mind, relax and float downstream', and the backing track designed to be reminiscent of a thousand chanting monks, it was clear nothing would ever sound the same again.

Despite what more hardcore psychedelic music fans might say, in my opinion, it is difficult to deny The Beatles had immense influence through- out the sixties and their creativity in psychedelic music was keenly felt. Admittedly, they weren't taking as much acid as many others and were not anything like as involved in the psychedelic culture as the San Francisco bands, but pop artists throughout the globe looked to them for sonic inspiration, and their arrangements and instrumentation were copied everywhere.

In truth, so many bands fed off one another. The Byrds can link their roots back to Dylan just as The Beach Boys do to The Beatles, and The Beatles, in turn, themselves pay tributes to The Byrds. In the final analysis, they all look back to Little Richard, Muddy Waters and Robert Johnson. But it was the production techniques and creativity of The Beatles that so many musicians picked up on, including psychedelic bands from coast to coast. *Sergeant Pepper's Lonely Hearts Club Band* was the album most obviously leaning towards the use of LSD, but, in fact, the albums *Magical Mystery Tour* and *Yellow Submarine* contain the most classically psychedelic songs. One way or another — and I'm no Beatles expert — once the lysergic bug had been caught, by 1967 it was catapulted everywhere; the concept of psychedelia spread worldwide and made everyone sit up and listen.

It is fair to say that almost every well-known pop band at the time made at least one album or single that leant towards the cosmic angle (even Cliff Richard went mildly weird on a couple of his 1968 singles), such was the mainstream appeal of psychedelia at the time. One simply *had* to wear flowers and scarves, burn incense and talk about the inner world — just as kids today wear… whatever it is that kids today wear. The English approach was always slightly more whimsical and tongue in cheek than the serious mind-benders coming from the States — just as Ronald Sandison's gentle psycholytic therapy technique contrasts with Leary and Grof's high-dose peak experience approach. Throughout the songs of The Beatles, The Small Faces, The Pretty Things, Traffic, Cream and even Hendrix's early stuff there is the very English sentiment that one can take a trip, stroll through heavenly gardens of delight then come down and be home for tea, clear-headed and ready to meet the wife. But the American approach was considerably more mystical (Country Joe and The Fish, Love, JK and Co., HP Lovecraft, etc.) or just plain 'out there' sixties punk, as in the 13th Floor Elevators, The Moving Sidewalks and The Seeds. (Note that I quite transparently claim The Jimi Hendrix Experience here as an English band. The better part of their career, the band's management, and record label, all came from England. Sorry if that offends American readers keen to hold on to Jimi. He's ours! In return, you can keep one of our TV talent show winners.)

Psychedelic music got heavier as the decade progressed towards Woodstock and Altamont, and then fell into the seventies in a screech of rock as artists began turning down the little orange pills or sugar cubes and reached instead for the bottle, the mirror or the brown. But the psychedelic tradition was kept alive in the burgeoning 'acid folk' scene, which took us nicely into the free festival scene and the hippie bands resisting the norm.

Lose Your Mind — But Be Sure You're Home for Tea

It's true that, in general, the psychedelic revolution came to the UK late. We didn't have the gradual emergence out of the 1950s Beat Generation to the same extent as they did in the States. Nor did we have the Vietnam War to stir up protest, or such a healthy CIA government-testing program of LSD as existed over there (though there were a few important studies done on British troops, films of which have become rather popular on YouTube)[19]. In America, there was a larger grassroots development of a jilted generation of poets and writers who slowly adopted the use of the mind-expanding drugs leaking from Leary's set. There were a few notable characters spearheading the way in the UK, but in general the British psychedelic scene emerged instead from a well-established popular culture. Kings Road and Carnaby Street were already exploding with style and popularity by the time LSD came flooding in.

A big part of that flood was the result of Michael Hollingshead, who, in 1965, returned from the States where, since 1961, he had been cavorting with Tim Leary and his large mayonnaise jar of LSD. On his return to London, he brought back with him a huge stack of Leary's guide book, *The Psychedelic Experience*, and set out on a personal mission to 'turn on' the UK. He formed the World Psychedelic Centre in his Belgravia flat in Pont Street, and invited all and sundry (well, all those from the exclusive trendy set) to learn what the Americans had been doing for the last four years. He had with him 5,000 doses of Czechoslovak LSD, which he dispensed in 300-microgram doses injected into grapes for a host of willing invitees, including Clapton, McCartney, Polanski and The Stones.

Psychedelic clubs sprang up all over London, of which the UFO Club in Tottenham Court Road, The Roundhouse in Chalk Farm and the Middle Earth Club in Covent Garden were the most famous[20].They became the hotspots to watch the jangly groups of the 'British Invasion blues' sound lay down their hard riffs and pick up sitars and beads. All the garb was available from the boutiques of London, including the *uber* fashionable 'Granny Takes a Trip' (immortalized by the Purple Gang's song in 1967), 'Hung on You', 'Biba' and, a little later, 'The Apple Store' (and we are not talking iPads). An influential figure of the day in London was the American producer Joe Boyd whose deft ears brought us Pink Floyd, Fairport Convention, The Incredible String Band and, later, Nick Drake. For an excellent review of The Incredible String Band's ground-breaking album *The Hangman's Beautiful Daughter* — as well as many other illuminating essays on the undulating portraits of psychedelic history in the UK I can highly recommend Andy Roberts' new book, *Acid Drops* which provides a telling glimpse at how these fascinating drugs have influenced our cultural landscape in this country — and for which I proudly wrote the foreword[21].

In the 1960s artistic and literary influences emanated from the Indica Gallery and Bookshop in Soho, owned by John Dunbar, Peter Asher and Barry Miles, and were keenly supported by their neighbour Paul McCartney. It was in the Indica Gallery that John Lennon first met Yoko Ono who was displaying her artwork at the time. One of the Ono installations involved climbing a ladder and using a dangling magnifying glass to read a tiny word written on the ceiling. Lennon, who by then already had his eye on Yoko, had told himself that if the message was one of positivity then he knew that he and her would hit it off. He climbed the ladder, used the magnifying glass and strained his eyes to see what was written. The word was 'Yes'.

Another centre of cultural influence in the London psychedelic scene was the London Free School in Notting Hill, set up in part by John 'Hoppy' Hopkins in 1965. He and Barry Miles of the Indica Gallery also helped to propagate and disseminate the printed psychedelic word with their paper *International Times*, which, together with *Oz* (founded initially in Sydney by Richard Neville and which then had its second lysergic outing in London in 1967) brought limited print-run colourful acidic words to the kids in capes tearing round London in their Mini Mokes. For a lovely description of this period of underground publishing history in London, check out Richard Neville's book *Hippie Hippie Shake*[22]. Richard sadly passed away in 2016.

Wales, London, Goat-breeding and a WPC Called Julie

In 1977 a major police operation made the UK's biggest ever LSD bust and 'rescued' the streets from six-and-a-half-million doses of the 'killer' drug. This happened after an elaborate undercover police project called Operation Julie, named after one of the female officers working in the team of 28 'undercover hippies', which must have been quite a sight.

The story began nine years earlier when Richard Kemp, a chemist, met American David Solomon who by then was already something of a vintage name on the psychedelic circuit, having written a popular book on drugs earlier in the decade and who later founded the British LSD Club. By

1969 Kemp was producing LSD from his flat in West London. By far the hardest thing about making LSD in those days, and today, is getting hold of the base ingredient ergotamine tartrate, which, although not itself psychoactive, is also a controlled drug. But Solomon sorted out a sure supply. The chain from chemistry set to acid tab included another key player in Henry Todd, the distributer. He was joined later by Leaf Fielding, ex-student of Reading University who initially acted as tableter. Also involved was another mysterious character who was strangely both omnipresent and conspicuously absent throughout the whole psychedelic period: Ronald Stark; a man with connections to the world's major producers and suppliers of the drug, The Brotherhood of Eternal Love.

Operations moved out of London and into a secluded spot in Wales in 1973. This major LSD production, tableting and distribution network was by now churning out acid for the UK, European and American markets and for several years had stayed completely under the police radar. The acid was readily swallowed-up at the mushrooming circuit of free festivals that burned all summer long throughout the early seventies in Britain. In 1974, Kemp and Todd fell out. Kemp carried on making acid but didn't have a distribution network. He recruited another chemist and their lab on Seymour Road, London supplied most of the acid taken almost anywhere in the world between 1974–1977; microdots for the UK market and volcanoes (tiny conical-shaped tablets) for the European and wider international scenes. Kemp and his girlfriend, Christine Bott, kept themselves to themselves in their Welsh cottage, playing the part of dropped-out hippies running a smallholding but in fact churning out vast quantities of LSD. They grew their own vegetables and generally kept a low profile, though Christine emerged occasionally to parade one of her prize-winning goats at local shows.

In 1975 Richard Kemp was involved in a serious car accident that tragically resulted in the death of a local vicar. When the car was searched, the police found a vital clue: a piece of paper that had been ripped up but when put back together spelled the words 'hydrazine hydrate', one of the ingredients necessary for making LSD. The undercover operation was underway.

The police camped out at a nearby Welsh farmhouse and kept watch on Bott and Kemp for almost a year before swooping simultaneously on them and on the lab in London. The British LSD ring was busted, and the festival circuit LSD dried up. The cost of a tab went up from 50p to over a pound thereafter.

Most of the main players went to prison for long sentences. Christine Bott had nothing to do with making acid but she was busted for conspiracy. As the other chemist later said: 'I got eleven years for making LSD, Christine got nine years for making sandwiches!'

The defence of these LSD producers — and many other suppliers of the drug since — was that theirs was not a major profit-making industry but, rather, a mission to spread the positive effects of their chosen sacrament to the masses, a defence that never works with the judges. Leaf Fielding kindly helped me with this section of the book and he came and spoke about his Operation Julie experiences at Breaking Convention in 2013. Since his release from prison in 1982, he has since gone on to be an educator and philanthropist, setting up a school home for orphaned AIDS children in Malawi. And he has recently released a great book about Operation Julie, *To Live Outside the Law*, which is well worth a read for an insider's view of this fascinating piece of UK memoir[23]. There have been many other books about Operation Julie, from both the producers and from the police involved in this wonderful piece of English psychedelic history[24].

Haight, Collapse and Blame: It's All LSD's Fault

Of course, as mentioned, by the time London had swallowed the pill in 1967, the Haight-Ashbury area of San Francisco was already in psychedelic decline. This artsy neighbourhood perched on top of a hill (as is most of San Francisco, depending upon which angle one is lying) with its wide streets and beautiful wooden houses was where the hippies congregated because it was cheaper than the surrounding San Francisco neighbourhoods. In 1966, when the LSD bomb exploded, tens of thousands of kids, waifs, strays and runaways flooded into the area hoping to find those famous people with flowers in their hair. But by then many of the early pioneers already owned large properties out of town, drifting upwards to the serenity of Marin County or south to LA, where we later saw the move away from psychedelia and the emergence of the singer-songwriter introspection — a natural 'come-down' from the trip.

It seems the hippies were unable to stop the Vietnam war, which grumbled on with increasing casualties into the mid-seventies (when will we learn? — Bush, Reagan, Thatcher, Blair, Cameron, May, Trump, whatever). LSD was made illegal in 1966 and soon became maligned by 'The Man' as public enemy number one, blamed for the total moral collapse of the idealistic 1950's vision of the American family and the American Dream. The shopping malls had won. Charles Manson's grizzly version of psychedelic reality ended in a horrific bloodbath with the murders at the Polanski residence. The part LSD played in this was obviously seized upon by the media and used as justification that acid was a machination of the devil. Polarisation of the issue allowed politicians to deflect attention from their own killing spree in South East Asia and blame the whole of society's degeneration on a humble molecule derived from mouldy rye.

Timothy Leary was convicted of two very minor cannabis offences and, by 1969, was on the run from the authorities, who were determined to get his guts one way or the other for spoiling the kids' saccharin youth. Nixon dubbed Leary 'The Most Dangerous Man in America' and, in 1970, he was jailed for *30 years* for the possession of two dead roaches (as in joint ends, not the insects). He rightly escaped from jail in an elaborate plot involving The Black Panthers, the Weathermen and those international purveyors of underground acid, The Brotherhood of Eternal Love, which absolutely must be made into a film some day. Travelling in various disguises and with both formal and informal political and cultural asylums from many sympathetic — and a few unsympathetic — offers of help from Algeria to Beirut, Switzerland to Kabul, and eventually London, he found himself back in the clutches of the authorities in the USA.

The sixties were over, and to quote again from Danny in *Withnail and I:*

> 'The greatest decade in the history of mankind is coming to an end, man, and as Presuming Ed here has so consistently pointed out, we have failed to paint it black.'

By the early 1970s the Haight neighbourhood had declined into a quagmire of amphetamine and heroin abuse. Homelessness — which today in the Haight (and other districts of San Francisco and elsewhere) has become a national movement worthy of its own sovereign state — quickly set in.

But It's Not All Doom and Gloom

California remained very much the centre of the psychedelic, consciousness-expanding, countercultural cyclone thanks to Esalen, San Francisco and the music scene. But the hippie generation morphed with the times. For those serious-minded folks for whom the psychedelic experience was much more than just a hedonistic thrill, representing instead a true journey out of the humdrum consumerism of the growing modernity, they began to organise themselves into new communities with lifestyles centred around communal living.

As some of the more stalwart believers would have said, one-million years ago psychedelics propagated through the galaxy as alien spores clinging onto meteorites from distant stars, bringing about human spiritual development by feeding our cave-dwelling ancestors with mind food. This event catapulted early humans from cabbage-munchers into sentient god worshippers. Such believers would also claim that the 1960s and the resulting cultural explosion, propagated a cultural renaissance of equally important gravity and magnitude. Many of today's psychedelic community would consider themselves the enlightened 'Children of Aquarius', the Indigo Children. They have drunk the elixir and *know* with absolute certainty that the key to human and, indeed, the entire planet's survival, is through the transcendence of the ordinary limits of human consciousness with the help of psychedelic plants and fungi. There are a great many people who believe this. Well, a few anyway.

LSD, Computer Geeks and Green Activists: A New Age of Social Enlightenment

Today, we have roughly the same genome as we enjoyed 100,000 years ago. And if one subscribes to a purely reductionist viewpoint, this means we have the same physical machinery in our bodies and brains with which to invent our gods, form our religions, download our apps, develop social structures and work out how to best have relationships with the ones we love and the ones we cannot stand. Despite the external trappings of culture our brains are unevolved and may as well still be shuffling across the grassy plains of Africa from where we only very recently migrated.

But what *has* evolved is the transmission of ideas and knowledge — information conducted not as genes through DNA, but as memes through collected knowledge recorded in songs, pictures, laws, writing, drama and dance. Psychedelic drugs, and the maelstrom of influence they whipped up in the 1960s and beyond, are the primeval soup in which these memes swim, pushing forward and carrying in their wake information about art, music and fashion.

It is no surprise that the ecology movement sprang directly from the psychedelic scene. A spontaneous and fundamental phenomenon of the psychedelic experience is that of getting close to nature. Under the influence of LSD, one feels in tune with the waves and the wind in the rustle of the trees. These are the feelings that appear to intrinsically entangle one's own cells with the cells of those living and natural phenomenon all around. Everything is carried forward in an incessant flow of energy, a vibrational dynamism that feels, at least, as if it is part of something deeper than oneself and not of this age. There is a natural inclination to hark back to archaic times before newspapers, televisions, cars and frappuccinos. In 1953, Huxley lost his mind in the petals of a rose in a vase on the table, gazing dreamily with tear-filled eyes at the pure unadulterated beauty of God, made physical before him. He felt an immediate and natural connection with nature and saw in the flower himself and his place in the world. Yet when Osmond led him out into the Californian sunlight to stroll through the garden he collapsed into hysterical laughter at the sight of the car in the driveway. The absurdity of human invention! How ludicrous and false, how grotesque a mockery of nature is such a thing as a car! It jarred instantly with the feelings of connectivity he had with nature.

So, in the 1960s, the hippies naturally fed into and developed these beliefs. Saving trees, saving whales, vegetarianism and veganism, hugging trees and recording the screams of flowers as they were picked: these cultural peculiarities, that have since marched with alarming necessity into mainstream political circles as we face the prospect of global ecological disaster, are direct descendants of the LSD experience. Perhaps it is going too far to thank LSD for the Kyoto Agreement (which the US didn't sign up for anyway), but the roots of the green movement certainly owe a lot to the oceanic boundlessness of the psychedelic experience, if you can dig it.

And San Francisco certainly kept its cultural charm, remaining a centre for all things hippie-like — from a commercial point of view at least. In 2010, 2013 and 2017 I was fortunate to be invited to present updates on British Psychedelic Research at the Psychedelic Science Conferences held in and around San Francisco by the Multidisciplinary Association for Psychedelic Studies (MAPS). After the meeting in 2010 I found myself becoming happily stranded, unable to get out even if I had wanted to because of a most generous volcanic explosion from Eyjafjallajökull in Iceland. I stayed in the Red Victorian Hotel on Haight Street — a classic San Franciscan Victorian building, now home to Sami's World Peace Center and representative of all things hippie. I had a wonderful time playing my tunes in the bar for Sami and the staff, and staying in the 'Summer of Love' room for 14 days. By complete coincidence, my April stay that year also took in the famous annual '4/20' celebration in Golden Gate Park, which saw thousands of modern-day hippies congregate on 'Hippie Hill' dancing to reggae under clouds of smoke, giving me a little taste of what it might have been like back in 1967. Thank you Eyjafjallajökull for that.

It's Not All Over Yet

In the late 1970s and early 1980s, there were still bands emerging from the post-punk era, which harped back to the sounds and the drugs of the 1960s for their inspiration. One of the first bands I ever knew and owned the recordings of was The Soft Boys, courtesy of my sister's then boyfriend, the bass player. They were formed in Cambridge around the enigmatic front-man Robyn Hitchcock, were influenced by 'the four B's' — Beatles,

Barrett, Byrds and Beefheart — and their jangly tunes took their listeners back to the 1960s. The genre of 'neo-psychedelia' endured throughout the 1980s with many other bands like Echo and the Bunnymen and The Teardrop Explodes emerged on the fringes of 'goth' music and certainly burned a flame for the creative imagination offered by LSD (not that I realized it at the time). In recent years, contemporary psychedelic rock is back in vogue again, with the likes of Tame Impala finding fabulous mainstream success with their lysergic sounds. But what brought back all the culture of the 1960s, in all its Technicolor glory, was a different substance altogether, one based not around the tryptamine molecule, but around that of another endogenous brain chemical: phenethylamine.

Ecstasy is Upon Us

In 1988 the UK witnessed a new cultural phenomenon: the rave scene. The drug Ecstasy (3,4-Methylenedioxymethamphetamine, or MDMA) became prevalent at large music events, where it's stimulant and mildly hallucinogenic effects were favoured for all-night dancing. The drug has remained immensely popular ever since. Now in the UK around 750,000 people take Ecstasy every weekend, and over 100 million tablets are consumed annually[25].

MDMA was first synthesized and patented by the German pharmacological company Merck in 1912, not as a known psychotropic substance but as a precursor for other chemical reactions. Some sources have suggested MDMA was developed as an appetite suppressant for the German army but this is not accurate. In the first and second World Wars Germany favoured methamphetamine as its chosen appetite suppressant, whilst the allies used amphetamine sulphate on their troops (commanding governments have always drugged their soldiers to make them sleep less, eat less and fight harder) and MDMA never went into the mass production stage[26]. It is interesting to imagine what might have happened in those world wars had it gone in that direction!

Instead, MDMA was shelved by the 1920s and little more was mentioned about it until the mid-fifties, when it resurfaced again alongside a host of other psychotropic drugs being tested by the US military as possible 'truth serums' or weapons of war. Now, the CIA had a secret operation called MK-ULTRA, in which they tested hundreds of substances, including psychedelic drugs such as LSD, on hosts of people in dangerous and unethical circumstances. There are reports of agents giving people drugs without the subjects knowing they had been dosed in order that the agents could watch them surreptitiously. Suffice to say neither LSD nor MDMA made much progress when used in this way by the army. The subjective effects of the psychedelic drugs can become meaningless and unpredictable when no attention is paid to set and setting.

The 1960's drug culture came and went with very little mention of MDMA — most hippies preferring LSD. There was some limited use of the methylated amphetamine MDA, which has similar properties to MDMA, though less empathogenic and longer-lasting. Again, we can only wonder what the cultural, artistic, political and social landscape might have looked like had MDMA been discovered in large quantities in the 1960s instead of LSD; maybe the rave scene of the 1990s would have come early. Woodstock with bleeps?

The Grandfather of MDMA Meets His Grandson for the First Time

In 1967 Alexander 'Sasha' Shulgin was introduced to MDMA by one of his graduate students. Shulgin was a very successful organic chemistry graduate from Harvard who had since worked for the chemical company Dow. He left Dow in 1965 to pursue his own private business testing drug samples for the DEA. Impressed by MDMA, which he called his 'low-cal Martini', Shulgin continued to take the drug himself — together with whatever new chemical invention he had cooked up that month in his laboratory — with

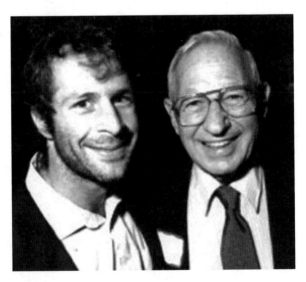

Picture 44: Pioneering MDMA Therapist Leo Zeff — with a young Rick Doblin.

a small group of chosen friends throughout the late 1960s and 1970s. This monthly study group, in which he and his friends methodically tested his new psychedelic discoveries, has become a thing of legend, and Sasha wrote a great book about the experiments, *Tihkal*[27]. Shulgin developed a neat system of rating scales to judge the effectiveness of his new creations, which many psychonauts still use today. Check out any 'trip reports' on *Bluelight* or *Erowid* to see Shulgin's rating scale in action, which rates the drugs' effects from Plus One (+), which is a just noticeable effect, to Plus Four (++++), which is a full-blown spiritual experience.

In 1976 Shulgin developed a new method of synthesis for MDMA, thus bypassing the Merck patent, and then introduced it to psychotherapist Leo Zeff. Now Zeff was a retired psychedelic psychotherapist who had given up his work with LSD some years earlier, disheartened that he could no longer use it in his practice. But as soon as he experienced MDMA, Zeff came out of retirement and began travelling around the States and Europe telling hundreds of people about the drug.

Many of these converts went on to use MDMA themselves as a tool for psychotherapy. As described in chapter two, it is impossible to ignore the potential that MDMA has for psychotherapy. The unique effects of the drug are almost as if it was invented for this purpose. A new legal alternative to LSD for psychedelic therapy had been discovered.

MDMA Becomes Too Popular, Gets Banned and MAPS is Born

What happened to MDMA next is broadly like the path taken by LSD, in that what had been developed through careful and judicious study in the clinic could not help leaking into the wider community. By 1980 there were reports of this new substance turning up in trendy Dallas nightclubs, which (as the TV show *Dallas* bears testament to), was a burgeoning culture of wealth and decadence. Some described the acceptance of this new drug (then called 'Adam') to be 'more popular than cocaine'. Being primarily a stimulant, like cocaine, but with a delightful added mild psychedelic effect, it was perfect for partying and dancing. People began calling it 'Empathy', in line with the positive mood effects when used clinically[28].

Of course, as soon as it became apparent that mass interest was around the corner, the next step was inevitable. In 1984 the DEA took steps to make MDMA illegal. It called for emergency legislation to have the drug placed in Schedule One, which meant it was defined as having 'no medical uses'. The small but vociferous band of psychotherapists who by then had developed effective and evolving psychotherapy regimes with MDMA protested this measure. A hearing took place and the judge took testimony from both sides. The government hired scientists against MDMA who submitted claims about its danger, suggesting it had a high toxicity profile (such claims have since been discredited). And in favour of MDMA, those therapists who had been using it effectively for the previous five years argued their case that it can be used safely to relive many forms of mental disorder. The judge saw reason and placed the drug in Schedule Three (equivalent to Class C in the UK), which meant it was available to bona fide therapists to use with caution. But the government/DEA overruled the judge (which, let's face it, makes a mockery of the judicial process if governments can do such a thing) and MDMA was placed firmly into Schedule One, where it has stayed since. This wasn't the last time that a government would over-rule the testimonies of scientific experts in order to legislate against MDMA, as David Nutt experienced in 2010.

For those therapists for whom this new drug had held such promise as a tool for psychotherapy, there was much disappointment. A pressure group was set up to strive for more research to try to convince the regulatory authorities that there were important medical uses for the drug. From this group emerged Rick Doblin and the formation of the Multidisciplinary Association for Psychedelic Studies (MAPS). MAPS has since campaigned furiously for evidence-based research to fight the corner for clinical MDMA and other psychedelic drugs. But it has been an uphill battle all the way, caught as it is in the Catch-22 situation whereby there is not enough data out there to support MDMA as a medicine so it remains banned, and because it is banned it is very difficult to get a licence to carry out the studies to prove it is safe to lift the ban. It was this frustration that dogged MDMA research for the last 30 years, though it is now thankfully beginning to shift. My own experiences of negotiating this bureaucratic nightmare to set-up my UK MDMA studies has bordered on the insane at times. More of that later.

Banning MDMA Gives Birth to Ecstasy and Rave

Meanwhile, in the early eighties MDMA was picking up as a recreational drug. Legend has it that around this time an entrepreneurial dealer of MDMA decided that the name 'Empathy' would not be such a good selling point, so changed it to Ecstasy, which clearly did the trick.

In the mid-eighties, it came to Europe via a small band of followers of the Indian style-guru, Bhagwan 'Osho' Shree Rajneesh[29]. Osho's American commune in Oregon had been shut down in 1984 and his followers had disseminated across the globe, many going to Ibiza, which by now was a popular hippie hang out for those still coming down from the 1960s. The

Osho-ites spread their message of love and sex using meditation and MDMA and, by 1987, when DJs Danny Rampling, Paul Oakenfold and Nicky Holloway went there for a holiday and experienced the embryonic nightlife, the links between Ecstasy and house music had well and truly been made[30].

The DJs returned to the UK and set up the club *Shoom* in South London (the name derived from the feeling one gets when coming up strong on MDMA), which gave birth to rave music and took the movement nicely into the so-called Second Summer of Love in 1988. A double-stranded approach to the use of MDMA meant the craze sped off in two rather separate directions: one being the dance scene and the other being the sounds coming out of Manchester propagated by the likes of The Stone Roses and The Happy Mondays — whose drug of choice was the same little pills stamped with pictures of doves that were being sold to the ravers in Ibiza and London. Ecstasy became incredibly popular in the UK in the last years of the eighties, and by the early nineties was second only to cannabis as the young people's illegal drug of choice.

Raves sprang up everywhere. Initially they were small-scale collective party gatherings born out of the 1960s Free Festival circuit. The Free Festivals had rolled along throughout the 1960s, and expanded in the mid-seventies fuelled by an enormous production of LSD and the continuing rock scene. Massive gatherings at Stonehenge took place every year and attracted an ever more diverse crowd as punk influenced the crowds. The Peace Convoy provided an opportunity for free-spirited folk to take to the road and live an itinerant lifestyle, travelling from party to party and rejecting the grimness of the 1970s British existence.

Modern Raving, Festivals and Shamanism: Come Together

Many scholars, sixties hippies and contemporary ravers alike have compared the modern concept of partying on psychedelic drugs to the archaic work of the shaman. Both occur mainly at night, when the shadows and hidden crevices of the dark jungle night are mimicked by the darkened corridors of a nightclub or festival scene; both encourage the imagination to fill in the gaps and expand the possibilities of what might be out there looking on; and both raving and shamanistic rituals tend to go on all night long: participants are in it for the long haul. It is not like having a couple of stiff drinks; there is a far greater commitment than that.

Shamans and DJs both rely on the trance-inducing qualities of repetitive music. Beats from drums that loop repeatedly, drawing the listener in, removing the opportunities for complex melody and inducing a vacant stare into the hidden gaps between the notes. But that is not to say the music is mindless or lacking in beauty; on the contrary, it is these primeval sounds that connect one with nature. Everything is cyclical; tribal drumming emphasises this point.

Psychedelic parties have a powerful cohesive, group bonding effect on those experiencing the shared altered state of consciousness, just as they do for the village participants in a shamanic ceremony. Participants are not merely being told about *someone else's* experience of the spiritual realms as happens in a traditional European church service. Instead, every single person in the room, under the trees, or on the dance floor, is an active participant up there, in front of Mother Nature, staring Her in the face and directly experiencing the power and wisdom of Her.

At a rave the shaman is the DJ and MC. He or she is directing the ceremony, leading the crowd along with their breakdowns, the tweaking of the cerebral EQs and controlling the lights. Strobes flash, lasers and smoke machines pump out their gushing of mind-clouding material onto the dance floor as directed by the Master of Ceremonies. Everyone is safely in his or her hands. The DJ will challenge you. They will not let you get away lightly; you are there to experience the peaks of the drug's effects and this will not be a walk in the park — if it were there would be nothing to learn from the experience. But you know they will keep you safe and keep your eyes open so you will not miss a beat.

The group psychedelic experience at a rave or in a festival is the modern day Western version of a shamanistic community ritual. It is more than just a hedonistic act, more than a mere 'acute confusional state'. It requires hard work, diligence and careful guidance. And when these factors are followed it may result in spiritual and personal growth, and play an important role in social cohesion and stability.

Kids on E

For an excellent first hand description of a young person taking his or her pioneer Ecstasy tablet and experiencing the positivity, the highs and the lows of their first rave, try a careful listening to the song Weak Become Heroes by the band *The Streets*. Few artists describe the impact of the early rave scene on UK youth better.

In the UK, it all came together big time at an infamous gathering of tribes for the Castlemorton Common Festival on May Bank Holiday in 1992. It was here we saw a coming together of Ibiza ravers with the hardened crusty travellers from the old Stonehenge-Peace Convoy-Free Festival circuit of the 1980s; these disparate tribes combined for a vast

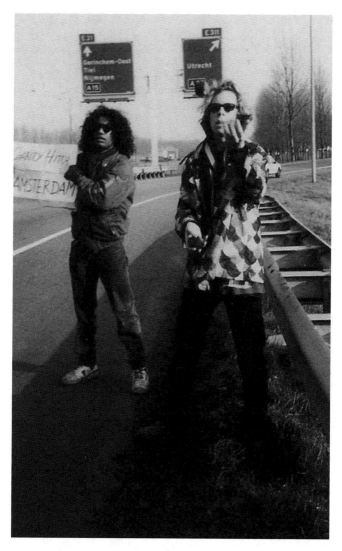

Picture 45: A couple of psychedelic ravers in 1991. With nothing better to do of a weekend than juggle and hitch their way to Amsterdam. With Manas Sidkar. Picture courtesy of Sarah Sessa.

anti-authority event, united by Ecstasy and dance music. The skanky psychedelic garb of the travellers met the trendy London neoprene of the ravers head-on and everyone realized they had a common purpose: to stay up all weekend long, peak and dance. While the post-punk travellers' favourite intoxicant of the past had been psilocybin mushrooms, amphetamine and high-strength canned beer both groups shared their love of cannabis and MDMA, and the marriage made in Castlemorton was born. The huge illegal party raged on whilst a bemused local population looked on incredulously. The police were unable to stop the event for five days and it eventually made front pages everywhere and was probably the single most important event that lead to the eventual Criminal Justice Bill in the UK[31].

DJ sound systems took over everywhere in the nineties, such was the general dross on offer in the popular music scene. Dance music rarely crept into the mainstream except in its most insipid form. The parties were in the custody of the kids and always one step ahead of the police.

Demonization of Ecstasy

Over the course of the 1990s, Ecstasy became the new public enemy number one (it seems like there must always be one — not sure what it is now... bankers perhaps, which, I suppose, is a progression in the right direction!). But things started going wrong, just as they had with LSD twenty years earlier. The quality of Ecstasy tablets plummeted and people began using nastier drugs. There were several high-profile tragic deaths of young people who took E for the first time in unsafe circumstances, and far too many people were over-indulging.

What happened next, quite inevitably, was that rave went mainstream, perhaps best characterized by the London group The Shamen, who sampled Terence McKenna's drones above a trancy beat. The band stormed the charts with 'Ebeneezer Goode' in 1993; "Eezer Goode, 'Eezer Goode. . . . He's Ebeneezer Goode!'[32].

Much to the chagrin of the UK drinks industry, kids in clubs stopped drinking booze and chose to supplement their E's with bottles of water instead. The drinks industry fought back with its development of 'Alcopops' — an obvious tip in the direction of the 'instant hit' but applied to ethanol rather than MDMA. This was a successful drive and we saw the UK drinking culture climb back to its ferocious position again. More recently, fruit flavoured ciders have been formulated, to capture the younger person market for sweet alcohol. The state-sanctioned legitimate alcohol peddlers have always been keen to put down illegal drugs. That is the trouble with keeping drugs illegal: there is no money to be made from it for governments. I liken the British drinks industry to our version of America's National Rifle Association. The NRA have for generations managed, somehow, to maintain the US's ludicrous gun laws despite the wealth of evidence against them. There are shady links between big money and politics. And in the UK, it is the drinks industry, more than any other, that is most staunchly opposed to any change in our non-evidence based drug laws.

In 1994, the British government made its greatest hit back at rave with the introduction of the Criminal Justice Bill, with its famously ridiculous description of electronic music as *'sounds wholly or predominantly characterised by the emission of a succession of repetitive beats'*. The new legislation meant police had increased powers of 'stop and search', and could more easily break up gatherings of people and confiscate sound systems without having to gain advance consent. My friends and I marched through London in our best rave regalia and partied all day up against police barricades in Hyde Park in October that year. It was a true 'fight for your right to party' moment, dancing to mobile sound systems in scenes reminiscent of the sixties, but to no avail. The Man had won, again. And to this day there continues to be an orchestrated system of fear projected onto ravers. As mentioned earlier, in 2016 we saw the local authority witch-hunt close the legendary London club *Fabric* on the grounds of drug use. The real reason for its closure was clearly because of the real estate value of the club's position and the growing tide of gentrification in London. I note that the 'normal' phenomenon of alcohol and cocaine related deaths in Mayfair clubs don't lead to their closure.

MDMA Research on the Ropes and Labels On the Wrong Bottles

As the 1990s drew on, Rick Doblin and the Multidisciplinary Association for Psychedelic Studies, MAPS, were struggling like mad to re-establish psychedelics' role in medicine. The demonization of Ecstasy was effectively grounding all research just as the backlash against acid in the mid-sixties did for LSD research 30 years earlier. And in much the same way as for LSD, the illegalisation of Ecstasy did nothing to reduce its recreational use, which continues to this day to be immensely popular, but was very effective at stopping bona fide medical research.

Reagan's presidency between 1981 and 1989 carried on Nixon's all-out War On Drugs just as blindly, steamrolling its way through the media and the courts, blocking Doblin at every opportunity. Reagan was followed by George H. W. Bush, 1989–1993, and he was certainly no better.

Between 1986 and 1988, Doblin submitted to the FDA (the Food and Drinks Authority, the American organisation which oversees the licensing of medicines required) five different applications for permission to conduct human research with MDMA and all five were rejected[33]. The FDA said there was too much risk of neurotoxicity from MDMA. But Doblin persisted. He knew the rejections were not for objective scientific reasons but because of an underlying cultural prejudice. The authorities simply could not see, or did not *want* to see, that an illegal recreational drug could have any clinical benefit. It would send the wrong message to the kids. Doblin was rightly concerned that the same thing that happened with LSD at the end of the sixties was happening again with MDMA. A socio-politically motivated cultural backlash was threatening to stop medical research in its tracks and the result was that patients would lose out. This could not be allowed to happen again. Surely the only message to send is the truth? But MAPS was caught in the imposed Catch 22^3. There was an insufficient amount of data, and MAPS wasn't allowed to go out and get it[34].

In the late eighties and early nineties, MAPS continued to do what it could, funding animal toxicity and Phase One human studies at Stanford and Johns Hopkins Universities in the States. Then Doblin's perseverance began to pay off. In 1992 Dr. Charles Grob, Professor of Child and Adolescent Psychiatry at UCLA, submitted a protocol for a clinical MDMA study on patients with terminal cancer. The FDA started to see sense, and said they would consider this protocol only after a further Phase-One safety study was conducted on MDMA to test its toxicity at the doses proposed for therapy. The safety study was approved and subsequently completed in 1995. It demonstrated — just as everyone at MAPS expected — that MDMA did not present any significant risks to humans at the doses and patterns of doses proposed for psychotherapy[35]. The FDA, however, remained cautious for the rest of the decade and continued with a level of bureaucracy that made it very difficult for Grob's study to progress.

Meanwhile Dr. Jose Carlos Bouso in Spain, who has also been planning a MAPS-sponsored MDMA for PTSD study, eventually obtained approval in 1999, which got underway in 2000. But just over a year after starting, Bouso's Spanish study began to falter. After just six of the planned 29 patients on the study have received their initial dosing with MDMA the Spanish government — fuelled by a political backlash influenced by negative media pressure — bears heavily on Bouso and the study is shut down. It is 2002, some 17 years since MDMA was banned, and clinical research is still a very distant dream. Everything seems to be against the clinical study of MDMA. There is just too much erroneous negative pressure filling the newspapers, augmented by media scare stories about reckless ravers and international drug cartels. Despite the fact these issues have nothing to do with the medical use of MDMA in therapy, governments everywhere dare not back the research for fear of unwanted political fallout. And this attitude of fear and bias is even infiltrating the scientific community, with a host of methodologically unsound and even, possibly, downright scandalously flawed data sets supporting the entrenched position of the governments who wish to continue their War On Drugs — even when it flies in the face of medical necessity.

As mentioned earlier, there was a famous incident in 2002 which illustrates well this farcical debate, when Dr. George Ricaurte, working for a US government-sponsored MDMA project, published a study that apparently unequivocally demonstrated severe neurotoxicity in primates who had been given only moderate amounts of MDMA. The study appeared in the highly influential journal *Science* and Ricaurte's damning results were beamed all over the world. Here was the smoking gun. The international media and governments jumped on the story and used it as clear justification for their heavy restrictions on MDMA research and on those troublesome clubbers. But then, in 2003, it transpired that Ricaurte's research had been highly inaccurate. His team had not given their primates MDMA at all, but rather *methamphetamine* — a highly toxic compound that bears no resemblance to MDMA. Although Ricaurte subsequently retracted his study from *Science* and offered an apology, the damage was done and governments clung on to that smoking gun for many years — perhaps they still do. I am no conspiracy theorist but Doblin has certainly continued to pursue exactly what went on there. Possible speculations include someone in Ricaurte's lab switching the bottles by accident, or on purpose, or even that the DEA themselves were implicated at the original source of the drug. One way or another the erroneous result caused an enormous amount of damage to genuine MDMA research and the apparent 'accident' fitted in well to the malevolent political agenda against MDMA[36].

Doblin Meets Mithoefer at a Conference for the Spiritual Vine

In 2000 Doblin met Michael Mithoefer at an ayahuasca conference in San Francisco sponsored by Leary's old colleague Ralph Metzner. Mithoefer, a psychiatrist from South Carolina with a lifelong interest in MDMA and an experienced practitioner with cases of severe PTSD, believed strongly that MDMA might offer a desperately needed new therapeutic approach for his patients. Unfortunately, by this point Dr. Grob's study looking at patients with end-stage cancer was not happening at all, due to the DEA's continued barriers to using MDMA; so he decided to use psilocybin instead. He went on to produce a ground-breaking clinical study with psilocybin, which we will come to later.

By the turn of the new millennium, dance music and Ecstasy use had moved to a new level. Perhaps because of the Criminal Justice Act, what used to happen in small clubs and dingy warehouses at an underground level now filled arenas and supported a whole legitimate industry on both sides of the Atlantic. In 2000, the ubiquitous direct drive Technics 1210 turntable — the standard hardware set-up for any self-respecting disc jockey — was outselling guitars for the first time as the teenage Christmas present of choice. Vinyl was back on the shelves, and now everyone wanted to be a DJ. MDMA had saved the vinyl record industry.

Things Start Looking Up for MDMA Research

With the turn of the new millennium, Mithoefer and Doblin gained approval for their PTSD study and over many further years of red tape and headaches it gets underway. However, recruitment and enrolment remain slow in the face of so many bureaucratic restrictions. The researchers apply to the review board to make an amendment, wishing to add a third MDMA session to the course of therapy, which takes a full three years to get approval but they keep going, slowly seeing 37 patients through the treatment protocol.

In 2004, I wrote my first editorial for the *British Journal of Psychiatry* on the state of international psychedelic research[37]. Although the movement was in full swing in the States by this stage, I felt disheartened that, for the clear majority of my generation of British psychiatrists, it was still an unknown subject. Rick Doblin was supportive of my work and encouraged me to cast the net wider to try to bring on board more psychiatrists

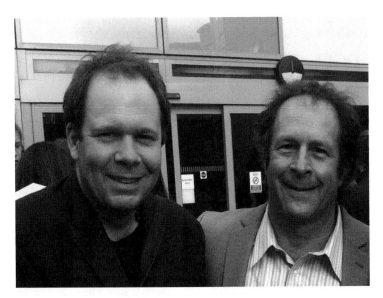

Picture 46: Rick Doblin at the first Breaking Convention at Kent University, Canterbury, in 2011.

from the UK. Through publication of my paper in the *British Journal of Psychiatry* in 2005, and while still in Oxford, I met Amanda Feilding. In 2007, after my work came to the attention of David Nutt, I put Nutt and Mithoefer together, and, in his role as president of the European College of Neuropsychopharmacology (ECNP), Nutt invited us both to talk on the state of psychedelic research at their annual meeting in Vienna and we got along fabulously. I invited him over to the UK, together with Charlie Grob, to speak at a symposium in Liverpool that I was chairing at the Royal College of Psychiatrists Annual Conference in 2009. This symposium was approved for the College by one of the UK's leading psychiatrists specialising

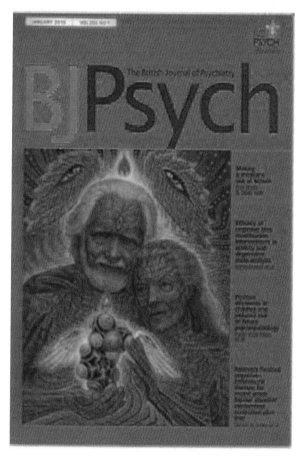

Picture 47: The British Journal of Psychiatry goes psychedelic in January 2015 with Alex Grey's 'The Shulgins and their Alchemical Angels' (2010) Acrylic on wood, 24x30 inches. Used with the kind permission of the artist.

in PTSD, Dr. Jonathan Bisson from Cardiff University, and would prove to be another important stepping stone in the story of MDMA research in the UK — but none of us knew it just yet.

Then, in 2010, Michael Mithoefer's study was fully written up. I was invited to review the paper for the *Journal of Psychopharmacology*, for which David Nutt was the chief editor. The data was in. MDMA therapy could be delivered safely and effectively to treat PTSD. The paper was approved and the world's first human clinical MDMA study was published — a whole 35 years after the substance was inappropriately banned in the first place. Rick Doblin, whose dream to see this happen dates to 1985, deserves a Nobel Prize for his perseverance.

Since the publication of Michael's pilot study with MDMA-assisted psychotherapy for treatment-resistant PTSD, MAPS has continued to lead the way in international MDMA research, with a plethora of new studies springing up throughout the world; including two in the UK starting in 2016, about which there will be more later.

In June 2014 the psychedelic research community — and lovers of chemistry and Ecstasy everywhere — heard the sad news that Sasha Shulgin passed away after some years struggling with dementia. He and Ann were always keen supporters of *Breaking Convention* and his inspiration to me and others in the field of MDMA science continues to resonate. Some months after his death I submitted a raft of papers and commentary to the *British Journal of Psychiatry* to celebrate Sasha's contribution to psychedelic science. Myself, Ann and psychonauts everywhere were thrilled and triumphant when the special edition of the journal came out in January 2015. It featured the famous painting of Sasha and Ann by US visionary artist Alex Grey on the front cover and two academic editorials on psychedelics — one piece written by David Nutt and myself on tackling the legal restrictions around MDMA research[38], and one by Dr Matthew Johnson of Johns Hopkins University and myself about using psychedelic-assisted psychotherapy to treat addictions[39]. And the final cherry on the cake was a brief piece Alex and I wrote in homage to Sasha[40]. It felt, at that point at least, as if the UK medical community was getting behind contemporary psychedelic science.

Sasha, like Albert Hofmann and his stance towards LSD, stood firm in his keen belief that MDMA can, and will, be an important force to be reckoned with in the future of medicine; whatever socio-political storms it needs to go through before general mainstream understanding of the usefulness of this important medicine is accepted by all.

CHAPTER 6

Psychedelic Creativity

Measuring the Influence of Psychedelics on Creativity

It is perhaps no surprise that John Lennon, after taking LSD, thought George Harrison's heavily chimney-stacked Berkshire mansion resembled a giant yellow submarine. LSD does stuff like that. The link between psychedelics and creativity is ancient, and, as Terence McKenna would have us believe, these peculiar compounds could account not only for brief excursions into creativity during the acute intoxication with the drug, but also for the entire development of human consciousness itself. Indeed, looking at the role LSD played in so many facets of human life in the sixties, one might conclude that never have so many fields of human endeavour, from art and architecture, to fashion, music and design, owed so much to such a small molecule.

Certainly, human creativity is difficult to define and measure. And it is such an important cognitive process that it becomes an interesting challenge for modern scientific exploration. There are clear similarities between the typical traits of creative people and the subjective psychological characteristics of the psychedelic drug experience[1]. This phenomenon — which may seem obvious to some people but ludicrous to others — was studied in a number of small trials and case studies in the 1960s but results were inconclusive, and the quality of these studies by modern research standards was merely anecdotal.

Nevertheless, with today's current renaissance in psychedelic drug research, we are beginning to revisit these studies with contemporary research methods and neuroimaging. Like many aspects of modern psychedelic research, this is an area of research long overdue. Many of today's contemporary psychedelic studies, as in the 1960s, focus on the drugs' potential clinical applications. But there are increasingly more research avenues for experiments with less obvious clinical applications, that are adding to our understanding of the aesthetic and creative elements of the human brain.

Creativity, Psychedelics and the Human Brain

The well-documented but erroneous 'left-brain versus right-brain' model of brain functioning polarises and oversimplifies an individual's cognitive and creative skills as either artistic, at the expense of language and mathematics, or vice versa. But modern functional neuroimaging challenges this popularly held belief and instead provides a three-factor anatomical model of creativity that focuses on interactions between the temporal lobes, frontal lobes and limbic system. The neuroscientist Robin Carhart-Harris at Imperial College London has shown the direct role psilocybin has in activating the area of the brain associated with the retrieval of emotional memories, providing an immediate link between creativity and expanded levels of consciousness. And Robin's more recent imaging studies with LSD have demonstrated that the classical psychedelic hugely increases the networking between otherwise largely disconnected areas of the brain; areas that were once talking to one another when the brain was in its childhood mode, but since adulthood such networks have become separated. It appears that LSD brings them together, recreating for a few precious hours, that childlike wonder and creativity[2]. These findings fit with the known observation that creative thinking requires more than just a general intelligence and specific knowledge, but also the ability to develop alternative solutions to a single question, requiring divergent thinking and the ability to form novel ideas.

Many psychedelic explorers come to entertain the view that mind/consciousness is present throughout the universe, and not just the by-product of brain activity. A reductionist point of view, on the other hand, postulates that highly creative individuals are able to store extensive specialised knowledge in their temporoparietal cortex, be capable of divergent thinking mediated by the frontal lobe and, crucially, can modulate the activity of the locus coeruleus (which fires in response to novel stimuli — and, under the influence of the drug LSD) via the norepinephrine system 'to understand and express novel orderly relationships'[3].

Since the Renaissance, creativity has often been measured in terms of examining the output of so-called creators. The sheer volume of works by Da Vinci and Michelangelo are frequently quoted as testament to their creative geniuses. However, defining objective measures for the process of creativity is notoriously difficult, especially when considering the subjective nature of an individual's aesthetic appreciation of a creation. It is arguable, of course, that creativity defies measurement, because all tests have predetermined correct answers and originality is a requirement of creativity — implying that any 'correct' answer in a creativity test could not be creative[4].

The psychological experience induced in humans under the influence of psychedelic drugs is multifarious and idiosyncratic. Nevertheless, a broad range of common characteristics are frequently identified. Alongside the alterations in the user's perceptions, there are also changes in the emotions and expansion of thought and identity, which is a feature of the psychedelic experience that has special relevance to the creative process. The psychedelic experience is one of a general increase in complexity and openness, such that the usual ego-bound restraints that allow humans to accept given, preconceived ideas about themselves and the world around them are necessarily challenged. Another important feature is the tendency for users to assign unique and novel meanings to their experience, together with an appreciation that they are part of a bigger, cosmic oneness. These experiences — like those features of spirituality which were described earlier in the book — are fundamental, and arise spontaneously for any users of psychedelic drugs, regardless of any pre-experience or social influence. The evidence for the universal nature of such experiences comes from the multi-cultural similarities of the experiences of users of psychedelic drugs throughout the world.

Unsurprisingly, there are many anecdotal examples of artists and writers describing the use of psychedelic drugs, such as LSD, to enhance the creative process (and a number of such accounts disputing this suggestion). The use of drugs to enhance artistic creativity is not new, illustrated when the Roman poet Ovid said, *'There is no poetry among water drinkers'*. There are examples of prehistoric art from all around the world that use optical illusions or entoptic phenomena to enhance the visual experience. This observation has been recently studied by a group of researchers including the anthropologist Luis E. Luna from the Research Centre for the Study of Psychointegrator Plants, Visionary Arts, and Consciousness, located in Brazil. Their paper, 'Enhancement of creative expression and entoptic phenomena as an after-effect of repeated ayahuasca administration', which I reviewed and approved for the *Journal of Psychopharmacology*, examines the frequency of entopic shapes reported as emerging in the visual fields of users of ayahuasca[5]. More studies of this sort will undoubtedly appear in coming years as we delve deeper into the quagmire of thought that links neuroscience with art. Dr. David Luke at the University of Greenwich, a passionate and informed proponent of psychedelics, creativity and psi phenomena, is a keen supporter of this direction of study[6].

Art, Music and Psychedelic Creativity

The links between artwork and the prehistoric use of psychedelic drugs is well established; it is described in the artwork of many ancient cultures from Ireland, Africa, France, and South America to as far afield as Siberia and the Arctic Circle. The use of opium (while not usually credited as a psychedelic drug) to influence creativity is also well recognised. Thomas De Quincey described the pleasures and the pitfalls of taking opium in early 19th century England[7], and the romantic poet Samuel Taylor Coleridge reported the vivid imagery of the opium experience in his poem *Kubla Khan*[8], as did Alexandre Dumas Pere[9] and Alfred Lord Tennyson[10]. In the 20th century, the French poet and playwright Antonin Artaud used opium extensively, as well as the peyote cactus[11]. More recent examples of artists using psychedelic drugs include Henri Michaux, the Belgian-born French painter, journalist and poet, who at the age of 56 started using mescaline and cannabis, and wrote about his experiences in his later works[12]. And, as we have seen, Huxley's famous account of his mescaline experience in 1953 secured his place as a centrally revered figure for the subsequent cultural drug revolution that followed.

Since the 1960s, the volume of modern Western art and music that attributes its influences to the psychedelic drugs is vast. Some of these artists and musicians categorically proclaim themselves to be 'psychedelic artists', whereas many others will frequently acknowledge the influence that psychedelic drug experiences have had on their work. I mentioned earlier the *British Journal of Psychiatry* showcasing Alex Grey's artwork in 2015[13]. The journal has also previously featured a front cover piece of artwork by visionary photographer Dean Chamberline, whose work is heavily influenced by the psychedelic experience, which appeared in 2006 to celebrate Albert Hofmann's 100th birthday[14].

Some of the finest and most original pieces of popular music to come out of the Western world in the last six decades have been directly influenced by the psychedelic experience; indeed, we have already touched upon the vast body of work attributed to LSD that forms the basis of the genre of psychedelic music. Suffice to say, there are hundreds of bands and thousands of tunes — from the briefest punkadelic explosions of cerebral damage to triple-gatefold albums of Prog Rock dirge about pixies, crystals and timeless voids — all of them striving to capture the essence of the psychedelic experience onto crackling vinyl. 'Pure tone poem imagery' is how George Martin described The Beatles' psychedelic period of musical influence.

Studying How Psychedelics Influence Creativity

An attempt to explore the value of the agent LSD in influencing artistic creativity was made in a remarkable long-term series of anecdotal case studies by the American psychiatrist Oscar Janiger[15]. Between 1954 and 1962, he facilitated LSD sessions for almost 1,000 people between ages 18 and 81 in a variety of professions, from doctors and nurses, lawyers, housewives and police officers to judges, truckers, students, and the unemployed and retired, including the film star Cary Grant. In contrast to the often highly controlled design of most other psychedelic research of this period, Janiger's experiments were largely unguided and took place in a naturalistic setting — his own home — with a view to exploring what might be the nature of the 'intrinsic, characteristic LSD response' (if indeed there was one). Unsurprisingly, the volunteer's reports varied widely. Adverse reactions were extremely rare, and the clear majority described the experience as valuable and sustaining. During this work with LSD, two experiential characteristics emerged repeatedly: those of spontaneous spiritual experiences, and those where there was a boosting of the subjects' experiences of creativity. These latter observations led Janiger to conduct a parallel study examining the effects of the drug on creativity in a controlled setting.

He subsequently gave LSD to a mixed group of 60 visual artists over a seven-year period, and they produced over 250 drawings that were later analysed by a professor of art history, who compared the artists' work before and after the LSD sessions. Because of the heterogeneity of the population and the aesthetic nature of analysing the results, making objective statements about how LSD effected the artists' creativity is impossible. That said, the drug did appear to enhance certain aspects of the artists' work; namely, there was a tendency towards more expressionistic work, a sharpening of colour, a greater freedom from prescribed mental sets, an increased syntactical organisation, a deeper accessibility of past impressions and a heightened sense of emotional excitement. However, perhaps the most valuable aspect of Janiger's study is the many qualitative reports from the artists themselves, who without exception found the LSD experience artistically and personally profound.

Further experiments in creativity and psychedelics include those of Stanley Krippner in the early 1970s, and a much earlier study by Berlin in 1955 in which four prominent graphic artists were given mescaline and LSD and encouraged to complete paintings under the influence of the drug[16]. A panel of art critics judged their subsequent paintings to have 'greater aesthetic value' than the artist's usual work. In the mid-sixties, the American psychologist Frank Barron gave psilocybin to creative individuals and recorded their subjective impressions[17], and the psychiatrist McGlothlin gave LSD to graduate students who subsequently described a greater appreciation of music and the arts, but no actual increase in creative ability[18]. Many of the creativity psychedelic studies of the 1960s paid little attention to the importance of set and setting, those two very important factors that have been shown to radically alter the outcome of individual's experiences under psychedelic drugs.

A Nice Study by James Fadiman and Colleagues

A study in 1966 by Harman and Jim Fadiman from the Institute of Psychedelic Research of San Francisco State College deserves closer attention[19]. The researchers took care to select individuals already engaged in creative industries (engineers, theoretical mathematicians, physicists, architects and designers) and 'primed' them with a pre-drug session in which they were encouraged to select problems of a professional interest that required a creative solution. The researchers, who told the subjects that the drug would enhance their creativity and help them to work more productively without distractions, therefore encouraged a positive mind-set. At the psychedelic sessions (using mescaline) a few days later, subjects were encouraged to work in groups and as individuals to tackle their chosen problems and were subjected to psychometric tests. Afterwards, subjects submitted a written subjective account of their experience and were then interviewed by the researchers eight weeks later. All participants showed enhanced abilities on all tests when under the drug compared with the previous non-drug tests and, in the subjective written accounts, all the participants described subjective enhanced effects of the drug on their creative process. From these qualitative reports the researchers formulated a mechanism by which psychedelic drugs can enhance creativity:

1. Reduced inhibition and reduced anxiety.
2. Improved capacity to restructure problems in a wider context.
3. Increased fluency and flexibility of ideas.
4. Increased visual imagery and fantasy.
5. Increased ability to concentrate.
6. Increased empathy with objects and processes.
7. Increased empathy with people.
8. Subconscious data more accessible.
9. Improved association of dissimilar ideas.
10. Heightened motivation to obtain closure.
11. Improved ability to visualize the completed solution.

Although this study is limited by not being double-blind and placebo-controlled, it reports the power and importance of set and setting, and its potential implications for the creative industries is highly significant.

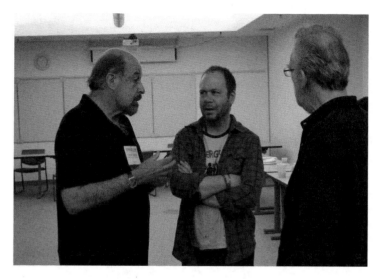

Picture 48: Jim Fadiman talking with psychedelic psychotherapist, Andrew Feldmar, in Oakland, California 2013.

Jim Fadiman is a respected and deeply open-hearted veteran of the psychedelic research who continues to inspire today's generation of young researchers. These days he is working with the concept of micro-dosing with LSD and psilocybin as a tool for enhancing cognition. Micro-dosing — using sub-threshold doses that do not cause a significant psychedelic effect but, much more subtly, enhance thinking and alertness — is very much flavour of the month in the States. Watch this space to see where that anecdotally-driven pastime drives research in the coming years.

Commercial and Design Applications for Psychedelic Creativity: LSD Architecture

A better understanding of creativity and how best to enhance it has vast implications for commercial industry. Above and beyond the artistic and neuroscientific interest in the creative process, practically all aspects of modern industry rely to some extent on the concept of product design — particularly in the advertising industry, where creativity is arguably the most important element of success. Despite the enormous amount of money and energy invested in such commercial industries, the scientific concept of how creativity is enhanced remains poorly understood. This makes the neuroscientific understanding of these processes particularly relevant.

There have been some notable historical examples of designers using psychedelic drugs to improve their skills. One such example from 1965 is when the architect Kyoshi Izumi was asked to design a psychiatric hospital in Canada and decided to take LSD and perform extensive visits to old mental institutions to see the wards in a new light[20]. He found himself terrified by the standard hospital paraphernalia such as the tiles on the walls, the recessed closets and the raised hospital beds. There was no privacy, and the sense of time was nil, because of the absence of clocks and calendars. After his LSD insights, Izumi could design what has since been called 'the ideal mental hospital'. The first was built in Yorkton, Saskatchewan, and five others have since been modelled upon it elsewhere in Canada[21].

From Double-helix DNA to San Franciscan Hippies and Geeks with Mice

Another example of the creative influence of psychedelic drugs — though almost certainly more psychedelic legend than reality — comes from the alleged use of low doses of LSD by the Nobel Prize winner Francis Crick, who discovered the double-helix structure of the DNA molecule in Cambridge in the 1950s. Although LSD was indeed available as a tool for psychotherapy at that time (with Ronnie Sandison having started his work with LSD at Powick in 1952), there remains considerable debate about whether Crick used it *before* publication of his famous double-helix paper that won him the Nobel Prize, and therefore whether LSD creativity can be credited for such an important discovery[22]. His family have always denied that LSD played a role in the discovery of the structure of DNA. What is undeniable, however, is that Crick become a notable psychedelic enthusiast later in his career. He was a well-known admirer of Aldous Huxley and went on to campaign for the legalisation of cannabis in the 1960s. So one way or the other, I suppose one could say that psychedelics were always in his DNA.

Another example of, unambiguous, psychedelic drug-induced creativity from the scientific community comes from the Nobel-Prize-winning chemist Dr. Kary Mullis. He invented the Polymerase Chain Reaction (PCR) process, which has become a staple method of chemical analysis of DNA. Mullis is quoted as saying: 'Would I have invented PCR if I hadn't taken LSD? I seriously doubt it. . . . I could sit on a DNA molecule and watch the polymers go by. I learnt that partly on psychedelic drugs'. A further striking example of psychedelic drug-enhanced creativity in industry comes from the computer industry in California. The liberal atmosphere and loose approach to creativity fostered by the 1960s use of LSD on the

West Coast of the United States spawned a population of creative post-hippie entrepreneurs. Pioneers such as Steve Jobs and Steve Wozniak, founders of the Apple computer industry, were both products of the LSD-fuelled counterculture setting out to turn computers into a means for freeing minds and information[23].

Clinical Applications for Psychedelic Creativity: Autism

Clinically, how can we use this creativity phenomenon associated with psychedelics? Perhaps an obvious area is that of autism. Patients with autism are often unable to see the intrinsic and abstract connectivity between people and objects. And one of the central features of the psychedelic experience is the improved ability to find new meanings, and see associations, through feeling as if one were participating in an enhanced part of the abstract connectivity of the universe. Although these are subjective effects enhanced acutely only during the psychedelic experience, they are experiences always enjoyed by most people to a lesser degree, but in autism, such experiences are frequently impaired.

This phenomenon was explored in the early part of the 1960s in a small number of studies using LSD on children with autism, as previously discussed in chapter five of this book. One study looked at subjects between 6 and 10 years old, all severe cases of autism who had failed to respond to other forms of treatment. Consistent effects of the psychedelic drugs included improved speech in otherwise muted patients, a greater emotional responsiveness to other children and adults, increased positive mood with frequent smiling and laughter, and decreases in obsessive-compulsive behaviour. After a long hiatus, there are now researchers looking again at the role for psychedelics as a treatment for autism.

The researcher Alicia Danforth and others working with MAPS have been carrying out such a study in recent years. The drug MDMA, with its known empathogenic effects, is being researched as a tool to enhance psychotherapy for people with Autism Spectrum Disorder.

But all research into the links between psychedelics and creativity struggle with measuring the extent to which creativity is being altered. It is often difficult to get meaningful data because subjects frequently become engrossed in the subjective aspects of the drug experience and lose interest in the tasks presented by the investigators. Understandably, psychological tests are often seen as absurd or irrelevant by the subjects, illustrated well by this quote from the psychologist Arthur Kleps:

If I were to give you an IQ test and during the administration one of the walls of the room opened up, giving you a vision of the blazing glories of the central

galactic suns, and at the same time your childhood began to unreel before
your inner eye like a three-dimension colour movie, you too would not do
well on an intelligence test[24].

The Future Looks Creative for Psychedelic Research

With psychedelic research's current renaissance, the current political climate is beneficial for exploring the therapeutic possibilities of such drugs that have hitherto been considered off limits simply because they have been used recreationally. In recent years, we have seen Walter Pahnke's famous Marsh Chapel Experiment re-created by Roland Griffiths' team at Johns Hopkins University, providing measurable evidence of the spiritual experience under the influence of psychedelic drugs.

In today's modern psychedelic research renaissance, it was only a matter of time before some brave researcher decided to recreate the previously mentioned study by Harman and Fadiman to provide similar data on the objective association between creativity and psychedelics to the neuroscientific community.

The researcher in question is Shlomi Raz, a New York entrepreneur with a keen eye on transforming how we see psychedelics working as tools

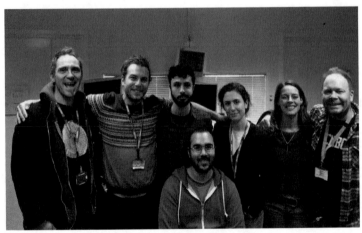

Picture 49: The Eleusis Clinical Trial Team on the day I participated in the study. London, 2015.
David Luke, Leor Roseman, Russell Shernoff, Guillerme Livera, Neiloufar Family and Maria Pap. This picture is in no way representative of the entire team, but rather just those covering the study on the day of my participation. Many other people, who spent countless hours at the research facility, played a vital role in this project; in particular, and not pictured here, study manager Luke Williams.

for the future of humanity. Since 2014 he has been carrying out some important studies in North London through his company *Eleusis Benefit Corporation*, Founded in 2013 to explore new ways of utilising tryptamine psychedelics, the main focus of Eleusis will be Alzheimer's Disease and depression. As part of the research towards developing psychedelic science to tackle these disorders, Eleusis carried out Phase 1 safety / tolerability studies in 2015 and 2016 with LSD. These studies also included a fascinating exploration of LSD cognitive effects in both naïve and experienced psychedelic users. I have had the great pleasure to be involved in these ground-breaking studies, alongside a host of other UK-based doctors.

We look forward to seeing the results emerge in the coming years.

In the meantime, we'll just have to take John's word for it that George's house looked like a submarine.

CHAPTER 7

Modern Uses of Natural Plant and Fungi Psychedelics

If we are to progress, we must break away from our restrictive Western view of what functions and what doesn't when it comes to improving our individual and societal health. The apparently instinctive model of unbridled greed simply does not work and it *will* kill us unless we experience a global transcendence of our current level of consciousness — not necessarily spiritually but, certainly, socially and behaviourally[1]. This need to go beyond current attitudes to health, politics and the organisation of society is no longer a fringe point of view held by the bearded and beaded, but, in recent years, has rather become the talk of mainstream politics[2]. Our exponential destruction of the world's ecosystems, since the advent of agriculture, and particularly through industrialization in the last 150, is shooting us in our Nike Air clad feet, when what we really need to do is re-learn how to slip off our sandals and start feeling the earth between our toes again.

We know for certain that the sacramental use of psychedelic mushrooms has been going strong in the last 5,000 years of recorded human history and there is no reason to believe it hasn't played an equally central role in human life since the dawn of humans themselves. Indeed, if the graph is extrapolated backwards from 5,000 years ago, there is plenty of evidence to suggest sacrificial mushroom consumption was more, rather than less, widespread the further back one goes.

Wasson All the Fuss About?

Perhaps an even more influential event than Huxley's 1953 excursion into his 'archipelagos of the mind' on mescaline is Gordon Wasson's 1957 excursion to Mexico in search of the psilocybin mushroom. Wasson's trip, which subsequently piqued Timothy Leary's interest in mushrooms, truly deserves a large part of the credit for kick-starting the massive cultural changes of the 1960s.

The American Robert Gordon Wasson was, believe it or not, yet another character from psychedelic history with a wide range of esoteric interests. And, like many others in the field, once the subject of psychedelic drugs seduced him they changed the direction of his life thereafter. He was initially a banker, the vice president of J. P. Morgan & Co., no less, who developed a sideline interest in mushrooms through his Russian wife, who was, incidentally, a child psychiatrist.

In 1955 the pair travelled to Mexico to carry out field research on the cultural use of fungi and discovered the locals using what Wasson referred to as 'magic mushrooms' (*Psilocybe mexicana*) as part of their spiritual practice (not to be confused with *P. semilanceata*). Wasson became the first known Western outsider to participate in a psilocybin mushroom ceremony when he was given the sacrament by the Mazatec *curandera* (local shaman) Maria Sabina[3]. When Wasson returned to the USA and published his results for *Life* magazine in 1957, along with pictures taken by the photographer Allan Richardson, the event became the first wide-scale mention of psychedelic drugs to occur in contemporary Western consciousness and it led to a wide interest in the subject[4]. Wasson went on to collect many other specimens of different mushrooms and plants such as *Salvia divinorum*. It was his specimens that Albert Hofmann used to first identify and synthesize the active psychedelic compound psilocybin. In Wasson's wake many others besides Timothy Leary followed his path to Mexico, and, by 1967, when the psychedelic revolution in the West was in full swing, Maria Sabina had reluctantly become something of a local celebratory. Visitors included Bob Dylan and Mick Jagger, travelling to meet Sabina and pay their respects. Albert Hofmann also visited Maria Sabina and gave her some of the newly developed Sandoz psilocybin pills to see what she thought of the synthetic alternative. She admitted that the little yellow pills did indeed appear to contain some of the spirit of the mushroom. But Sabina later came to regret allowing herself to be thrust into the limelight, saying that the foreign visitors, coming in their droves, had ruined the power of her holy sacrament.

Wasson's continued interest in the subject led to him making claims that mushroom cults were widespread throughout all parts of the world and that the *Amanita muscaria* (fly agaric) mushroom was the source of the mysterious Vedic soma — a belief that has been supported by many in the psychedelic community until very recently, though there are now some notable challenges to his ideas.

Mazatec Magic Mushroom Morning Mayhem

There is reliable archaeological evidence that the indigenous people of South and Central America have used psilocybin mushrooms for thousands of years. Mushroom shaped statues and paintings have been discovered in ancient tombs, which supports the view that the use of the mushroom for religious purposes is older than the Spanish conquistadors that tried so hard to eradicate it.

In Guatemala, mushroom-shaped stones have been discovered, which point towards a sacramental use by the ancient Mayans. As I student I travelled with two friends to Guatemala and, after sneaking past the nonchalant pot-smoking guards, we spent the night on the top of the tallest temple of Tikal after everyone else had left. At dawn we had the place to ourselves, looking down from our position above the canopy of the trees. We marvelled as the sky lit up the jungle and surrounded us with coloured birds — only to have our solitude destroyed by a busload of tourists shipped in like a colonial invasion, hoping to be the first people on the temple to enjoy the daybreak after having had a nice night's sleep in their hotels. What they thought when they climbed the steps to find three straggly hippies already there sitting strumming their guitars I do not know.

Psychedelic mushrooms are ubiquitous throughout Central and South America, and were well known to the Aztecs at the time of the Spanish offensive. The ancient pagan practices were viewed as deeply blasphemous and well worth eradicating by the wise and knowledgeable Christians, who did not share the Aztec's enthusiasm for a fungal based approach to altered states of consciousness as a channel to communicate with the divine.

In 1656, Dr. Francisco Hernandez had this to say of the hallucinogenic mushrooms: *'When eaten they cause a madness of which the symptom is uncontrollable laughter and all kinds of visions, such as wars and demons'*. This grated with the European version of spirituality, in which the orthodox Christian approach to religion does not allow for followers to actually, *experience* God first hand. Rather, that privilege is only for the priests, whose job it is to then transmit the message to the flock. In stark contrast, in the shamanic use of communal psychedelic ceremonies, the whole group of worshippers take part in the ritual and directly experience their gods.

Despite the efforts of the conquistadors, the practice of mushroom ceremonies was not eradicated entirely. Rather it was pushed into secrecy, surviving only in the most remote mountainous parts of the continent. Over time, in certain places Christian beliefs were embraced, adopted and incorporated into the mushroom ceremonies until we begin to see a peculiar crossover between pagan religion and Christianity. And where the practice of spiritual Mexican mushroom use persists today, we still see this hybrid Christian-pagan ceremony. Some of the cults today believe their mushrooms were a gift from the Christian God, and that the mushrooms grew from the earth in the spots where Christ's tears fell as he hung on the cross:

> We wait for our father, we wait for our Father,
> We wait for Christ.
> With calmness, with care,
> Man of breast milk, man of dew, Fresh man, tender man,
> And there I give account, the mushroom says,
> Face to face, before Your glory, the mushroom says,
> Yes, Jesus Christ says, there I have an answer[5].

Over Fields we go, Laughing all the Way . . .

We will now travel, astrally, from the steamy rainforests of Central America to the frozen wastes of Siberia. During the winter solstice, here we find a fascinating seasonal character, dressed in red with white plumage, a magical being with the power to fly. No, it's not Santa, it's the *Amanita muscaria* mushroom. Or are they in fact the same thing?

The role of the *Amanita muscaria* mushroom — or 'fly agaric', so called for its capacity to attract flies (it is used as a bait/insecticide in many countries) — has become the classic symbol of psychedelia, folklore and fantasy alike. It is the fat, bright red, spotted white toadstool that appears in children's stories. It also has psychedelic qualities as a result of the active components muscimol and ibotenic acid, which can cause nausea, drowsiness and low blood pressure as a result of its cholinergic effects. Despite its vivid 'warning' colour, the toxicity, as well as the psychedelic effects of amanita, are not too much to write home about. Certainly, though it can cause harm if not used correctly (as can staplers and chilli peppers), reported fatalities are rare indeed. Drying or boiling the mushroom can reduce the toxicity, as can drinking the urine of someone who has eaten it, in comparison to eating the raw mushroom.

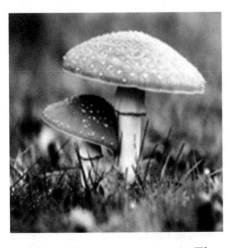

Picture 50: *Amanita muscaria* (Fly Agaric) mushrooms. The prototypical image of magical psychedelic fungus.

Use of *A. muscaria* for spiritual purposes is well known throughout northern Europe, and noted by many scholars, particularly James Arthur, whose book *Mushrooms and Mankind: The Impact of Mushrooms on Human Consciousness and Religion*, is well worth a read[6]. Siberia is particularly famed for its use of *A. muscaria*. There is a rich shamanistic tradition attached to the use of the mushroom, which still endures today. The Siberian shamans go out in search of their deity dressed in red and white to pay homage to their hunted prize, filling their sacks with the fruits when they find them growing at the base of pine, spruce, fir, birch and cedar trees. Siberian shamans believe these trees point upwards into the heavens, towards the Pole Star, and that eating the flesh of the *Amanita muscaria* mushroom is equivalent to climbing the trees to their summit and reaching the sky gods beyond the stars.

Reindeers feature heavily in the lives of these Siberians, which further ties in with the Santa analogies. The reindeer themselves also enjoy spontaneously searching for and eating the spotted mushroom, drinking each other's or even the human urine of those who have consumed the fruit[7]. Muscimol, the more psychoactive and also the safest of the two active ingredients, is excreted virtually unchanged in the urine and so effective is it at attracting reindeer that Siberian tribesmen will sometimes bottle post-mushroom human or reindeer urine and use it to attract back those beasts that have strayed from the vicinity.

Flying through the sky in a chariot pulled by reindeers, dressed in red, following a star that sits on top of an evergreen tree. It seems that when Coca Cola 'invented' Christmas in their 20th century advertising campaign, they knew more than a little about the shamans of Siberia.

Objections to the Mushroom Cult

R. Gordon Wasson made much of the Siberian mushroom stories, as well as believing the *Amanita muscaria* mushroom was the legendary *soma* of the pre-Hindu texts. He described a worldwide ancient mushroom cult and his ideas gained great popularity in the 1960s. But, more recently, scholars have begun to come up with opposing views. Certainly, in terms of *A. muscaria* being the mythical product *soma*, it seems an unlikely candidate simply because it is not strong enough as a psychedelic drug to produce the kind of mental states described in the *Rig Vedas* — unless (and this is quite possible, of course) those ancient Aryans knew of some tremendous purification techniques which have since been lost in the midst of time.

The British academic Andy Letcher goes a step further, challenging the view (longheld, since the sixties) about the widespread use of magic mushrooms in the United Kingdom. The sixties gave birth to a myriad of stories about pixies, druids and pagans from these isles, including many theories about the role mushrooms played in the building of and worshipping at Stonehenge and other ancient monuments. Despite the wishful thinking of many people, Dr. Letcher argues very persuasively in his book *Shroom* that there is no evidence — either archeologically or, more importantly, *culturally* — to support the idea that magic mushrooms played any part whatsoever in British history until very recently[8]. Even as recently as Victorian times, the mention of liberty caps was rare, with most mushrooms being understood simply as either edible or poisonous. Some conspiracy theorists would argue that this is because of the Christian anti-psychedelic propaganda of the Middle Ages and beyond, to effectively erase such data from the collective knowledge. But, as Letcher says, this has not been the case in South America, where, despite the extreme efforts of the conquistadors, the mushroom cults survived and continued. Letcher's argument about the informal cultural recording of such information is strong. We British are fantastic at preserving our cultural heritage through folk songs and stories, even in the face of powerful political or dogmatic religious forces that try and oppress such traditions. Yet there is no mention of magic mushrooms anywhere in a rich back catalogue of folk songs, drama and art from this country. Nothing, not a single psychedelic sausage. Shakespeare doesn't touch on it and nor does anyone else. Personally, I am inclined to share Letcher's opinion that this cultural omission from British history would be unfeasible if mushrooms were out there and people were indeed taking them.

On the other hand, (and I put this to Letcher when I invited him to talk at the *Breaking Convention* conference in 2011), how on earth did so many generations of Welsh hill walkers possibly miss the liberty cap mushrooms? It is impossible to walk more than 20 feet across the countryside in October and November without crushing them underfoot. Dr. Letcher wonders whether in fact the liberty cap mushroom is a relatively recent addition to our natural habitat, relying, as they do, on a particular climate and lots of rich grass-land that has only been available in abundance since the 17th century tradition of large scale deforestation, both for the practice of farming and in order to build fleets of wooden ships to defeat Spanish armadas[9].

Whenever the mushrooms arrived in Britain, what is certain is that since the sixties it has been very difficult to convince the psychedelic community of any point of view other than one that assumes the whole world revolves around psychedelic drugs.

The Long-standing Use of Peyote Cacti

We now look back across to the other side of the world to meet a small green cactus about which there is no dispute regarding the role it has played in the cultural development of southern Texas and Mexico. The peyote cactus is a slow-growing, spineless green button that peppers the desert scrub. Archaeological finds of the cactus, at least 5,000 years old, have confirmed that the native people of America — particularly the Huichol of Mexico — have used this plant as a tool for spiritual worship just as long as any other recorded psychedelic on the planet — despite its incredibly bitter taste![10]

The cactus' active component, mescaline, produces a long-lasting and intensely sustained psychedelic experience accompanied by rich visual phenomena that encourage spiritual searching. It provides a deep connectivity to the Earth for those that use it as part of their ceremonial worship, and it is a powerful unifying force for the community. Not only does it cause no demonstrable problems for the community, but recent evidence demonstrates that those tribes that use peyote have better general mental health than those that do not use the cactus. In particular, peyote-using tribes have reduced rates of alcohol dependency, which fits with our knowledge about the important role to be played by psychedelics as psychopharmacological tools to combat addictions. No doubt the anti-alcohol effect is partly attributable to the intense cohesive effect of the traditional cactus-taking ceremonies, which help the native users to resist the tide of Western trappings, of which alcohol is one of the more destructive elements[11].

As in South and Central America's traditional pagan use of the psilocybin mushrooms, peyote ceremonies have also now developed to incorporate aspects of Christian tradition alongside the ancient beliefs. This is exemplified by this quote from Quanah Parker: 'The white man goes into his church and talks about Jesus. The Indian goes into his tepee and talks *with* Jesus.'[12]

Parker, born in 1852, was an important figure in the history of the Native American people as he was arguably the most successful at demonstrating an ability to adapt to the changing face of white persecution. For many Native Americans, this means he sold out, but, nevertheless, he remains respected by both sides. Parker was a firm believer in the traditional use of peyote after it was used to heal his wounds when a bull gored him. He was a founder of the Native American Church, which combined Christian and ancient religious elements and kept peyote at the centre of the worship. While mescaline is a Schedule-One controlled substance in the USA and elsewhere, even today Native American members of the church can legally use peyote as part of their practice.

Ibogaine: Nature's Anti-addiction Plant

In the West African countries of the Democratic Republic of Congo and Gabon, many people follow the Bwiti spiritual practice. It is a form of

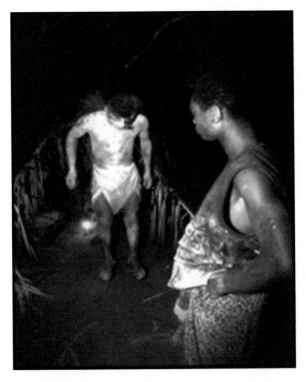

Picture 51: The West African use of ibogaine produces a trance state in which users meet with their spiritual ancestors.

religion in which the root bark of the *Tabernanthe iboga* plant is consumed for spiritual purposes[13]. The plant contains the drug ibogaine, which produces an intense psychedelic high with an accompanying strong dissociative effect, so users typically report visual hallucinations as well as out of body experiences. This mixed bag of psychoactive effects arises from the complex psychopharmacological profile of ibogaine.

The drug behaves as a partial 5-HT2A agonist — as does LSD, DMT and psilocybin — which explains its classical psychedelic effects. But it also acts to some extent as an NMDA-antagonist (like ketamine) and a kappa-opioid agonist (like *Salvia divinorum*), which explains its dissociative effects. The Bwiti incorporates the subsequent extremely dreamlike qualities of the experience into their functional use of the plant.

Used as part of a community ceremony led by an *N'ganga,* who occupies a shamanistic role of priest and respected village elder, the ceremonies have an ostensibly healing purpose in which individuals may seek to communicate with the dead, ask questions of the spirits of ancestors or seek the answers to meaningful personal questions about their health or future. The root bark is chewed or eaten in large quantities and the experience happens at night, accompanied by elaborate and colourful rituals of drumming, designed to enhance the altered state of consciousness. Many users also experience vomiting and nausea.

The Bwiti use the ibogaine ceremonies as an important rite of passage and it is a hugely significant moment when young men take the plant for the first time. As with other non-Western psychedelic shamanistic ceremonies, in many Bwiti tribes there is a mixture of Christian and more archaic spiritual practice woven into the ceremony.

What makes ibogaine stand out as a therapeutic tool, one that has attracted the attention of the West, is its capacity for treating addictions. It is uncertain how long the West Africans have been using ibogaine as a sacramental tool for their religious purposes, but the anti-addiction qualities have been known to the Western world for around 150 years. The drug appears to be effective at not only relieving the subjective unpleasant effects of withdrawal from dependent drugs such as alcohol and opiates, but also for producing a reduction in the long-term craving and reducing habitual, repetitive and obsessional behaviours that often accompany substance dependence. There is good anecdotal and epidemiological evidence for this, supported by the low rates of alcohol dependence by the Bwiti tribe people. Formal clinical trials are underway and will be described in the next chapter. For a vivid and personal account of ibogaine therapy used to treat a person with opiate dependence, see the work of film maker David Graham Scott[14,15].

Using ibogaine has been of tremendous importance in improving and sustaining community cohesion for the Bwiti. Its use has been credited as having helped Gabon and the Democratic Republic of Congo resist external Western influences such as widespread drug and alcohol use and consumerism. This has got to be a good thing, if only we in the West could recognise it.

The Eerie Effects of the Diviner's Sage: *Salvia Divinorum*

Those who know *Salvia divinorum* always refer to it in the female form, so I shall pay the plant the same respect. She grows in the forests of Oaxaca, Mexico, where she has been used for thousands of years by the Mazatec people as a tool for spiritual worship; and still is today[16].

She exerts her effects via the compound Salvinorin A, a potent kappa-opioid agonist, that, like ibogaine, causes dissociative states of altered consciousness. She is very low in physiological toxicity and very high amounts can be consumed. In her native country of use, she is almost always eaten or drunk, either by making a tea from the crushed and infused leaves (about 50 are required) or chewed in great rolled up bundles of leaves like a massive green cigar such that the psychoactive effects come on slowly and build insidiously over time. But when consumed in the West (bought most often by teenage hedonists on the internet), kids usually choose to smoke a purified extract of the plant through a bong, which produces an immediate and intense high.

Salvia is held in high esteem by the Mazatec shamans, who believe she is an incarnation of the Virgin Mary (more of that ubiquitous Christian influence creeping in here). The psychoactive effect is often trance-like. Some describe it as eerie or spooky, with peculiar visual distortions. She is used in order to produce a visionary state which may be useful for healing of specific ailments or as a tool to help the user gain a greater insight into whatever personal questions they choose to ask her when they start on their journey to the realms of insight opened up by consuming the plant.

A particularly well-known effect is the graceful afterglow that users experience after the more intense psychedelic effects have worn off, which has led some researchers to postulate whether salvia might have uses as an antidepressant — a clinical application that has also been explored for the dissociative psychedelic ketamine. More about this in coming chapters.

The Sacred Vine: Ayahuasca

Interest in this mysterious South American brew, which is found throughout the Amazonian basin in Columbia, Peru and Brazil, has grown exponentially, like a jungle vine, in recent years. The use of it now represents a major subject of research for university departments throughout the world. Ayahuasca studies encompass elements from chemistry, shamanism, sociology and ecology, medicine and legal issues. At our *Breaking Convention* psychedelic research conference in 2011, we dedicated an entire day's parallel track presentations to the subject, knowing how popular the subject had become. All the talks on ayahuasca were packed to the rafters, with delegates spilling out of the rooms and sitting in the corridors, such was the demand to learn more about this vine.

Interest in ayahuasca continues to grow, with publications on the subject weaving like vines through the academic and popular press. In recent years, there has been a significant industry of tourism to these countries for those soul-searching psychonauts inclined to taste its glories in its natural habitat. There are passionate opinions on both sides of the debate about whether such drug tourism is a good or bad thing. Many notable Hollywood celebrities have trekked to the jungles of South America (accompanied, no doubt, by large crews of bearers to carry their Louis Vuitton bags) and returned to tweet their experiences to the masses. Indeed, 'Ayahuascaphilia' has now reached such a jungle fever peak that there is something of a split occurring within the psychedelic community — much like the one that occurred when LSD entered the popular scene in the mid-1960s. Back then the question on the lips of anyone who was anyone was Are You Experienced or Not? There are those who have taken ayahuasca and rave about it, like born-again enlightenment bunnies, and those who (because they have not yet had the experience) don't. The issue is becoming somewhat divisive. Then when

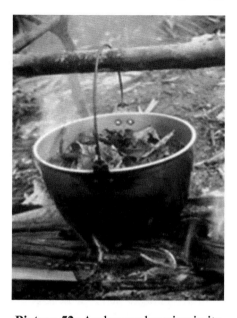

Picture 52: Ayahuasca brewing in its natural habitat. A specified mixture of MAOI and DMT containing plants; combined in a recipe handed-down to the curanderos by the plant spirits themselves.

one throws in the growing negative mainstream media reports — which must only be taken with a hefty pinch of shamanic snuff — about spiritually-absent drug tourists steam-rolling into the Amazon and leaving their physical and psychological litter behind, whilst unscrupulous pseudo-shamans take liberties with, at best your girlfriend and your money or, at worst, your life, we have ourselves a heady mix of controversy.

These conflicts are not new to psychedelia, of course. In the sixties stories abound about how "if only all the world leaders could just take LSD, there would be no more wars" For the 90s substitute 'Ecstasy' and for the early decades of the 21st century we can now say 'Ayahuasca'. There has always been a vying for spiritual authenticity when it comes to mass psychedelic use; one guru is kosher and another is a fraud. And there will always be the 'early pioneers' who so keenly pronounce that *their acid* back then was better than it is now and how *their trip* to San Francisco / the Amazon / Esalen / India was the *real deal*; whilst lamenting how sad they feel to see so many people flocking there now. Let's not forget that when it comes to being the first to trample through Amazonian jungles, whose magic is defined by their isolation from Western influence, such trail blazers are, by that very definition, also culture crushers.

One must not judge too harshly the rights or wrongs of global ayahuasca experiences and the growing commercialization that is emerging. One man's Western exploitation is another man's livelihood, after all. What is clear, however, is that safety and, something I feel passionately about, giving psychedelic users a good name, is paramount to the wider issue of how these chemicals and plants are going to be assimilated into the generations of the future. There is much good in ayahuasca and its potential for healing — both societal and clinical.

But What is It All About?

Ayahuasca (which means variously 'vine of the soul' or 'vine of the spirit') is the name for a psychedelic brew made from several key ingredients, the main constituents being at least one plant containing DMT and at least one plant containing the essential monoamine oxidase inhibitors (MAOI) required to allow the DMT to become psychoactive when consumed orally[17].

Usually the MAOI plant is that of the *Banisteriopsis caapi* vine, which contains, among other chemicals, harmine and harmaline. The DMT commonly comes from the *Psychotria viridis* (or chacruna) plant, although a number of alternative plant sources of DMT may be used, including *Diplopterys cabrerana* (or chaliponga).

Traditionally, the plants are chopped and ground, then boiled together by a shaman with intimate knowledge of the local jungle flora. Icaros are sung by the people processing the plants, and over the boiling mixture. There is wide variation in the exact ingredients. The leaves, flowers and bark of many other plants may be added to the brew, each with their own idiosyncratic and purposeful intent to provide particular effects. Contemporary scientists marvel at how the traditional shaman could have possibly known which of the many thousands of species of plants combine to produce the specific desired effects of the brew. The shamans say the spirits themselves told them how to make the brew. It seems there are many such revelations arising from traditional cultures that could teach us in the West a lot, if only we could open our eyes to the fact that just because it does not come from 'big pharma' doesn't mean it isn't important.

The Ayahuasca Ceremony

Ayahuasca is traditionally taken as part of a religious ceremony. The rite is led by the shaman, who sings songs periodically to enhance and guide the travellers on their inner journeys during which the consumer will engage with aspects of their personal, collective and communal spiritual awareness and pass through different dimensions of a spiritual reality. The intensity of the psychedelic experience is described by many as 'simply colossal', something that is no doubt influenced by the set and setting engendered by a necessary visit to a strange foreign country and a trek through the rainforest to where it takes place.

Ceremonies often involve several separate sittings, in which the drug is taken over the course of many days, and they also incorporate many non-drug rituals as part of the process. There is a strong element of purging — both mentally and physically — and users routinely spend many hours vomiting or passing diarrhoea in the early stages of the intoxication with the drug, all of which contributes to the overall intensity of the experience.

Participants will frequently encounter entities (a phenomenon also seen when DMT is smoked or injected), often in the form of jungle animals representing spiritual ancestors, who provide messages and instructions for the journeyer.

Ayahuasca Through the Ages

Ayahuasca was first brought to the attention of the Western world in the 1950s by the explorer and botanist Richard Evan Shultes, who is also credited as being the father of modern ethnobotany for his adventures with psychedelic plants and fungi amongst indigenous populations of the world.

The traditional practice of ayahuasca ceremonies amongst Amazonians has most likely been taking place for thousands of years. It was certainly known to the conquistadors of the 16th century who, just as they did with the mushroom ceremonies, dismissed and tried to eradicate the practice of ayahuasca use, believing the excited psychedelic states induced by the brew were akin to fornicating with the devil. Such was the skewed wisdom of those culturally-pure Catholic liberators of old.

William S. Burroughs famously travelled to South America in the 1950s in search of the plant, immortalised in *The Yage Letters*[18]. Similarly, it was the search for the magical properties of the sacred vine that set Terence McKenna on his pathway to psychedelic notoriety in the mid-1970s when he tracked through the jungle with his brother Dennis, resulting in his book *True Hallucinations*[19]. Dennis also describes those jungle moments in his own more recent book, *Brotherhood of the Screaming Abyss: My Life with Terence McKenna*[20]. Those South American experiences with ayahuasca and psilocybin mushrooms led Terence to discover his 'novelty theory', which holds that many connected strands of the

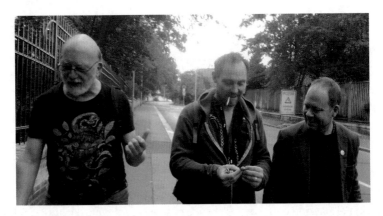

Picture 53: Walking in, early morning, to present our lectures at the Beyond Psychedelics conference, Prague, September 2016. I shared a house with Dave Luke, Robin-Carhart-Harris, Rick Doblin and Dennis McKenna. Plus, a spare room for the entities.

universe converge together towards an epoch 'eventually reaching a singularity of infinite complexity on the winter solstice in 2012, at which point anything and everything imaginable will occur simultaneously'.

When the first edition of the *Psychedelic Renaissance* was published in early 2012, it remained to be seen whether McKenna was right, and humanity and the multiverse were going to melt into a vortex of psychedelic apocalypse on 21ˢᵗ December 2012. But, here we are in 2017 and, as far as I can tell, that hasn't happened yet. Some (of the more hardcore believers) in the psychedelic community might still maintain that McKenna was correct, and that some vitally important event did indeed happen that day, about which we are yet to experience the manifestation of its meaning. Whatever.

Ayahuasca in Modern Times

As described earlier, many Westerners have well and truly latched on to the idea that ayahuasca represents yet another vital mind-tool worthy of exploring, and are now flocking into the Amazon basin, such is the righteous boredom with our modern TV living. But the growth of interest in ayahuasca has also blossomed amongst indigenous people in the Amazonian regions. And as with the Native American church's claim to use peyote in their ceremonies as an example of the right for religious freedom, several ayahuasca-using churches have emerged.

The Brazilian Santo Daime church was founded in the 1930s in the Amazonian state of Acre by Raimundo Irineu Serra. Serra first drank ayahuasca (or Daime) in the 1920s when he was working in the forest as a rubber tapper. He began conducting ceremonies for local people; using sung hymns alongside the ayahuasca medicine to provide a healing ceremony for sick people who could not otherwise access other medical treatments. The traditional Santo Daime ceremony — just like that of the contemporary Mazatec mushroom ceremonies — uses elements of Christianity, alongside more pagan imagery worshipping the natural elements and environment. The Santo Daime church has undergone several changes in the last 80 years, with different factions emerging and continuing alongside the original version.

Another religious organisation centred around the use of ayahuasca is the União do Vegetal (UDV), which translates as 'union of the plants'. Founded in Brazil in 1961 by José Gabriel da Costa, it has since spread throughout the world with around 20,000 members. Both the Santo Daime church and UDV have been subject to legal battles with authorities over their entitlement to use ayahuasca legally as part of their religious practice. In 2006 the UDV, quite rightly, gained approval from the US courts to practice their religious use of ayahuasca, under the Religious Freedom Restoration Act. Both the UDV and the Santo Daime church continue to fight legal battles throughout the world regarding the legal status of ayahuasca, which has become an interesting subject of its own.

In the last ten years, numerous organisations and individuals have sprung up, not affiliated with either Santo Daime church or the UDV, providing ayahuasca experiences for people on every continent on the planet. And the global network of ayahuasca interest now has a fine home in the World Ayahuasca Conference, which met in 2014 in Ibiza and Brazil in 2016. Organised by the ICEERS Foundation, these gatherings have provided the ayahuasca research and experiential community with a wonderful opportunity for multidisciplinary exploration of their work. Some exciting clinical projects with ayahuasca will be discussed later in the book.

DMT itself, in its pure form, is universally classified as a Class A and Schedule One substance. But, like the debate that continues to rage about psilocybin mushrooms, there remains considerable lack of clarity about whether plants that contain DMT are themselves illegal. After all, if they are that makes the waterways of the UK hotbeds of illegal drug cultivation, as Reed Canary Grass and the gardeners' favourite Ribbon Grass both contain high concentrations of DMT, as do the brains of many mammals (including humans). In short, the concept that vessels that contain DMT can be outlawed is surreally self-defeating. Nevertheless, the law generally stands that, as with mushrooms, as soon as one makes efforts to prepare the DMT-containing plants in some way — for example, by drying or boiling them — one is seen to be heading towards an interest in DMT, and one gets busted.

In 2011 in the UK, we had a sad situation in which a modern-day shaman from the west of England, Peter Aziz, was jailed for possessing and supplying DMT. He was offering ayahuasca to his clients as part of his well-established 35-year practice and got caught foul of the law when importing plant products from South America. Inevitably, the authorities (and the media) took issue with his atypical (meaning non industry-sanctioned) approach to pharmacology. Many others, myself included, wrote in his support at the time, but to no avail[21]. His legal defence was that of religious freedom, but this rarely satisfies the judge. It seems Christianity's cultural devouring of all in its path is not a phenomenon confined only to the 16th century.

Name and Shaman

In recent years, there has been an alarming increase in reports of unscrupulous pseudo-shamans, whose practices are unsound, unethical and unsafe. Some high-profile deaths have occurred and there are many stories of sexual assaults occurring in the context of ayahuasca ceremonies, around which participants are, by the very nature of the experience, at times highly vulnerable. The worldwide ayahuasca communities are, in my opinion, working hard to organise themselves into a network of support to tackle these problems. It is essential that they do this if the practice, which, as I said earlier could be an important force for good in the world, is to be recognised predominantly for its merits rather than its pitfalls. All psychedelic drugs are powerful, but ayahuasca particularly so — especially when it is delivered in far-off places with little opportunity for visitors to seek redress or access support. Basic checks and measures, such as appropriate psychological and physical screening to identify vulnerable users, and greater safeguards (given the disposition of some shamans — who, like any other group, are wide ranging in their personal ethics), must be established.

The Weed: The Risks, Benefits, Culture and (brief) Chemistry of Cannabis

Let us now move away from ayahuasca and on to another popular substance: cannabis. This subject is vast and mostly beyond the scope of this book. It encompasses so many strands of human developmental culture, from science and sociology to botany, law and medicine, that I will not begin to try and cover it all here. There are many other books I could recommend for the interested reader; going back as far as the mid-19th century for *The Hasheesh Eater,* some extremely psychedelic writing from Fitz Hugh Ludlow[22], countless books from the 1960s and 1970s and a detailed and sensitive revisiting in the early 1990s by Harvard's Lester Grinspoon and James Bakalar[23]. Another excellent contemporary tome about the green stuff is Julie Holland's *Pot*[24]. Holland is a learned and wise researcher of all things psychedelic, but particularly cannabis and MDMA (she also edited a great book called *Ecstasy: The Complete Guide* a few years ago)[25]. And there are even books about what a prohibition-free future in which cannabis is legally available through a regulated market in the UK might look like[26]. One can easily lose oneself in the smoky vapours of cannabis writings. Perhaps one ought to.

But is cannabis a psychedelic drug? My answer, of course, is yes. Used at low doses the psychedelic high is slighter than drugs like LSD or DMT, obviously, but at high doses — as one tends to see with the many hydroponic strains of cannabis that most people in the West now smoke — the effects can be extremely strong, bordering on the same sense of altered state intensity induced by the classical psychedelics.

Cannabis' link with humanity is an old as the hills. Queen Victoria was a big fan. She used the drug throughout her life to treat everything from labour pains to anxiety and epilepsy. Our knowledge of the medicinal uses for cannabis continues to grow every year. With the tremendous revolution in medicinal cannabis research in the United States in the last fifteen years — with accompanied promising

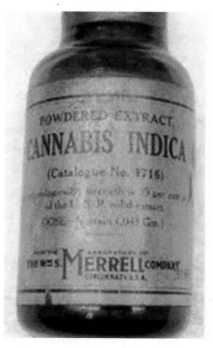

Picture 54: Let's not forget that the Western world's demonization of cannabis is a relatively recent phenomenon. For thousands of years up until the early 20th century it was globally recognised as a valuable medicine.

shifts in prohibition — the drug is increasingly carving a place in the pharmacopeia of modern clinical practice[27]. As with research on compounds like LSD and MDMA, research into cannabis has been difficult up until now because of restrictions on its use by doctors and scientists. Much of the research on its potential use in psychiatry revolves around the different constitutional chemicals found in the cannabis plant. There are many hundreds of active components in cannabis but two stand out as important. The first is delta-9 tetrahydrocannabinol, or THC, and the second is cannabidiol, or CBD. THC is generally considered to be the principal chemical that produces the psychoactive, more psychedelic, alerting and trippy effect of the high; and the CBD is the chemical that produces the more relaxed, bodily dreamy effect. Furthermore, whilst THC is illegal (in most places), CBD is legally available (in most places).

In the field of psychiatry, THC is generally thought to be a psychotogenic drug; that is, it can induce psychosis in people who have a genetic predisposition to the condition and it ought to be avoided by those people with schizophrenia. I can say this with relative authority as I, like all psychiatrists, have seen my schizophrenic patients coming back into hospital as a direct result of relapse secondary to heavy cannabis use. This does not mean that I believe cannabis will *cause* schizophrenia in people who don't have that genetic predisposition — if that were the case then we would see a great many more cases of schizophrenia than we do! After all, at least 10% of the population smokes the drug regularly and rates of enduring psychosis (schizophrenia) have remained relatively stable at around 1% all over the world since records began.

So, cannabis does not *cause* the condition to arise *de novo*, but it can certainly trigger an episode in those who already have it. In such cases, the most likely cause of the psychotic effects is the THC content of the plant. The cannabidiol on the other hand is another story. There is a general acceptance that CBD may have an antipsychotic effect[28]. Its presence in the natural form of cannabis (not the hydroponically grown and selectively bred strains of skunk weed, which are abnormally high in THC and low in CBD, but the pure 'grass', as grows in the ground of those countries where it is a native species) acts to balance the psychedelic effects of the THC and provide a calming effect. There are many researchers investigating whether CBD in its pure form can act as an anticonvulsant[29], an antidepressant[30] an antipsychotic[31] or an anxiolytic drug[32]. This is an area that deserves a great deal more research. In the meantime, as a psychiatrist, and this is what I tell my patients who have decided to continue to smoke, I would say avoid skunk and move on to unadulterated weed or low grade hashish, which would naturally have a higher CBD content, provide a more balanced smoke and have possible positive neuro-protective factors. But, as mentioned, if there is any personal or family history of psychosis it is best to avoid this drug altogether. Furthermore, in my experience clinically, most my patients with any degree of psychotic fragility usually do not need much reminding not to use cannabis; they readily state that weed scares the hell out of them at the best of times.

I am all-too-rapidly summarizing a vast amount of research and knowledge here, so do forgive me. Nevertheless, we shall briefly consider a few other aspects of cannabis in its context as a non-Western contemporary religious sacrament.

Indian Cannabis

Where does cannabis grow? The simply answer to this is that cannabis grows just about anywhere on the planet. It is one of the hardiest plants we know, which is why in the form of hemp it makes such good rope — and canvas, of course — from which the name derives. But cannabis is strongest, from a psychoactive point of view, in the hottest climates. It thrives throughout Asia: Thailand, Cambodia, India, Afghanistan, Pakistan, Nepal, Tibet, Mongolia, China, and so forth. It is also particularly strong in Africa, especially Malawi, where I went for my medical elective, just before graduating from med school in 1997, spending six weeks delivering babies in an isolated rural and badly resourced obstetric hospital. But that's another story.

It is well known that the ancient Chinese shamans used cannabis as a vehicle to communicate with the other worlds, and its use by the Greek, Roman and Norse societies is also well documented. But it was particularly central to the development of the Indian culture. The 4,000-year-old Vedas describe the Hindus use of cannabis very clearly, unlike their vaguer descriptions of the sacramental substance *soma*, which may have been a variety of different compounds — including cannabis. Cannabis was clearly a 'food of the gods' and was also venerated by the early Sikhs as a powerful ally in battle. Like the Chinese, who documented the

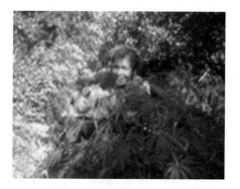

Picture 55: The author sitting inside a wild cannabis bush playing the guitar in Nepal in 1990.

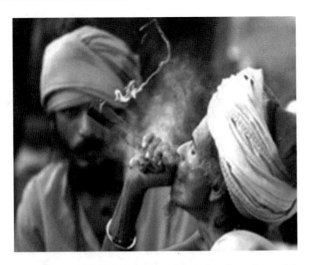

Picture 56: Hindu tradition describes how the churning of the oceans created the elixir of life, which Shiva then purified with cannabis, which he created from his own body. Sounds like a positive endorsement to me.

medicinal properties of the plant meticulously, cannabis has always played its part both as a healer of the sick in this world and as a sacramental substance for religious purposes.

Cannabis is at the heart of Vedic India[33]. Modern Hindu holy people, *sadhus*, still take their cannabis traditionally in the form of *charas* — a handmade resin, sometimes mixed with datura leaves, which they smoke in a tall clay pipe called a chillum. Their presence all over India is abundant. Millions of people chose this lifestyle (including people from professional business backgrounds), that of a solitary wandering monk without possessions or home, on the final leg of the Hindu journey towards *moksha* (liberation). One cannot turn a corner in India without seeing one of these old men (and sometimes women) adorned usually in rags, their skin smeared in white ash, contorted in impossible yoga poses and smoking a tall chillum. Smoking cannabis is a sign of devotion to Shiva for these Hindu holy people as they wander barefoot through their magnificent country from one holy site to another on their final pilgrimage (they get free travel on buses and trains), which ends at the banks of the Ganges in Varanasi. Their final opportunity to break the chain of reincarnation, if they haven't achieved *moksha* through their lifetime of devotion, is to be burned in a funeral pyre and floated down the river. India is truly a country out of this world. I can highly recommend a long visit with no set date or ticket for return, as I did for seven months as a young man. I believe I may have left various parts of my consciousness there. One day I might return to find them.

East African and Jamaican Rastafarian Religion and Cannabis

The Rastafarian way of life arose in Jamaica in the 1930s, but has its roots in East Africa and particularly Ethiopia. The Jamaican political activist Marcus Garvey did much to propagate the cohesion of Jamaican fervour for collective organisation and is venerated by the Rastafarian religion, as is the late Emperor of Ethiopia, Haile Selassie I, whose previous name before becoming royalty, Ras Tafari, after which the movement was named[34].

The hair is traditionally worn long in dreadlocks, and smoking cannabis is a powerful way of demonstrating dedication to god, or *Jah*. Cannabis is central to the life of Rastafarians, who are found all over the world. Whilst I was in northern Kenya a Rastafarian funeral was taking place, in which hundreds of devotees followed the procession and gathered at the graveside to smoke copious amounts of cannabis before throwing an eternity's supply of joints and growing plants into the grave for their brother to use in the afterlife's appreciation of Jah.

Like other psychedelic drug ceremonies mentioned earlier, there is a mixture of Christianity and traditional African religions in the Rastafari religion. Parts of the Bible are quoted by Rastafarians to validate the spiritual acts of smoking cannabis:
Genesis: 3:18 'Thou shalt eat the herb of the field.' Proverbs: 15:17 'Better is a dinner of herb where love is, than a stalled ox and hatred therewith.'

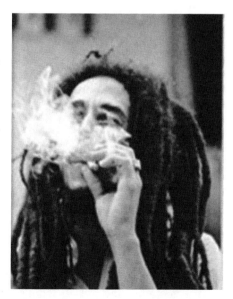

The Weed is Here to Stay

With whatever lens one chooses to look at the influence of cannabis through the years, there is no getting away from its universally abundant presence. It always has been, and probably always will be, the gateway drug of choice for generations of young people. This is not because it has some

Picture 57: It is fabulous that in 2015 after many decades of lobbying, those practicing the Rastafarian religion in Jamaica were finally granted permission to legally use the plant as part of their sacramental practice[35].

unique pharmacological trait that makes it lead on to harder things (as the politicians who wish to maintain its prohibition may tell us) but, rather, because it carries the mantle of being such a mild, safe and harmless prohibited substance, its very prohibition naturally makes questioning teenagers ask: *'What's so bad about this stuff? The government made out that if I smoked this I'd be out murdering my granny next week in order to sell her wedding ring for my next fix. What a load of rubbish! I've been lied to. Well, if they are lying to me about cannabis then they are probably lying about ecstasy and cocaine . . . and heroin . . . so I may as well try those too!'*

This prevalent reaction against current drug laws, which is well documented, is worrying indeed. If the laws are seen to be so unfit for purpose that they encourage young people to try harder drugs, then surely it is time to review them. There will be more commentary on the issue of the illegalisation of cannabis later in the book.

This is What I tell My Teenage Patients About Cannabis

By far the most dangerous aspect of weed is that it is illegal and to be caught with it can ruin your life. The next riskiest element is that it causes a degree of chilled relaxedness, or viewed another way demotivation and apathy — that is, after all, its *raison d'être* and why people take it. So forget trying to pass your exams if you're smoking a spliff on the way to school each day. Another important risk factor regarding cannabis is its potential to impair normal brain development in young people. Between the ages of around 12 years and 20 years old adolescents' brains undergo an important process of 'neuronal pruning', in which many of the myriad connections between neurons (called dendrites) that formed during earlier childhood are selectively 'cut back' until the brain is left in its most high-functioning adult state. This is a vital process for healthy adult mental health and intellectual functioning. There is reasonable evidence that heavy and persistent cannabis use between 12 years and 18 years old can impair this process of pruning; which has been shown to result in potentially life-long intellectual impairments[36]. However, some studies dispute the significance of long-term cognitive impairment from cannabis use[37]. Because of the potential risk I sometimes find myself telling my child or teenage patients that if they insist on being lifelong heavy cannabis smokers (something I would advise against; chronic daily use of any drug is bound to be destabilizing over time, not to mention boring), then I recommend they at the very least give up for a few years in their adolescence and wait until they are in their 20s before recommencing their use. They will then give themselves the best possible adult brain to later expose at their will.

So, cannabis is certainly not entirely without its risks — whatever the pro-cannabis lobby might tell you. But for most adults, moderate to low dose cannabis use is generally relatively harmless. Indeed, it is the smoking aspect of cannabis consumption that can be the most harmful for heavy users. Respiratory disease is bound to occur eventually if one frequently drags the smoke of burning plant material into the body's most sensitive and fragile tissue — the lungs. But this is the 21st century; there are now many excellent vapourisation options for cannabis consumption. Inhaling smoke is *sooo* last century, man. Pharmacology delivery methods have come a long way since the Middle Ages. Vape, man.

However, there are more serious risks for a small number of unfortunate people who use cannabis. For around 1% of people cannabis, like many other drugs, is a poison. That 1% is the same 1% that already have, or may be susceptible to developing, schizophrenia. For these people, it is best avoided. It is well recognized that cannabis use can trigger a psychotic episode in those unfortunate souls who carry the genetic and environmental risk factors for schizophrenia. The genetic risk factors are unavoidable; simply having a family member with a history of psychosis is all it takes. Environmental risk factors, such as stress induced by relationships, are multifarious and not at all specific to schizophrenia. Drug use is the most important of the non-genetic risk factors.

So, whilst cannabis is clearly a risk factor for acute psychoses in vulnerable people, (a phenomenon well-established in large systematic reviews)[38] does cannabis cause schizophrenia in people who don't have that pre-existing genetic vulnerability? As mentioned, it would seem not, or we would see especially high rates of schizophrenia amongst the Jamaicans in Jamaica, the Africans in Africa and the Asians in Asia — not to mention in the West — where cannabis is smoked copiously by large proportions of those populations. We do, incidentally, see increased rates of schizophrenia in black populations living in cities *in the UK* and other Western countries, but that is different, and due to the stress of social exclusion, poverty and frank racism — both from the wider community and from the medical profession who misconstrue their idiosyncratic and culturally-bound presentation as psychosis[39]. Hopefully, in future categorical manuals for psychiatric diagnoses we will include the category 'spiritual emergency', which will allow for certain people to behave in a fashion as befits their culture without having to pathologise them further. In the meantime, we remain restricted to the medical model, with all its shortcomings and gross prejudices.

Genetic vulnerability — in combination with environmental risk factors, including cannabis — remains the primary most likely cause of chronic schizophrenia[40]. Incidentally, some interesting findings from a recent study suggest that schizophrenia and increased use of cannabis may have a shared genetic aetiology; meaning people with a predisposition to use cannabis heavily also have an increased genetic risk of developing schizophrenia anyway[41].

She Who Controls The Spice...

In recent years, we have seen a worrying emergence of synthetic cannabinoids — called various names recreationally but generally lumped together under the term 'Spice'. These are drugs that are potent specific CB-1 and CB-2 agonists. Until the 2016 Psychoactive Substances Bill they could be bought legally in head shops or online and have rapidly become the scourge of healthcare, social and criminal justice services. Although they were initially sold as legal alternatives to cannabis, the effects of Spice are far different from weed. When Spice first entered the market its psychoactive properties were something of a mystery, because the herbs themselves were advertised as blends of benign plants such as Coastal Jack-bean, Blue Egyptian water lily, dwarf skullcap, lion's tail, lotus and honeyweed — all with little or no known psychoactivity. It then became apparent that these herbs were merely a vehicle for the sprayed-on potent synthetic cannabinoid chemicals.

There is a large range of synthetic cannabinoids. Some of the most popular forms of spice contain the naphthoylindoles JWH-018 and JWH-073, which act as a full agonist at both the CB-1 and CB-2 cannabinoid receptors. Like most research chemicals most of the new synthetic cannabinoids have not undergone any toxicity testing. And more arrived on the market every week to stay ahead of the legal restrictions.

The JWH novel cannabinoids were first synthesised by John William Huffman, professor emeritus of organic chemistry at Clemson University, South Carolina. Huffman himself, who says of the current misuse of Spice, "It bothers me that people are so stupid as to use this stuff", embarked on his research of synthetic cannabinoids to develop drugs to target multiple sclerosis and HIV/AIDS[42]. He therefore must not be blamed for any subsequent misuse of his discoveries; just as Shulgin and Nichols cannot be blamed for their role in developing so many new chemicals that have since been used irresponsibly by some people.

Spice in herbal form is added to a spliff or smoked in a pipe in the same way as traditional cannabis. The intoxication tends to be very extreme; with users describing high levels of paranoid psychosis, physical ailments including muscular pains, cramps, diarrhoea and — ironically, given that natural cannabis is an antiemetic — vomiting, which can then be associated with seizures. Spice is also highly addictive; with regular users rapidly progressing to daily use in large quantities to avoid frightening and painful physical withdrawal symptoms.

Significant numbers of psychiatric admissions are now associated with the use of Spice, with some researchers dubbing the condition "Spice-ophrenia"[43]. And the drug has also seen a proliferation in prisons, as the drug is currently not easily detected in bodily fluids using standardized drug testing kits, prompting Public Health England to publish an 'NPS Toolkit' in 2015 for staff to use when dealing with prisoners using Spice, among other NPSs[44]. In a potentially even more worrying recent development, users are now able to buy a liquid or powder form of CB-1 and CB-2 drugs, bypassing the herbal medium, which presents a whole new host of risks including injectable forms of Spice.

I am far from the sort of person to hold a restrictive or draconian view about drug use or dissemination; believing that for most drugs there exists a possibility of safe — even beneficial — use, that can be separated from examples of misuse. But I — and my colleagues in the field of addictions — am concerned about Spice. The therapeutic window between recreational and addictive use is narrow and Spice appears to becomes problematic very quickly for most habitual users. Nevertheless, this does not mean that I believe a blanket banning of the substance is the answer. Spice is arguably the main target in the sites of the new Psychoactive Substances Act, which, as I have already stated, will not work to reduce the usage or harms of the drug. What is clear, however, is that the very existence of Spice is the greatest example of the utter failure of the War On Drugs. The fact that, when it first emerged, it could be bought legally resulted in some people preferring to risk their health with harmful Spice rather than take the risk of breaking the law and use the tried and tested, low toxicity natural cannabis that has been taken safely taken for thousands of years. What a startling illustration of the folly of drug prohibition laws.

Being a 'Psychedelic Consultant' for MTV

In 2008 a producer at MTV contacted me. She needed a doctor with knowledge and experience of psychedelic drugs for insurance purposes, to consult on a new show she was planning. *Dirty Sanchez* entailed a group of young Welsh chaps travelling the world quaffing local psychoactive plants. It was a less culturally highbrow version of the Bruce Parry programme *The Tribe* that was quite popular at the time. From what I knew of *Dirty Sanchez* (and I'll leave the reader to look up what that name means), the

Welsh fellows in question were famed for their brashness. I was wary of getting involved and spent some time stressing to the producer that if the presenters were planning on meeting shamans and partaking in spiritual ceremonies they must pay attention to the local customs and behave with respectful deference and humility. I happened to know they had a habit of nailing their scrota to planks of wood in the past.

I was sent their travel itinerary and a list of the substances they had in mind. With assured safeguards in place they set off and I responded to the updates as they came in from distant shores; providing trans-Pacific and trans-Atlantic psychedelic consultation. The producer told me what country they were visiting next and drawing references from Stafford's *Psychedelics Encyclopedia*[45] and Hofmann and Schultes' *Plants of the Gods*[46], I suggested which indigenous psychedelic flora were worth sampling. Some of my notes to the producer are reproduced below.

If in South Africa, One Must Try *Sceletium*

Sceletium tortuosum and *Sceletium expansum* — also known as *mesembryanthemum, kanna* or *channa* — have been used for millennia by Hottentots as a vision-enhancing hallucinogen. Smoked, chewed or absorbed through the mucous membrane of the mouth, the plant contains the psychoactive alkaloid components mesembrine and mesembrenine. The main effect is a mild simulative intoxication not unlike cocaine, with elevated mood, and energy. In higher doses the user enters a prolonged state of sedation.

When in Australia You May Wish to Consider Cane Toad Licking?

There are no mentions of indigenous use of cane toad venom as a sacrament. The toads were introduced to Australia in the 20th century to eradicate pests in sugar cane crops. The most popularly used variety by Australian hippies is *Bufo alvarious* and the active components are 5-MeO-DMT and bufotenin. The toads are not actually *licked*. Rather, the venom from the parotid gland behind the toad's ear can be gently 'milked', then dried and smoked in a glass pipe. The toad's store of venom replenishes within a month so there is no need to kill it. But sometimes the toad is killed, dried and eaten, smoked or boiled into a foul-tasting tea and drunk. The effects of smoking the venom come on quickly and may be strong — similar to psilocybin or LSD.

If in Tonga, Check Out the Kava

Kava (*Piper methysticum*) is an evergreen shrub with large heart-shaped leaves and woody stems. The mashed up roots make an intoxicating drink with active ingredients called kavalactones. The effects lasts for up to eight hours, with mouth numbness, nausea and a lot of falling over. It produces reduced social inhibitions, much like drinking alcohol. Popular in Pacific Polynesia, it is enjoyed in the evenings as part of a communal activity. (The MTV producer wanted her boys to snort their kava. I warned her that unless they were using a concentrated extract they would need to snort so much material they could get serious sinus problems). There is no historical tradition of snorting kava. Though it's probably superior, as a recreational high, than nailing one's scrotum to a plank.

Next Stop India: for Indian Snakeroot

Also called serpentwood or rauwolfia, this evergreen shrub found in forests in springtime is peppered with white and pink flowers. It is not especially psychedelic. The alkaloid reserpine produces a sedative and depressant effect and has been used in Ayurvedic medicine for thousands of years to treat everything from poisonous reptile bites to insanity.

Calamus! Calamus! Will You Do the Fandango?

Calamus — also known as sweet flag, sweet sedge, sweet root and myrtle grass — grows in wetlands as leafy stems bearing yellow-brown flowers. The chewed stems taste horrible and contain the active components, alpha and beta-asarone, which increase energy, reduce hunger and provide a calming sensation. It has been compared to LSD by some; but those familiar with the effects of LSD may disagree.

If You Stop in South East Asia, Be Sure to Ask for Kratom

In South East Asia Kratom is called mambog. It can be found throughout Thailand, Malaysia, Borneo and New Guinea. The dried leaves are smoked or chewed and contain many indole alkaloids, including mitragenine, which can be simultaneously stimulating, like cocaine, and soothing, like morphine. It has been used as an opium substitute to cure opiate addiction and has become popular in the West in recent years, with many internet based suppliers. One of the best being *Kratom Frog.*

Nonda Mushrooms

Boletus manicus and *Boletus kumeus,* Papua New Guinea's Nonda mushrooms, are famed for causing what psychiatrists call Lilliputian hallucinations; visions of miniature people and animals. Natives claims the mushrooms cause violent rages and sometimes take them before planning to kill another person. Not one for Glastonbury Festival then.

The 'Rubbish' Bird

Also from New Guinea, the pitohui bird is referred to as 'rubbish' by locals because of its foul taste if eaten. Pitohuis produce a defensive endotoxin, homobâtrachotoxin, that comes from their diet of choresine beetles. The taste is extremely bitter. There are no reports of it being psychedelic (except to look at; beautiful plumage) but some 16th century Aztec documents mention a bird that "induced visions". This could be the pitohui bird, at a stretch.

New Guinea's Fierce Agara

The colossal *Galbulimima belgraveana* tree grows up to 90-feet tall. When the bark and leaves are boiled together with another plant, *ereriba,* over twenty alkaloids combine to produce a deep, vision filled slumber. The people of the Okapa region use Agara leaves to make men fierce against the malevolent power of a variety of illnesses.

The Visionary Plants of Africa

Africa is splendidly mystical; oozing with spirituality just as much as, though less overtly, perhaps, than India. Every rock, tree and river in Africa breathes a spiritual history. My travels there have been more contemplative than the screeching rancour of the East, but certainly no less spiritual. The concept of African 'witch doctors' is well known and Western doctors struggle with the idea of people practicing medicine without the proper evidence-based methods. Time will tell who offers the best therapeutic interventions for full holistic well-being.

Ubulawu is the Zulu word for visionary plants; the hundreds of barks, bulbs, vines, pods, roots, leaves, seeds and flowers that are chopped to make the white frothy mixture. Plants incorporated in *ubulawu* are often those growing near to rivers and include African dream root (*Heimia salicifolia*), *Acacia xanthophloea* and *Dianthus mooiensus*. Unlike the South American *ayahuasca*, *ubulawu's* effects are wildly idiosyncratic. Dreams are enhanced and certainly full-blown psychedelic experiences are possible. African shamans use the medicine as a divine tool:

> *Ubulawu belongs to the ancestors. It opens your brain to work. It is used to induce or clarify dreams of ancestral spirits and opens minds to receive the messages of the ancestors.*

(Of note: In 1997 when I was working in Malawi I was getting a lot of arthritic pain from my distant childhood fractures, so was recommended to visit a local shaman for treatment. Adorned in animal skins, he shuffled about his hut, fussing over plastic pots, bits of tangled defunct electrical equipment and animals that wandered in and out during the afternoon session. I was not aware that he had given me any visionary plants (but he may well have been on something or other himself). Rather, he held my ankle tightly, murmured, tossed runes and bothered the ashes in the fire, creating billowing sparks. When we left I asked my Malawian guide to translate what the man had said about my foot. Although he had been talking to me constantly for over two hours during the session, all she said, with a smile was, 'He says when you die, you will still have both your legs'. Very reassuring.)

The Zulu's Strawflower Smoke

Strawflower is tall, being of the sunflower family, and it produces clusters of golden-yellow flowers. It grows in Africa and the Zulu traditionally smoke the dried herb. Although native doctors use it to induce trances, the active ingredients, coumarins and diterpenes, are not known to have any psychedelic effects.

Jenkem

Jenkem is allegedly fermented human faecal matter and urine. The active ingredients are methane and ethanol, which, when inhaled, is like a mild version of sniffing glue. Some people say that the whole concept of jenkem is a hoax designed to humiliate drug tourists. Perfect.

Pandanus Nuts

Screw Pine grows along the coast in salt marshes. Huge quantities of these pine nuts, which contain dimethyltryptamine (DMT), must be eaten to get any psychedelic effect whatsoever. Used in folk medicine and for ceremonial purposes, Pandanus nuts are attributed to outbreaks of 'irrational behaviour' called Karuka madness.

Whatever Happened to the Dirty Sanchez Boys?

The producer never sent me a DVD of the series. But several years later, I saw a late night program featuring two Welsh boys sitting respectfully in meditation with a shaman. I was impressed to see they were displaying appropriate reverence to the local customs. Then, sure enough, at the end I realized it was *Dirty Sanchez* and there I was in the credits: *'Psychedelic Consultant — Dr. Ben Sessa'*. Job well done.

CHAPTER 8

The Psychedelic Renaissance Part One:
Movers and Shakers

The next two chapters will focus on the contemporary research projects, and the people behind them, that have emerged in the last 25 years.

For those of us in the field, it is exciting that today's society and medical profession are deciding to look again at psychedelic compounds. At the end of the 1960s, when these drugs were demonised, a wealth of knowledge about how to work clinically with psychedelics as tools for healing was at risk of being lost; cast aside onto the scrap heap of historical medical follies alongside a belief in humorism and the use of leeches. But all was not lost. Although a 20-year relative hiatus has since ensued, in the late 1980s the socio-political climate changed. At first there was just a trickle of interest, but this soon built into a great flood of re-visitation to the psychedelic studies of the past. Since the dawn of the 21st century, the contemporary psychedelic research community has become well established again. But this time the medical profession's slant on psychedelic drugs is different. Unlike the virginal approach to mind-expansion that characterised — and eventually killed — LSD's mass discovery in the 1960s, both the clinical and the popular psychedelic community since the late 1990s have been coming from a different place. Today there is less novelty about psychedelia and, for most people in research, less emphasis on using psychedelics to change the world.

Society has also changed in its general perception of pharmacology. By the 1990s the public had a much better handle on different forms of drug use and misuse than when they were first bombarded with the anti-drugs message 30 years earlier. We have passed beyond the psychedelic sixties, through the cocaine excesses of the seventies and the Ecstasy rave explosion of the late eighties and nineties. People these days have a much more sophisticated understanding about the distinctions between those drugs (such as methamphetamine, heroin, crack cocaine and alcohol) that create ghettos, cause dependence and restrict living opportunities, and those (such as psychedelics) that are aligned with artists, musicians and philosophers. Drugs like LSD, psilocybin, cannabis and MDMA need not be tarred with the same brush as those other, more dangerous drugs. Now, well into the new millennium, the public are simply too savvy to keeping falling for the superficial *War On Drugs* message of 'All Drugs are the Same and All Drugs Are Bad'. People, and drugs, have moved on.

This enlightenment about the true risks and benefits of different psychotropic drugs, together with tremendous advances in neuroimaging that allow us to not only visualise the anatomical architecture of the brain but also watch directly the development of physiological changes as the brain carries out functional tasks, sets the stage perfectly for a class of drugs that can be used to fine-tune a bespoke approach to neuroscience.

No one knows how far we might have travelled in the field of psychiatry and in our understanding of human consciousness had we continued to study the psychedelic drugs at the rate they were being explored between 1950 and 1966. We have sadly wasted at least 30 years, but now we have a chance to make amends and reintroduce these tools into our clinical armoury again. However, in some respects, perhaps history had to happen in this way. Water has needed to go under the bridge in order that we can now set our sights on the true medical applications for the psychedelic chemicals, unhindered by the need for associated socio-cultural revolution. And perhaps this way, if we progress carefully and cleverly, keeping the right people on side this time rather than intentionally marginalising them for 'not being experienced', we may even find a way for psychedelic drugs to provide humanity with a shift in global values for the better. God knows we could do with something like that now — far more than we ever did back in the sixties.

A Coming Together of Disparate Tribes

Like all groups who feel somewhat on the fringes of the mainstream, the psychedelic research community has always been good at organising itself into cohesive collectives and affiliations in which like-minded folk can share ideas and disseminate their findings. Their members also tend to be those sorts of people who like writing, feel an urge to organise the minority and enjoy staying up late. The result is a lot of words being written and spoken.

Under the auspices of Timothy Leary's *International Federation for Internal Freedom*, the journal *The Psychedelic Review* ran from 1963 to 1971. It started out with a scientific slant, encouraging a melting pot of ethnological, botanical, sociological, medical, psychiatric, cross-cultural and anthropological perspectives to discuss psychedelic drugs. But by the end of the sixties, the journal had begun to slant away from the academic focus, and gravitate towards the hippie cultural values predominant at the time. Today, original copies change hands for large amounts of money on eBay, but all the journal's editions are now also available online to read for free[1].

The Entheogen Review was a similarly targeted quarterly publication. Edited by David Aardvark and K. Trout, it ran from 1992 to 2008, and was host to the best of both old and newly emerging psychedelic devotees. It is now also available to everyone online at Erowid and psychonautwiki.

As in all fields of study, the internet has hugely increased the coming together of widely disseminated psychedelic interest groups. This has been particularly important for exploring multinational non-Western perspectives, and has allowed a mixing of medical and popular cultural movements to stay in close contact. There have been some fascinating gatherings, conferences and festivals in recent years in which the boundaries between medicine, art, cross-cultural studies and partying have been blurred, presenting unrivalled opportunities for multi-disciplinary and multi-dimensional learning.

Below are a few of the current groups, conferences, affiliations and websites operating right now that I know of.

Some Important Contemporary Psychedelic Organisations

1. The Multidisciplinary Association for Psychedelic Studies (MAPS)

MAPS is an immensely important psychedelic research organisation, formed in America in 1986 because of Rick Doblin's insistence to fight the rushed criminalization of MDMA by the US government. MAPS employs a skilled team of psychedelic researchers and media-savvy event organisation experts. With a clear educational strategy, a code of free access to information and Doblin's inspirationally motivational style at the helm, MAPS reviews papers, sets-up, runs, organises and funds clinical and non-clinical research and provides a platform for all aspects of psychedelic happenings all over the world. It also publishes books on psychedelic healing and culture, and maintains an important presence at international conferences and gatherings exploring the subject of psychedelic drugs[2].

Whilst MAPS supports a wide range of psychedelic research topics, from medical cannabis (or marijuana as they call the plant in the US), to LSD, psilocybin and ibogaine, in recent years they have focused increasingly — especially financially — on the specific topic of developing MDMA-Assisted Psychotherapy for PTSD. Having spear-headed the

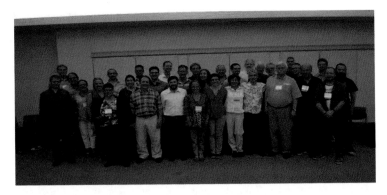

Picture 58: International Psychedelic Researchers at the Psychedelic Science Conference in Oakland, California, in April 2013. Including: Jordi Riba, Michael Mithoefer, Annie Mithoefer, Amy Emerson, Ilsa Jerome, Dana Blu Cohen, Thomas Kingsley Brown, Rick Doblin, Ingmar Gorman, Peter H Addy, Colin Hennigan, Marcela Ot'alora, Nese Devenot, Katherine MacLean, William Richards, Mary Cosimano, Matthew Johnson, Dave Nichols, Bob Jesse, Roland Griffiths, Andrew Feldmar, Tom Roberts, Luke Williams, Ken Tupper, Jim Fadiman, Darrick May. Photographer: Brad Burge.

Phase II studies in this field all efforts in the next six years are now concentrated on Phase III, and seeing MDMA-Assisted Psychotherapy licensed for use in treating PTSD. I owe an enormous personal debt to Rick and always enjoy seeing him and hanging out whenever our paths meet, which seems to be increasingly often these days.

2. The Heffter Research Institute

Founded in 1993 by David Nichols, George Greer, Mark Geyer, Dennis McKenna and Charles Grob, the Heffter Research Institute is named after the German psychopharmacologist who first studied the compound mescaline. With research centres in Los Angeles, New York, Arizona and Baltimore in the US, and at the University of Zurich in Switzerland (where, under the auspices of Franz Vollenweider many of the Phase I psychedelic studies of recent years have emerged), the Heffter Institute incorporates an impressive board of high-level clinical and research scientists from around the world. They design and oversee clinical, pre-clinical and socio-cultural research concerning psychedelic drugs and provide education to the medical profession, policy makers and the research community[3]. In 2013 Heffter joined forces with MAPS to hold the hugely successful international Psychedelic Science conference in Oakland, California.

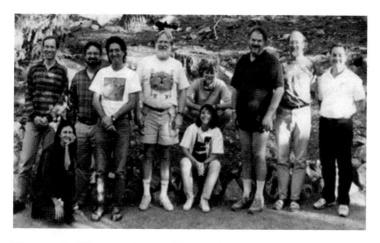

Picture 59: The very first Heffter Institute board meeting at their formation in 1993. With George Greer and his wife and co-therapist Requa Tolbert, Phil Wolfson, Charles Grob, David Nichols and Dennis McKenna.

Like MAPS, Heffter, whilst broadly supportive of any well-designed psychedelic research, have primarily focused on one substance; in their case psilocybin. Closely affiliated with Johns Hopkins University as well as New York University, they have been pushing back frontiers in the areas of psychedelic therapies for treating end of life anxiety, addictions and the use of psychedelics to explore spirituality and finding ways of tackling rigid and maladaptive personality traits.

3. The Beckley-Imperial Research Programme

Founded in 1998 by Amanda Feilding from the UK, the Beckley Foundation operates from beautiful surroundings in rural Oxfordshire. Since its inception, the foundation has been lobbying for changes to international drug law policy[4].

When in 2005 Amanda Feilding teamed-up with David Nutt – then at Bristol University – the collaboration of such high-powered individuals was bound to be fruitful for psychedelic research. Then David moved to Imperial College London, the partnership continued and since then we have seen some of the world's most innovative and significant psychedelic studies emerge. The programme allows for funding for PhD students and interns to take part in the ongoing studies conducted at Imperial College. The relationship between David Nutt and Amanda Feilding started when David was in Bristol and has since transferred to Imperial. The studies

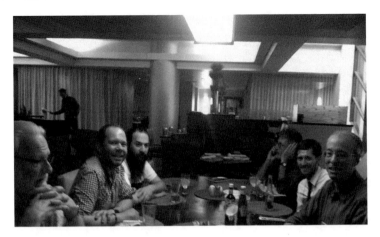

Picture 60: An historic meal bringing together old and new psychedelic scientists. The Heffter research crew meet the Imperial College crew. At Psychedelic Science in Oakland, California, 2013. David Nichols, Luke Williams, Charles Grob, Robin Carhart-Harris, George Greer and the arm of (off camera) David Nutt.

carried out have pushed the boundaries of contemporary neuroscientific research, with neuroimaging exploring the mechanism of action and therapeutic potential for drugs such as LSD, psilocybin, cannabis, DMT and MDMA and as well as other international projects.

4. Council of Spiritual Practice

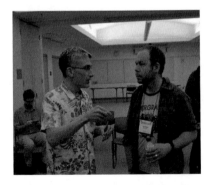

Picture 61: Bob Jesse, a gentle man with a bold vision and a determined spirit. At Psychedelic Science in Oakland, California, 2013.

This is an organisation convened in 1993 in San Francisco by Bob Jesse. Its mission is to increase people's access to 'direct experience of the sacred'. The council aligns itself with many methods and practices to do this, including psychedelic drug use and meditation. It provides a strong support for the use of entheogens as a vessel through which to connect to a greater sense of cosmic unity. The council supports psychedelic events. Together with MAPS and the Beckley Foundation, it co-hosted the 2011 and 2013

Psychedelic Science conferences in San Jose and Oakland, California, and is keen to propagate the work of past and present psychedelic studies, particularly those that pertain to the spiritual aspects of the experience[5]. Eyjafjallajökull volcano. It was at this point that I realized there truly is a god.

5. Breaking Convention

This is the UK-based conference that had its first gathering in 2011 in Canterbury, Kent, UK. Since then we have had meetings in Greenwich University, London in 2013 and 2015[9]. It has been a privilege and pleasure

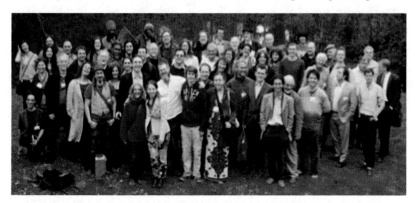

Picture 62: Great shot by Jonathan Greet of the speakers at the first Breaking Convention Meeting, Kent University, Canterbury, UK, in 2011. Including: Cameron Adams, Caspar Addyman, Brian Anderson, Ali Beiner, Friederike Meckel Fischer, Marianne Kaspersen, Jonathan Hobbs, Kilindi Iyi, Nikolas Karalis, Joseph Bicknell, Rick Doblin, Henry Dosedla, Robert Forte, Nick Giagnoni, Arfan Iqbal, Andy Letcher, David Lee, David Dupuis, Mike Jay, Amanda Feilding, Axel Klein, Reka Komaromi, Ras Binghi, Congo-Nyah, Cara Lavan, Konrad Fischer. Evgeny Krupitsky, Petra Bokor, Bia Labate, Robin Carhart-Harris, Neal Goldsmith, Merjin de Boer, Ivan Casselman, Caroline Chatwin, Jon Cole, Mike Crowley, Kevin Feeney, Liam Cummings, Paul Devereux, Jonas Di Gregorio, Stan Grof, Graham Hancock, Halvard Hårklau, Val Curran, Roland Griffiths, Ram Dass, Robert Dickens, Danny Diskin, Dave Luke, Luis Eduardo Luna, Edward MacRae, Torsten Passie, Thomas Teun Meijer, Ralph Metzner, Peter Oehen, Isabella Oliviera, Andy Parrott, Leonardo Rodriguez Perez, Vit Pokorny, Dirk Proeckl, Engelbert Winkler, Ffion Reynolds, Andy Roberts, James Rodger, Donal Ruane, Kalliopi Tavoulari, Diana Trimble, Charlotte Walsh, Manuel Villaescusa, Angela Voss, Ken Williford, Franz Vollenweider, Anna Waldstein, William Rowlandson, Neşe Şenol, Victor Petrone, Nexus, Max Freakout and Opaque Lens.

to be part of the fabulous group effort involved to make this organization a reality. Breaking Convention was set up by Dave King, Cameron Adams, Anna Waldstein, Dave Luke and myself in 2010 after experiencing the MAPS 2010 conference in California and realizing we had a simultaneous desire to see a similar psychedelic conference in the UK. The Breaking Convention summer meetings have gathered up to 800 delegates and speakers from over 30 different countries. We provide a broad range of topics for debate, which reflect the multidisciplinary backgrounds of the organisers. We have covered subjects from ethno-cultural-botany and sociology, to binaural beats, receptor profiles of psychedelics, clinical innovations and historical accounts of experiential moments in psychedelic history. The conferences are colourful affairs, with not only academic talks but also films, artist exhibitions, drama productions, bands, dance, flowers, incense, smart drinks and video links to some international speakers who cannot be there in person.

In collaboration with the publisher Strange Attractor Press, we also produce a book of proceedings at each conference, containing contributions from the previous year's conference. After our 2015 conference we used our profits to set-up the Breaking Convention Awards Foundation scheme, whereby we encourage budding psychedelic researchers to submit applications of their work for cash prizes. The plan is to continue, alongside other organisations, building a secure base of academic and artistic psychedelic researchers for the future. Since 2013 we have expanded the organization committee to include Aimée Tollan and Nikki Wyrd, plus a host of other committee roles to assist in the ever-growing complexity of this brilliant gathering[10]. Breaking Convention is repeated every two years, with the next meeting planned for summer 2017 — where we launch this 2nd edition *The Psychedelic Renaissance* book.

6. The Gaia Media Foundation

Dieter Hagenbach and Lucius Werthmueller founded Gaia Media in Basel in 1993. In 2006, they hosted the most special of all recent psychedelic conferences, the tremendous 'LSD Conference' in Basel to celebrate the 100th birthday of its illustrious board member, Albert Hofmann. In 2008, a follow-up event was staged: The World Psychedelic Forum. Gaia Media is a forum for artistic expression, constellation of ideas and dissemination of information about many esoteric aspects of science and the arts, including the clinical, spiritual and personal use of psychedelic drugs[6.] The book by Hagenbach and Werthmueller, *Mystic Chemist,* published in 2013, offers the most wonderful description of Albert Hofmann's life and works, together with a host of colourful pictures, by two of his closest friends and allies[7]. It is well worth a shmoozle. Dieter's death in 2016 was a sad loss for the psychedelic community.

7. The Psychedelic Society (UK)

In November 2014, there emerged — rather suddenly, it seemed — a vast network of people across the country signing up to attend the inaugural event of the Psychedelic Society in London. Set up by the highly talented activist and media manipulator, Stephen Reid, the Psychedelic Society now has branches in Edinburgh, Manchester, Leeds, Birmingham, Bristol and London. They put on regular lectures on a range of topics to do with psychedelics and organise local action group events, gatherings, film showings, parties and political activist happenings[14]. Committed to normalising the psychedelic experience and increasing accessibility for all, Stephen takes groups of enthusiasts wishing to partake in a safe, legal, guided experiences on regular retreats to Holland, where they can take psilocybin truffles in a ceremonial, healing context.

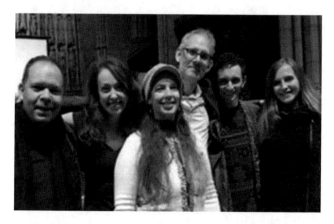

Picture 63: With Maria Broderick and Kevin Burns of the Brighton Psychedelic Society, Stephen Reid, Anna Waldstein, and Rita Kočrová of the Czech Beyond Psychedelics organisation.

8. The Beyond Psychedelics conference

This wonderful gathering of scientists, hippies, hipsters, psychiatrists and psychonauts took place for the first time in September 2016 in Prague, Czech Republic[18]. A great many of the big names in historical and contemporary psychedelic research attended and took part. It was tremendous fun and we look forward to Rita, Bara, Alex, Eva and the rest of the crew's next gathering in springtime 2018.

9. Horizons: Perspectives on Psychedelics

Originally set up by Kevin Balktick in 2006 in the wake of the Gaia Media Foundation's hugely popular LSD conference, this New York-based annual conference covers the social, political, clinical and multicultural aspects of psychedelic drugs. Neal Goldsmith, a multitalented speaker, organiser of people and author of *Psychedelic Healing*, curates the annual meetings and holds year-long lecture series gathering minds together[8]. In 2016 the conference celebrated its ten-year anniversary with a special event; it is ten years that has seen seismic changes in the field of psychedelic research.

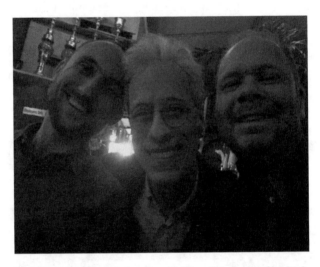

Picture 64: Neal Goldsmith in a bar in New York, April 2016, with Jag Davies, formerly of MAPS and now working at the Drug Policy Alliance.

10. The Open Foundation

The Open Foundation arose, like New York's Horizons conference, out of the success of the 2006 LSD Conference put on by the Gaia Media Foundation. A Dutch-based group, philosopher Joost Breeksema and anthropologist Dorien Tatalas founded Open. Their mission is to stimulate research, educate and encourage debate about psychedelic drugs and the psychedelic experience[11].

They have held major international conferences in Amsterdam: in 2010, The Mind-Altering Science conference, in 2011, the European Aya-huasca Research Symposium and in 2012 and 2016 the International Conference on Psychedelic Research (ICPR), all of which have been splendid. Amsterdam, after all, is always a fine place to visit for a psychedelically-minded researcher.

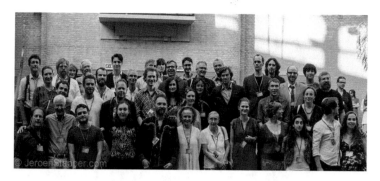

Picture 65: The speakers at Open's ICPR, in Amsterdam, in June 2016. Including: Matthew Clark, Rick Doblin, Elizabeth Nielson, Roland Griffiths, Peter Sjöstedt Hughes, Iker Puente, Amanda Feilding, Patrick Everitt, Bill Richards, Leor Roseman, MauriCio Dia, Raphael Milliere, Nese Devenot, Draulio Barros de Araujo, Pieter Skittonk, Shanna Wielinga, David Luke, Alex Belser, Alicia Danforth, Marcela Ot'alora G, David O'Shaughnessy, Andrea Langlois, Bia Labate, Athanasios Snapopoulos, Moni Wielo, Erwin Krediet, Ben De Loenen, Bradley Vines, Sarit Hashkes, Chiara Baldini, Jonathan Hobbs, Luis Fernando Tófoli, Mendel Kaelen, Ariadne Talot and Friederike Fischer.

11. Erowid

Erowid is an extraordinary online library resource, quite like no other, with detailed information on the pharmacology, history, effects, chemistry, legality, politics and cultural aspects of hundreds of psychoactive substances[12]. The lovingly nurtured creation of Fire and Earth Erowid, it is an impressive piece of technology. There is more on this website than one can read in a lifetime, with a dynamic emergence of users' trip reports and the latest breaking news about every known psychotropic drug, new and old. The Erowid crew is also a popular presence at the major psychedelic gatherings and conferences, dishing out their unbiased and measured important advice for psychonauts, drug-geeks and naïve learners everywhere. I frequently direct my patients or trainee doctors to Erowid as a source for contemporary knowledge about drug issues, as it is far more likely to provide answers about acute drug issues to patients and doctors than any 'official' government-based information service.

12. The Psychedelic Press (PsyPress) UK

Formed by Mr Robert Dickins in 2008, PsyPress started out as a humble home-produced platform for a journal for UK contributors of psyche-delic writings. It has since grown splendidly and now produces a thick bimonthly journal showcasing the latest scientific publications alongside psychedelic short stories, poetry, artwork and commentaries. PsyPress is also the publisher of several books, which have enjoyed wide readership. The organization works closely with Breaking Convention to disseminate new ideas and psychedelic events around the UK[15]. UK psychedelic writer Andy Roberts is a frequent co-editor.

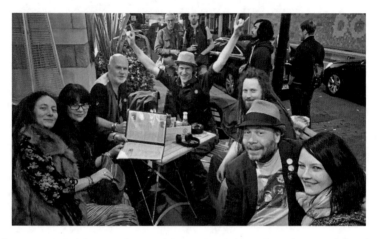

Picture 66: Taking on the world, one book launch at time. Celebrating the launch of PsyPress' Andy Roberts' *Acid Drops*, London May 2016. Left to right: Nikki Wyrd, Mandy & Andy Roberts, Jon Atkinson, Robert Dickins, Adam Malone, Cavan McLaughlin and Petra Kiviniemi.

13. Bluelight

This is a Dutch-based online resource for psychedelic drug users all over the world to share their experiences about drugs, doses, developments and happenings. Thousands of posts are collected, moderated and disseminated by a crew of active psychonauts with a keen eye on latest developments. They pride themselves on providing freely available information to all drug users as a means of reducing the harm caused by careless and misinformed use of drugs. There is a focus on MDMA/Ecstasy use, and resources include information about pill testing, and education and careers advice as well as access to the artistic and musical worlds connected with the psychedelic experience[13].

14. Psychonautwiki

This web resource has recently become the go-to place for information on the physiological effects of substances (for research purposes). Launched in August 2013, it presents similar info to Erowid but in a clear, consistent and objective style. https://psychonautwiki.org/

15. Ecology, Cosmos and Consciousness

This UK-based group, hosted by David Luke, has been running since 2009 from the October Gallery in London. A great many esteemed guests have spoken under the hollowed roof over the years on all kinds of weird and wonderfully esoteric subjects above and beyond psychedelics[16].

16. Reality Sandwich

This New York based internet magazine was founded by Ken Jordan, Daniel Pinchbeck, Michael Robinson and Jonathan Philips. It is a beautifully conceived online resource for many aspects of ecology, consciousness expansion, art, music, protest and shamanistic openings, with a particular emphasis on psychedelics. As it says on Reality Sandwich's website: 'Evolving consciousness, bite by bite'[21].

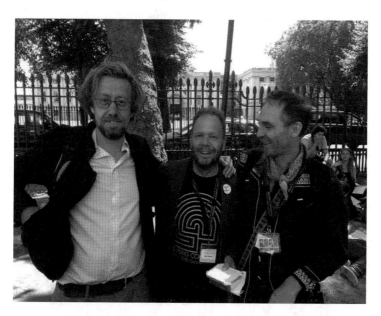

Picture 67: Daniel Pinchbeck, founder of Reality Sandwich, writer, popular cult figure and a good person with some bold visions of a positive future for humanity. Here at Breaking Convention 2015 with Dave Luke.

17. The University of Kent Psychedelic Society

Canterbury has always been a site for psychedelia, not least the university campus. The Kent Psychedelic Society predates the first Breaking Convention conference, and continues to provide a platform for speakers to inspire the students at Kent University[17].

18. Neurosoup

Founded and hosted by the ever-popular Krystal Cole, this website provides an exhaustive flow of regular video clips and podcasts in which Cole interviews users and experts, and describes experiences with just about every psychedelic drug imaginable[19]. Her site provides useful insights and education for psychedelic voyagers, with a strong emphasis on harm reduction, assistance for addictions and encouragement of careful use. In 2008, I had the pleasure of contributing a chapter to her *Neurosoup Yearly Review*[20].

19. Students for Sensible Drug Policy

An American organisation founded in 1998 by and for students all over the world, SSDP is primarily concerned with campaigning for a more fit-for-purpose, evidence-based approach to the international drug laws. It fights against the War on Drugs, based on the clear understanding that the War on Drugs is harming, not protecting, young people from the physical, societal and legal dangers of drug abuse[22].

20. Feed The Birds

This is a wonderfully creative activist group from Britain, set up in 2014 by the online alias Finn Hemmingway. As a means of highlighting the folly of cannabis prohibition in the UK, the group's message and method is very simple: scatter cannabis seeds (which are entirely legal to buy, sell and possess as they contain no THC until they germinate) throughout the country as food for birds[23].

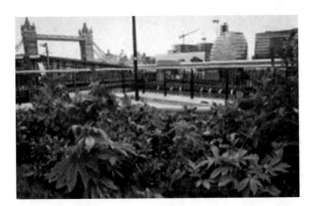

Picture 68: Feed the Birds adorn the UK streets and parks with a proliferation of cannabis plants growing in public places, which are then photographed and put online for all to see. Here they are growing quite happily in Central London.

21. Muswell Hill Press

This North London publishing house is not being included here simply because they are the publisher of this book! But rather because directors, Mark Chaloner and Tim Read, have created in recent years a broad range of important publications of a range of texts with psychedelic themes, including *Where Shamans Go* (Zoë Bran), *Walking Shadows* (Tim Read), *Therapy With Substance* (Friederike Meckel Fischer) and *Out of The Shadows* (Robert Dickins and Tim Read (Editors))[24].

22. The Tyringham Initiative

From his wonderful home in rural Buckinghamshire Anton Bilton operates this far-reaching project. His primary interest is consciousness research, and Anton has been an important figure in several contemporary UK studies (not least my own in Cardiff). A most welcoming fellow, with a keen eye on bringing people together, the house in Tyringham, which is set in majestic grounds including a unique chapel for ceremonial activities, has hosted recent UK meetings of leading lights in DMT and MDMA research[25]. We also had our last Breaking Convention committee meeting there, which was fab.

And many others!

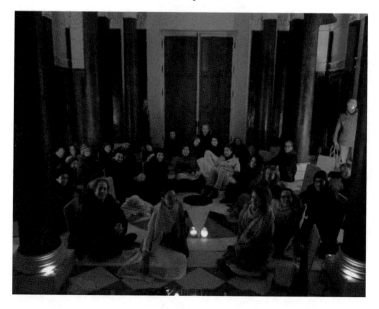

Picture 69: A ceremony of sacred music held in the unique chapel at Tyringham Hall, during the MAPS Training course in December 2014.

In the last five years, there has been a proliferation of social media-based groups providing click-fodder for all aspects of interest in the psychedelic experience, recreational use, philosophical ideas and experiential happenings. I will list a tiny number that I know about:

- Shroom With a View
- Psychedelic Spirituality Forum
- Psychedelic Parenting
- Entheogenic Anthropology
- Entheogens for a More Enlightened World
- Psychedelic Group Organizers
- Primary Sources for Psychedelic Research
- Psychedelic Supper: Psychedelics, Gender & Sexuality
- The Psychedelic Shadow
- The Psychedelic Community Learning Project
- Advanced Psychedelic Chemistry

Some Important Contemporary Psychedelic Researchers

There are many people worldwide who have contributed significantly to the renaissance of clinical, anthropological and social psychedelic research. There are, of course, many more from the old guard: Aldous Huxley, Terence McKenna, Albert Hofmann, Humphrey Osmond, Timothy Leary, Ronald Sandison, R.D. Laing and, very recently, Alexander Shulgin, who have now departed their mortal forms and will not be found on this list below. Such figures are well known and well-documented elsewhere.

Rather, the list below, which is not by any means exhaustive[26], represents some of the current working professionals in the field — some of whom have been in the game since the first wave of psychedelic interest in the 1950s and '60s, and some of whom are young and vibrant, working at the cutting edge of contemporary science. It is some of these lesser known youngsters that truly represent the psychedelic renaissance. It is their contributions to research in recent years that are spearheading a new generation of interest in the psychedelic compounds, stimulating new researchers to take up the mantle and enter the field.

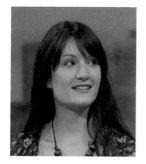

Aimée **Tollan** is a graduate from Kent University, Canterbury, UK, where she became involved in the local psychedelic society. Her organizational and personable skills transferred easily into the executive committee of Breaking Convention where she currently represents the role of treasurer. A lifetime in psychedelic research now seems inevitable, I hope.

Allan Badiner is a faculty member of the California Institute of Integral Studies, Transformative Studies Department. He is a popular and talented writer and activist. He has edited three books: Dharma Gaia: A Harvest of Essays in Buddhism and Ecology, Zig Zag Zen: Buddhism and Psychedelics, and Mindfulness in the Marketplace: Compassionate Responses to Consumerism. And a keen supporter of Breaking Convention.

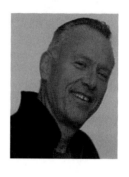

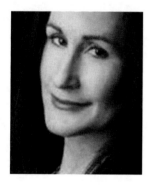

Alicia Danforth is a clinical and transpersonal psychologist from the United States. She has had an impressive start to her psychedelic career and has an assured future ahead of her in the field. Alicia, pictured here in Amsterdam in 2016, assisted Charles Grob in his Harbor-UCLA cancer-anxiety psilocybin study and her current research is looking at whether there can be a role for MDMA in managing social anxiety in people with autism[27].

Amanda Feilding is the founder and director of the Beckley Foundation. She is a popular and well-known figure in the psychedelic community; always rousing great crowds of admirers wherever she speaks. With a fascinating and colourful history going back to the swinging sixties of London, Amanda has been a figurehead for psychedelic research since its earliest beginnings. In recent years, her collaborations with Imperial College London and other academic institutions puts her at the centre

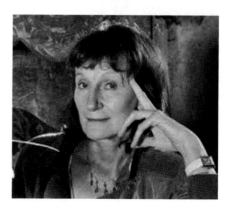

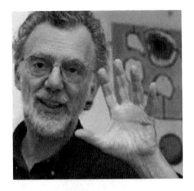

of the psychedelic renaissance — past, present and future.

Andrew Feldmár is a psychologist with 45 years' experience as a psychotherapist practicing in Vancouver. He has been writing about the benefits of psychedelic therapies since the 1960s and more recently has been part of the Vancouver team conducting MAPS-sponsored MDMA Therapy for PTSD.

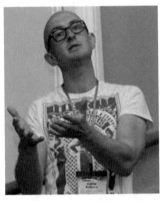

Andrew Gallimore, neurobiologist and chemist, is the author of several articles on DMT and the psychedelic state. He was the first to explain the effects of psychedelics within the framework of Tononi's 'integrated information theory', and is currently performing the first detailed phenomenological analysis of the subjective reports of the volunteers in Rick Strassman's landmark human DMT study.

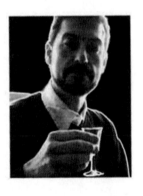

Andrew Sewell was a USA-based psychiatrist and neurologist working at Harvard Medical School. He was a pioneering and deeply sensitive researcher, with an interest in the role psychedelic plants, fungal alkaloids and LSD might have for alleviating cluster headaches. Together with John Halpern he investigated this phenomenon[28]. Always supportive of my own work, and the only non-living person in this list, he sadly passed away in 2013.

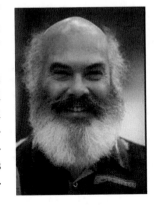

Andrew Weil studied at Harvard in the 1960s with Richard Alpert and Timothy Leary and has since became known for his interest in ethnobotany and complementary and alternative medicine. He is an advocate of integrative medicine; straddling the boundaries between evidence-based practice and alternative methods.

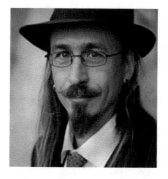

Andy Letcher is a UK-based folk activist and writer. His 2007 book, *Shroom,* has opened an interesting debate about the extent (or not) to which magic mushrooms have played an important part in shaping the culture of Britain[29]. He is a prolific writer about folk culture and plays an impressive number of traditional musical instruments.

Andy Roberts is a UK-based writer, investigator of all things mysterious and offbeat and general all round good egg. A lover of nature, psychedelic music and folk history, in 2008 he published an important book, *Albion Dreaming: A Popular History of LSD in Britain*[30] and in 2016 published a collection of memoirs, tales, and interviews with several psychedelic luminaries, *Acid Drops*[31]. He continues to provide insights into the role psychedelics have played in shaping this nation and humankind in general.

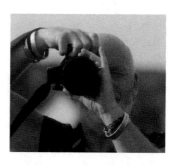

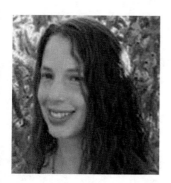

Anna Waldstein is a medical anthropologist who studies herbal medicines as a form of empowerment and/or resistance to bio-medical hegemony. Her research interests include self-medication with cannabis and the relationship between cannabis and identity. She is also interested in the role of psychotropic substances in human evolution and biocultural constructions of addiction. She works at the University of Kent, Canterbury, and as co-chair was a driving force of organisation, inspiration and spiritual awareness for the 2011 Breaking Convention conference in the UK.

Anton Bilton is an inspiring individual who has provided valuable resources for various research projects as well as generously providing a base in the UK for fertilizing and growing consciousness exploration projects. His home at Tyringham Hall, Buckinghamshire has been the venue for several important academic meetings in recent years.

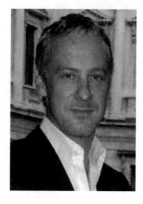

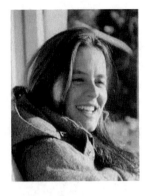

Bia Labate is a social anthropologist from Brazil with an impressive following and wide influence on the fields of drug policy, shamanism, ritual, and religion. She is co-founder of the Nucleus for Interdisciplinary Studies of Psychoactives. She talks widely throughout the psychedelic and scientific communities about ayahuasca.

Bob Jesse, whose formal training is in electrical engineering and computer science, is the gently enigmatic foundation stone of the Council of Spiritual Prac-

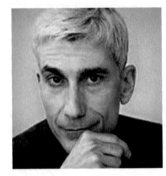

tices. The CSP operates from a broad base of tolerance and acceptance of all imaginable approaches towards mystical states, religious experience and psychedelic consciousness. He is also co-convenor of a spiritual community formed around ecstatic dance and, like me, has a leaning towards the pacifism and integrity of the Society of Friends.

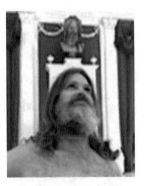

Cameron Adams is a medical and ecological anthropologist from Arizona with an interest in psychedelic medicine and ecological consciousness. Until recently he was a lecturer at the University of Kent where he was conducting web-based research on virtual communities. In 2011, he co-founded and co-chaired the UK's Breaking Convention conference, is now a central member of the executive committee and is now the chief editor of Breaking Convention Publications. Pictured here looking suitably resplendent at the Breaking Convention executive crew committee meeting at Tyringham hall in 2015.

Candice Monson is professor of psychology at Ryerson University, Toronto. She is currently working with MAPS to develop a version of cognitive behavioural conjoint therapy using MDMA-assisted sessions to treat couples in which one member has PTSD.

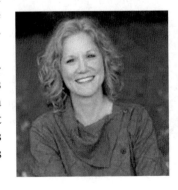

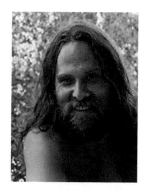

Casey William Hardison is an American chemist whose commitment to the concept of cognitive liberty and freedom of thought contributed to a nine-year custodial sentence when he was imprisoned for the production, possession and exportation of psychedelics. From his home-based clandestine lab in Brighton, UK, he produced 2C-B, DMT and LSD. He was released from prison in 2013 and continues to be an inspirational activist for many people around the world seeking the right to safely use psychedelics for personal and communal growth and development.

Celia Morgan is a researcher at Exeter University. She started working with ketamine and MDMA alongside Val Curran at UCL and has produced some illuminating work on the naturalistic behaviours of ketamine users[32]. She is currently carrying out a novel study exploring ketamine therapy as a treatment for alcohol dependence.

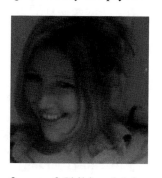

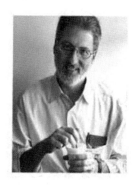

Charles Grob is a professor of Child and Adolescent Psychiatry at UCLA and on the board of the Heffter Research Institute. He has contributed widely to psychedelic research for many years[33]. His important studies have covered the mechanistic, sociological and clinical aspects of MDMA, psilocybin and ayahuasca, including a landmark project exploring the role of psilocybin as a tool to manage the anxiety and existential issues associated with end-stage cancer. His professional position as a child psychiatrist provides inspiration to those of us juggling our own clinical and research roles.

Charlotte Walsh is a lecturer at Leicester University, UK, where she teaches law and criminology. She has produced important work highlighting the legal aspects of the war on drugs, particularly pertaining to psychedelics and the issues of civil liberty and religious freedom.

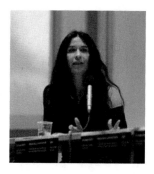

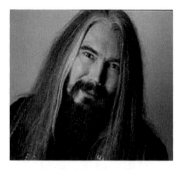

Christian Ratsch is a German anthropologist and writer. He's been around for donkey's years and leads the world's literate community on topics such as ethnopharmacology, psychoactive plants and animals. His seminal work *The Encyclopedia of Psychoactive Plants: Ethnopharmacology and Its Applications*[34] has enthralled the green-fingered and purple-minded for decades.

Christopher Timmerman is a PhD student at Imperial College London. He is currently heading a team conducting what the Imperial College psychopharmacology unit do best; multimodal neuroimaging with psychedelics. Chris' project (which involved injecting my brain, ouch!) is examining DMT; applying the same rigorous examinations with EEG, MEG and fMRI that Imperial have previously used to study psilocybin and LSD.

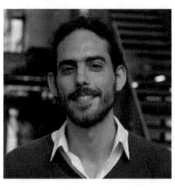

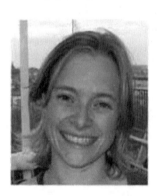

Claire Durant, from Imperial College London, is included in this list simply because she is the most incredible research associate on the planet and exactly the person one needs when trying to traverse the Kafkaesque task of a contemporary human psychedelic drug trial.

Clark Heinrich lives in the coastal mountains of California and specialises in comparative religion and ethnobotany. His book *Magic Mushrooms in Religion and Alchemy*[35] describes the role that *Amanita muscaria* has played in various mythologies. He represents a deep pool of knowledge on all things fungal and photographic.

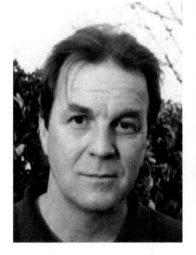

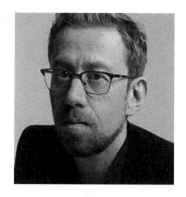

Daniel Pinchbeck is one of many writers and professional psychonauts, meticulously recording his journeys through the psychedelic landscapes, mapping the inner cosmos as he experiments with new mental states and beats the path providing cartography for others to follow. Forming his viewpoints from an alchemical mixture of his own experiential journeying as well as established science, Daniel's popular works emphasise the importance of sifting through all these concepts when it comes to understanding psychedelic drugs, consciousness and spirituality in their entirity[36,37,38]. He latest book, *How Soon is Now?* is an important text exploring the future options for humanity 2.0.

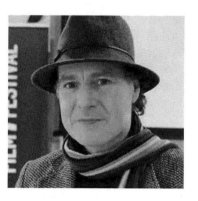

David Graham Scott is a Scottish film maker who has contributed significantly to the public understanding of how ibogaine therapy can assist a person to overcome the pain of opiate detox with his moving and highly two personal documentary films, *Detox or Die*[39] and *Ibogaine Nights*[40].

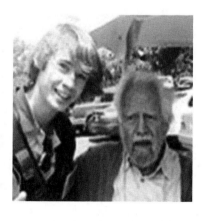

David King is an anthropologist from the University of Kent, UK. He has an impressive knowledge of the medical uses of psychedelic plants and fungi in the development of human culture. As co-founder, King has been instrumental in the origins and maintenance of the UK's Breaking Convention conference, and did time at the Beckley Foundation. Having lived in Singapore attempting to explore drug policy in what is one of the harshest environments on the planet for this field of research, he is now to be found in London studying medicine. Keep an eye on this lad. Pictured here with Sasha Shulgin in 2014, for whom he organized a highly successful online sale of blotter art in support of Sasha's medical costs.

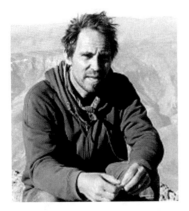

David Luke is a UK-based academic psychologist and Senior Lecturer at Greenwich University, London where he teaches an undergraduate course on the psychology of exceptional human experiences. He is also president of the Parapsychological Association and a past research associate at the Beckley Foundation. Voluminously published[41] and staggeringly well-connected with the global psychedelic community, Dave is also co-founder and spiritual leader of Breaking Convention as well as chair of the Ecology, Cosmos and Consciousness lecture series at the October Gallery in Bloomsbury, London. His special interests include the links between altered states of consciousness, paranormal phenomena and hexagons. He will not be pictured here as there are too many shots of him in this book already. He is a renowned collector of antique mandrake roots.

David Nichols is Professor of Medicinal Chemistry and Pharmacology at Purdue University, USA. He is the co-founder and director of the Heffter Research Institute[42]. He has contributed numerous works to the preclinical study of psychedelic drugs and acts as consultant to NIH, NIMH and NIDA advisory groups. His laboratory manufactured the original kilo of MDMA that Rick Doblin used in the early studies in the 1980s; of which 900 grams remains unused and locked in a safe. He is a Fellow of the Academy of Pharmaceutical Sciences and American

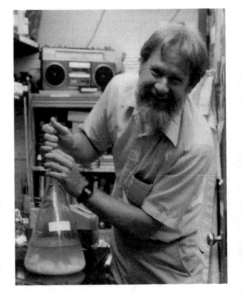

Association of Pharmaceutical Scientists. He has always keenly supported newly emerging talent in the field of psychedelics and gives great lectures that render the mysterious worlds of chemistry and neurotransmitters accessible to all.

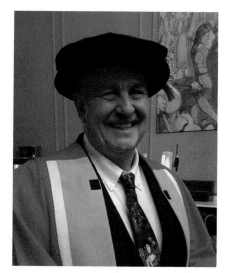

David Nutt is a British psychiatrist and one of the UK's leading neuropsychopharmacologists, having held senior positions at the British Association of Psychopharmacology and the Presidency of the European College of Neuropsychopharmacology. He specialises in addiction, anxiety and sleep disorders. Until 2009, he headed up the psychopharmacology department at Bristol University and now holds the post of Edmond J. Safra Chair in Neuropsychopharmacology at Imperial College, London[43]. He has an enormous popular following throughout the world; in recent years becoming well known for speaking out in favour of his patients against biased government interference in medical research. He is an enthusiastic critic of drug laws with limited evidence-based validity that are no longer fit for purpose. He runs a vibrant research department and is always keen to nurture new talent and fresh ideas. I and many others in UK psychedelic research owe a lot to David for his support and enthusiasm within this field of science.

Deborah Parish Snyder has been the CEO of Synergetic Press since 1984, which has been publishing a wide range of esoteric texts and paradigm-shifting concepts from biogeochemistry, consciousness and psychedelics for over 30 years[44]. Her connections with the legendary Biosphere 2 project since the 1980s, which explored methods by which humanity could learn to live within a sealed, self-sustaining environment fit for extra-terrestrial colonisation, illustrate her keen ability to think outside the box whilst living within one.

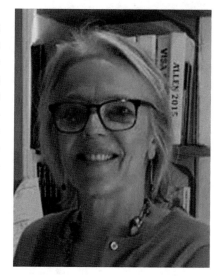

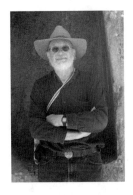

Dennis McKenna is a celebrated botanist, ethno-pharmacologist and author. He is a highly respected orator on ayahuasca and sits on the board of directors at the Heffter Research Institute. Together with his brother, Terence, he co-authored *The Invisible Landscape: Mind, Hallucinogens & the I Ching*[45] and is a popular writer, commentator on shamanism and altered states of consciousness in his own right. He has investigated Amazonian ethnomedicines for the treatment of schizophrenia and cognitive deficits.

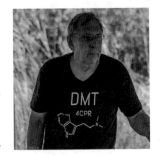

Ede Frecska is a psychiatrist at the University of Debrecen, Hungary. His earlier research was on schizophrenia and affective illness before developing an interest in the potential endogenous role of DMT, 5MeO-DMT, and bufotenin. Ede has published on the effect of ayahuasca on creativity, aggressive behaviour, and binocular rivalry. He has recently been central to the publication of the new Journal of Psychedelic Studies.

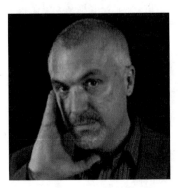

Emanuel Sferios is an activist and vigorous campaigner for MDMA harm-minimization and science. Having set up the renowned *Dancesafe*[46] organisation in 1998 his work on MDMA harm-minimization has reduced risks for millions of users around the world. He is currently working on the much-awaited: *MDMA — The Movie*.

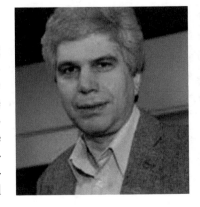

Evgeny Krupitsky is a psychiatrist from St. Petersburg, Russia with a special interest in addictions. Inspired by the work of Osmond with LSD in the 1950s, Krupitsky led the world in ketamine psychotherapy research in the 1990s, applying this substance to treatments for alcohol and opiate dependence[47]. He used the depth and powerful influence of the ketamine psychedelic experience alongside individual and group psychotherapy to achieve impressive abstinence results in chronic substance misusers.

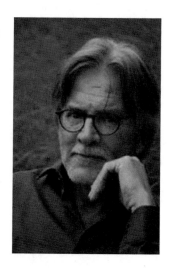

Franz X. Vollenweider is very much one of the super brains of the psychedelic research world. Franz is director of Heffter Research Centre Zürich for Consciousness Studies (HRC-ZH). Vollenweider is also Vice-Director of Research and Teaching and Director of the Neuropsychopharmacology and Brain Imaging Research Unit of the University Hospital of Psychiatry Zürich East and Professor of Psychiatry in the School of Medicine. His contribution to the pre-clinical understanding of psychedelic drugs in recent years is invaluable, and he has published voluminously on their neurophysiology[49]. He also gives marvelous lectures about neurotransmitters wherever he goes.

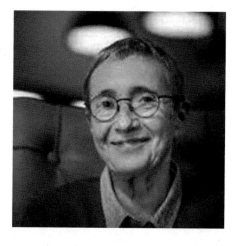

Friederike Fischer is a medical doctor from Germany who became a psychotherapist in Switzerland. Together with her husband Konrad, she has contributed enormously to contemporary psychedelic research, though in a somewhat unconventional manner. Trained as part of the psycholytic study group that formed legally in Switzerland between 1988 and 1993 (which also provided training for other psychedelic researchers Peter Oehen and Peter Gasser), Friederike went on to provide several years of underground psychedelic therapy to patients using LSD, MDMA and 2C-B. She described her work in the 2015 book *Therapy with Substance*[49]. And we also wrote a paper together, published in 2012, for the inaugural issue of David Nutt's new journal, the Independent Scientific Committee on Drugs, edited by David Nutt[50].

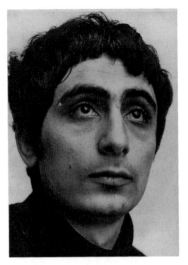

Gabor Mate is a Hungarian-born Canadian psychiatrist whose work with ayahuasca has brought him to the attention of the psychedelic community. But for those of us in the field of addictions his influence reached far greater. His book *In the Realm of Hungry Ghosts* speaks directly to the heart and mind in equal measures; describing perhaps better than any other medical book with mass popular appeal, just how and vital are compassion, patience and creativity when working with this terribly challenging but challenging group of patients.

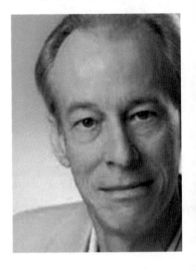

George Greer is a US psychiatrist from New Mexico who was the first person to publish data of the uses of MDMA-Assisted Psychotherapy in the 1980s before the drug was banned. He subsequently went on to be a founding member of Heffter and together with his wife and colleague, psychiatric nurse, Requa Tolbert, George remains an important inspiration for MDMA scientists and therapists today[51]. He's also a big fan of the psychedelic band, Fever Tree.

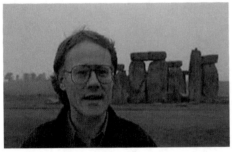

Graham Hancock is a UK-based sociology writer and researcher of many unusual aspects of human history. His interests include ancient civilisations, aliens, myths and legends and the role for altered states of consciousness in the evolution of human consciousness[53]. His books are incredibly popular and he draws big crowds for his talks — as when he spoke at Breaking Convention in 2011.

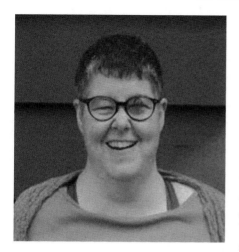

Ilsa Jerome is an academic genius from the USA, whose knowledge of MDMA studies is arguably the greatest on the planet. She reads and reviews thousands of articles on MDMA and distributes them across the globe to interested parties. Not a single paper, article, study or commentary about MDMA can avoid her gaze. She is therefore an invaluable person to know and befriend if thinking of starting an MDMA project — and was a major contributor to the MAPS mammoth MDMA Investigators Brochure, which had over 600 referenced scientific papers on MDMA. Her boundless knowledge of MDMA is matched only by her fastidious love of obscure electronic music and ice cream.

Ingrid Pacey is a psychiatrist working in Vancouver, Canada on one of the MAPS-sponsored MDMA-PTSD studies. She had her first introduction to psychedelic therapy with LSD in Australia in 1964. That is a lot of flight hours since then.

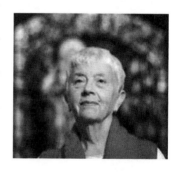

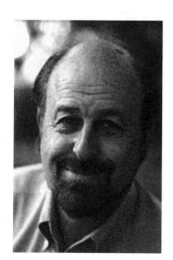

James Fadiman is a psychologist and writer and one of the respected old guard of psychedelic research. He is one of the co-founders of the Institute of Transpersonal Psychology and continues to research the field of LSD microdosing. He first came across psychedelics in Paris when introduced to psilocybin by his friend and former professor, Ram Dass, who at that time was Richard Alpert. With over 50 years' experience in this game, Jim has been a supportive and inspirational mentor to myself and other researchers.

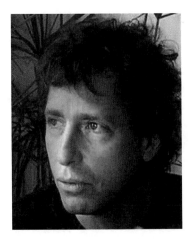

Jeremy Narby is an anthropologist and writer who has worked extensively in the Peruvian Amazon helping combat ecological destruction. He has written widely about ayahuasca and his book *The Cosmic Serpent: DNA and the Origins of Knowledge* (1995) and now directs the Swiss NGO, Nouvelle Planète. He studied history at the University of Canterbury, the venue for the first Breaking Convention conference in 2011.

John Halpern is an Assistant Professor of Psychiatry at McLean Hospital Harvard Medical School. His projects since the mid-1990s have included looking at cognitive functioning of MDMA and ayahuasca users, the use of psilocybin and LSD to relieve cluster headaches, and the Native American Church use of peyote. He started a clinical project examining the use of MDMA as an agent to treat anxiety in patients with end-stage cancer but this was shut down because of participant enrolment difficulties. He continues to play an important role in psychedelic research.

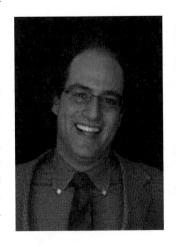

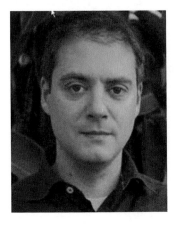

Jordi Riba is a Spanish pharmacologist working at Sant Pau hospital in Barcelona. He has conducted numerous studies on the clinical and neurophysiological aspects of ayahuasca, and has recently carried out some potentially staggeringly important studies demonstrating ayahuasca's potential capacity for boosting neurogenesis[54]. This could have profound implications for the development of future medicines for treating Alzheimers and Parkinsons.

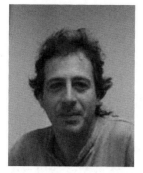

Jose Carlos Bouso is a clinical psychologist, with his PhD in Pharmacology. He has published studies on the safety and efficacy of MDMA Psychotherapy for PTSD and is currently conducting research on the long-term effects of ayahuasca use in the Spanish and Brazilian communities. He began one of the first clinical MDMA for PTSD studies outside the USA, which was regrettably shut-down for political reasons before completion.

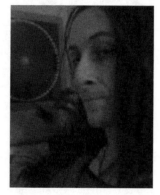

Julian Vayne is an occultist, and a writer[55], with a particular interest in the use of psychedelics within spiritual contexts. He has written several books and essays exploring this area, and presented talks to a wide range of audiences. He is also a museum and learning consultant, and is currently setting up The Psychedelic Museum. He is an active, charming and uncharacteristically sensible member of the Breaking Convention committee.

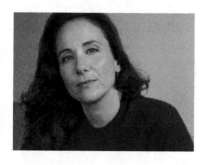

Julie Holland is a New York psychiatrist with extensive experience working at Belleview Hospital (and author of *Weekends at Bellevue*)[56]. She has an impressive curriculum vitae, spanning all aspects of the renaissance of psychedelic research. She has edited major works on MDMA[57] and cannabis[58], and continues to broadcast on the importance of recognising the relative risks and safety of psychedelic drugs as tools for medical, personal and societal development. She is also skilled at tapping into intra-familial emotional vibrations through the medium of music.

Katherine MacLean is a therapist who has worked with the Johns Hopkin's psilocybin-assisted psychotherapy team in Baltimore since the beginning of the project[59]. Katherine has sat in on more psychedelic sessions that she might care to remember; watching patiently as her subjects soar, twist and turn

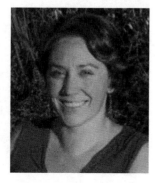

through their internal mental mindscapes. A stable figure providing mental containment is essential under such circumstances, which is what Katherine represents.

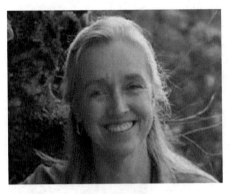

Kathleen (Kat) Harrison is an ethnobotanist exploring the relationship between plants, mushrooms and human beings. She weaves scientific and historical stories between psychedelic culture, rituals of healing and those artistic creations that illustrate the plant-human relationship. Kat, who came to Breaking Convention in 2015, founded Botanical, founded Botanical Dimensions[60] in 1985, with her then-husband, the late Terence McKenna. She delivers wonderful lectures about her shamanic use of the *Salvia divinorum* plant teacher; whom she lovingly refers to as 'She'.

Laurie Higbed is a clinical psychologist from Bristol, UK with a passion for working with people who suffer with addictions. Like me, she is interested in advancing a better understanding of the developmental pathway from childhood trauma to adult mental disorders. She is the co-therapist on the Bristol-Imperial-

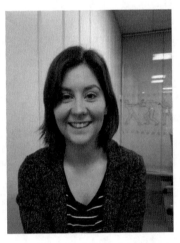

MDMA Alcoholism study and looks set to become a big name in the future of MDMA science. I just need to convince her to help me open a Bristol-based psychedelic clinic in the next few years.

Levente Móró works at the Centre for Cognitive Neuroscience in the University of Turku, Finland. He works in the Consciousness Research Group on the topic of altered states of consciousness, and specialises in the study of dreaming,

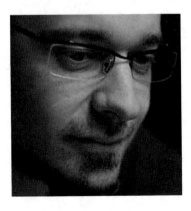

hypnosis, hallucinations, and psychedelics. He is committed to online drug information providing, drug policy reform advocacy, and drug-related harm reduction work.

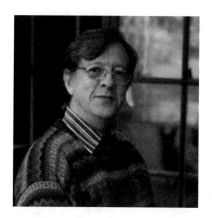

Luis Eduardo Luna studied comparative religion at Stockholm University and now works and writes extensively about shamanism, particularly as it pertains to South American culture[61,62,63]. He has published books on ayahuasca and is Director of the Research Center for the Study of Psychointegrator Plants, Visionary Art and Consciousness in Florianópolis, Brazil.

Luke Williams is a UK academic working at Imperial College London and senior manager with Eleusis Benefit Corporation. He has been at the helm of numerous UK psychedelic studies of recent years for Imperial College London, nurturing subjects through their experiences with LSD, psilocybin, DMT

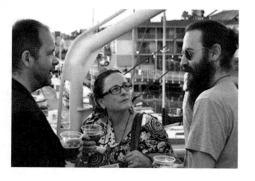

and MDMA. His lifelong career in psychedelic research of one sort or another now seems well cemented. Pictured here, with Annie Mithoefer, at the Psychedelic Science boat cruise on San Francisco Bay in 2013.

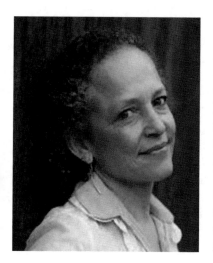

Marcela Ot'alora is a deeply inspirational MDMA Therapist working on the MAPS-sponsored MDMA-PTSD study in Boulder, Colorado, USA. Having received a B.A. in Literature and Art, an MFA in painting and an MA in Transpersonal Psychology her broad training and practice models reflect how it takes a lifetime

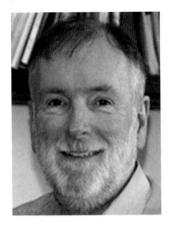

of work and experience to move so seamlessly as a therapist working within altered states of consciousness.

Mark Geyer is one of the co-founders of the Heffter Research Institute and contributes to work carried out at the Heffter's research facility based at Zurich University. He specialises in translational research and looks at the links between the behavioural effects of psychedelic drugs and cognitive processing in humans and animals.

Mat Hoskins is a trainee psychiatrist from Cardiff. With myself he is part of the team carrying out the world's first study giving MDMA to patients with treatment-resistant PTSD whilst they are in an fMRI scanner. The plan is to mildly traumatize the subjects and then demonstrate that when on MDMA, compared to placebo, they have a reduced fear response that is matched by reduced amygdala activation and a boosted prefrontal cortex response. We are assisted in this work by Chrissie

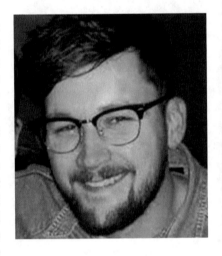

Turner Wilson and UK PTSD expert Professor Jonathan Bisson. It will, I think, be the start of a long career in MDMA science for Mat.

Matthew Johnson is a psychologist from Johns Hopkin's Medical School in Baltimore. Having worked alongside Roland Griffith's team for many years he is now turning his attention to the use of psychedelic-assisted psychotherapy as a tool for tackling addictions[64,65]. With the fabulous results of a recent pilot study in which psilocybin-assisted psychotherapy resulted in improved rates of abstinence amongst cigarette smokers, he looks well on the way to developing a viable treatment for one of the world's greatest public health problems.

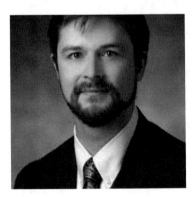

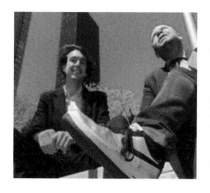

Maximillian von Heydon is a researcher from Berlin. He is the editor of the forthcoming *Handbook of Psychoactive Substances* (2017). We spent time together at Tyringham Hall in 2014, when he undertook the MAPS MDMA video training course. With an interest in psychedelic drug policy, he also attended the global

drugs strategy meeting, UNGASS, at the United Nations in New York in April 2016, (pictured above), where we hung out together again.

Mendel Kaelen is a PhD student at Imperial College London who has published some important research looking at the links between the psychedelic state and the subjective experience of music appreciation. Using fMRI, he has demonstrated the neurobiology of musical aesthetics when under the influence of psilocybin, LSD and, more recently, DMT.

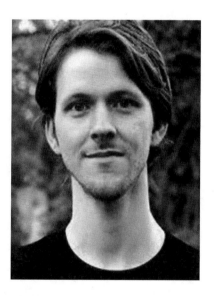

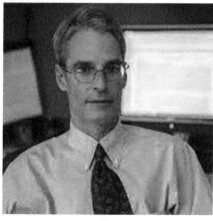

Michael Bogenshutz is a psychiatrist from New Mexico who has written extensively about the value of the psychedelic experience in tackling addictions. He recently published a pilot study testing psilocybin-assisted psychotherapy as a treatment for alcohol dependence[66]. We have modelled aspects of our own Bristol study using MDMA-assisted psychotherapy for alcoholism on aspects of Michael's study with psilocybin. Important work with a potentially vastly important future.

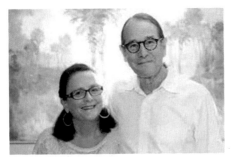

Michael and Annie Mithoefer are a psychiatrist and nurse pair of MDMA therapists from Charleston, South Carolina, with a life-long special interest in PTSD and psychedelic therapy. Michaels' research led him to meet Rick Doblin in 2000, which began their relationship to instigate the world's first randomised, controlled, double-blind clinical study with MDMA, published in 2010[67], with a long-term follow-up study showing the positive effects are sustained for up to four years[68]. Mithoefer and Annie continue to work closely with MAPS, currently running further trials with MDMA-assisted psychotherapy. They have also been responsible for training the world's next generation of MDMA therapists. They are pictured here in their clinic in Charleston, South Carolina, the day after facilitating my MDMA-assisted therapy session as part of my training to be an MDMA therapist. It was one of the most memorable experiences of this, if not the next, life for me.

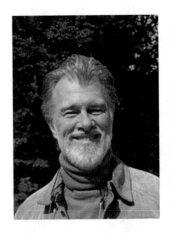

Michael Winkelman, PhD, has contributed widely to the field of shamanism, medical anthropology and neurotheology. His research has applied principles of shamanic healing in treating people with substance misuse problems. Amongst his large number of publications[94] is the recent two-volume *Psychedelic Medicine*, which he has edited together with Thomas Roberts[95].

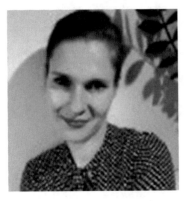

Monika Bartczak is a PhD student from Canterbury University, UK, now specialising as a Clinical Psychologist. She has completed an important project looking at the subjective psychological drug effects amongst recreational Ecstasy users and is set to become a trained MDMA Therapist in the coming years – hoping to be part of the forthcoming MAPS Phase Three studies in the UK.

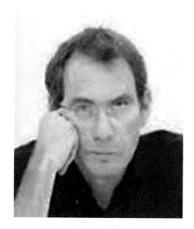

Moshe Kotler is the principal investigator for the MAPS-sponsored MDMA-PTSD study taking place in Beer Yaakov, Israel. Moshe is chairman of the Israeli National Council for Mental Health and former chief psychiatrist for the Israeli Defense Forces. Developing robust psychiatric treatments for severe PTSD is essential in all communities, but particularly in those where an on-going state if war contributes to high levels of psychological trauma.

Myron Stolaroff was an author and psychedelic researcher with a wide range of interests. He founded the International Foundation for Advanced Study in Menlo Park in 1960 and over ten years conducted clinical studies with LSD and mescaline, particularly in the field of exploring psychedelic creativity. Another peculiar sideline was his interest in sound recording. He co-designed the Ampex Model 200A reel-to-reel tape recorder, which became an important piece of kit for a generation of innovative recording artists. In 2004 he authored the book *The Secret Chief*[69], describing the pioneering work of early MDMA therapist Leo Zeff. Myron passed on to another level of psycho-spiritual energy in 2013.

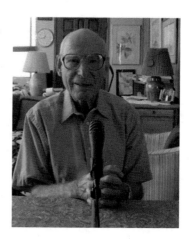

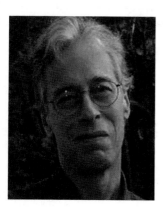

Neal Goldsmith is a psychotherapist from New York and the author of a recent book *Psychedelic Healing*[70]. He is the curator of New York's Horizons psychedelic conference. His clinical practice incorporates elements of transpersonal, humanistic and Eastern traditions and is particularly useful for adults undergoing existential crises, or couples coping with significant changes in their lives. Neal's gentle and persuasive approach to the study of psychedelic drugs and people in general as healing agents is an inspiration to all.

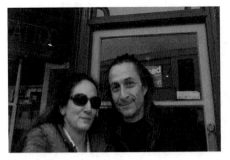

Nikki Wyrd has a BSc in Ecology, and is a magickal practitioner extraordinaire. Together with Julian Vayne (with whom she is pictured here), Nikki is author of *The Book of Baphomet*[71]; she now edits the Psychedelic Press Journal, as well as publishing and copyediting books, many of which feature psychedelic experiences. She is, perhaps, the most organised and together member of the Breaking Convention Executive Committee — but we won't hold that against her. Nikki lives on the edge of a city, with a river at the end of her garden.

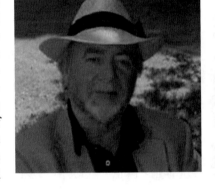

Paul Devereux is a UK-based commentator on anthropology and archaeology and a Fellow with the International Consciousness Research Laboratories (ICRL) group at Princeton University, USA. He has a special interest in the role psychedelics have played in the development of human culture and speaks, broadcasts and writes on a wide range of esoteric subjects including UFOs, ley lines and dowsing.

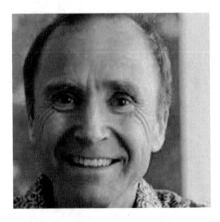

Peter Gasser is a Swiss psychiatrist with prior training in psychedelic psychotherapy during the brief window of psychedelic activity that occurred in Switzerland between 1988 and 1993. Peter, who kindly sent me one of his original medicine pots, published the first, published the first clinical study with LSD in modern times, exploring the role for LSD therapy in treating anxiety associated with end-stage cancer[72]. Crucially, Peter's study, which heralded a return to mainstream medicine for LSD, provided Albert Hofmann with important validation that his vital discovery had regained its place in history; a Wonder Child within his lifetime.

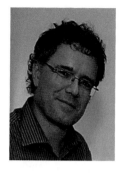

Peter Oehen is a psychiatrist and psychothera- pist in private practice in Biberist, Switzerland. He underwent training in psycholytic therapy during the 1988–93 period in Switzerland in which permis- sions were granted for several clinical professionals to work with LSD and MDMA. Peter is a member of the board of the Swiss Medical Association für Psy- cholytic Therapy (SAePT). He has been helpful in giving advice and inspiration in setting up our cur- rent UK-based MDMA studies.

Ralph Metzner is a US psychologist whose tow- ering status in psychedelic research was assured early on in his career as a founding member, alongside Timothy Leary and Richard Alpert, of the clinical team at Harvard University who in the early 1960s started the Harvard Psilocy- bin Project. The rest is, of course, history. Ralph has continued throughout his life to study, teach and learn about psychedelics; with an interest in ayahuasca. He is currently Professor Emeri- tus of psychology at the California Institute of Integral Studies in San Francisco and continues to inspire new generations of followers to take up the mantle of psychedelic research.

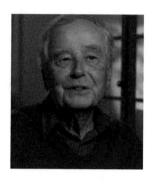

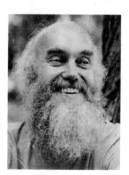

Ram Dass (aka Richard Alpert) was one of the founding members of the Harvard Psilocybin Proj- ect alongside Timothy Leary and Ralph Metzner in the early 1960s. From there he drifted Eastward into the spiritual maelstrom of India and became a deeply respected and warmly loved figure of inspi- ration for many millions of followers across the globe. A firm supporter of Breaking Convention — appearing by video-link at the 2011 meeting — he now lives in Hawaii and continues to spread love from there.

Rick Doblin studied psychology and policy stud- ies and founded the Multidisciplinary Association of Psychedelic Studies (MAPS) in 1986, which he continues to direct[73]. He remains at the forefront of psychedelic research as a popular figure inspiring new generations of young psychedelic researchers all over the world. Years from now, when MDMA and other psychedelics are commonplace and the

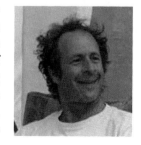

dust has settled after the end of the War on Drugs it is figures like Rick, who has encouraged so many young people to get involved, that we will see being erected as statues in town squares. A more dedicated yet humble person you would be hard pushed to find and I feel privileged to call him a good friend.

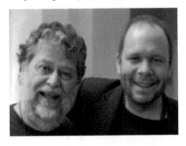

Rick Strassman is Clinical Associate Professor of Psychiatry at the University of New Mexico School of Medicine and president and co-founder of the Cottonwood Research Foundation, which is dedicated to consciousness research. In 1995, he published the first human psychedelic research study in modern times, paving the way for the resurgence of work since, when he studied the subjective psychological effects of DMT on healthy volunteers[74]. The subsequent publication of his book, *DMT: The Spirit Molecule*[75] in 2000, has enthused a whole new generation of interest in the subject of psychedelics and sent many people on searches into the pineal gland. Other publications include *Inner Paths to Outer Space* (2008)[76] and *DMT and the Soul of Prophecy* (2014)[77].

Richard Yensen played a vital role in psychedelic research during that 'dark ages' hiatus in the mid-1970s as a Research Fellow at the Maryland Psychiatric Research Center from 1972 to 1976. Richard (pictured left, in Oakland in 2013), studied psychotherapy extensively with the compound MDA[78] (which is related to MDMA) and is currently a licensed psychologist in California and director of the Orenda Institute in Vancouver and Cortes Island, British Columbia, Canada and president of the Salvador Roquet Psychosynthesis Association.

Rita Kočrová is a psychologist from the Czech Republic. She is the coordinator of the *Beyond Psychedelics* international psychedelic research conference, which had its first outing in Autumn 2016. She has studied the important role played by Dr Milan Hausner's long history of LSD therapies provided by the Sadska Hospital in Prague[79] and she now works on the ongoing psilocybin studies underway in the Czech Republic.

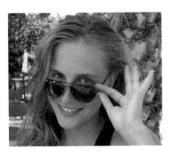

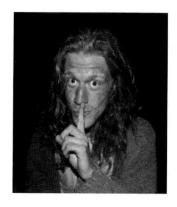

Robert Dickins is a UK academic who formed the Psychedelic Press in 2008 as a website, that has since grown into a successful publishing company housing many books and producing a bi-monthly journal[80]. Rob has an extensive knowledge of psychedelic literature and he brings this love of the subject into his highly successful business. The PsyPress journal provides an essential platform for UK and international showcased talent; from established researchers and writers to up-and-coming psychonautical enthusiasts. His book *Out of the Shadows* published in 2015 is a fascinating collection of greatest hits from the PsyPress journal. He is also a writer in his own right and is integral to the Breaking Convention organizational committee.

Robert Forte is a professor at the California Institute of Integral Studies. Having worked with both Mircea Eliade and Stanislav Grof, his qualifications for understanding the role of psychedelics and society are considerable. He is the editor of several recent important books on psychedelics: *Entheogens and the Future of Religion*[81], *Outside Looking In*[82] (about Timothy Leary) and *The Road To Eleusis: Unveiling the Secret of the Mysteries*, by Wasson, Hofmann and Ruck. Robert has a deep and influential interest in the power of entheogens to inform our social, spiritual,

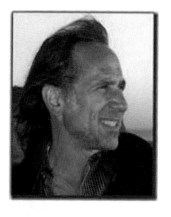

creative and athletic development; including some interesting ideas about how magic mushrooms can improve our understanding and mastery of golf. He is appropriately suspicious of governmental influences on human creativity and psychospiritual growth.

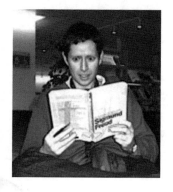

Robin Carhart-Harris is a psychopharmacologist from the UK, with an unusual training in rather separate fields. His dual degrees in psychoanalysis and psychopharmacology have prepared him perfectly to be the person to explore the neural apparatus, with a keen eye on both the physiology and the psychology of brain function. Having met him in

Basel in 2006 and then worked beside him in Bristol University psycho-pharmacology department, we have become close friends. Carhart-Harris's contributions to psychedelic research in this country have been prolific from the beginning. His recent work exploring the neurobiological mechanisms of action of psilocybin, MDMA and LSD and psilocybin's potential for treating depression has given the field of neuroscience plenty to think about. He now works at Imperial University, London[84]. There is certainly far more to come from Robin and his window boxes.

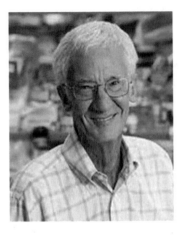

Roland Griffiths is Professor of Behavioral Biology and Neuroscience at Johns Hopkins University School of Medicine and a senior board member of the Heffter Research Institute[85]. As a doctor with an interest in alcoholism and psychopharmacology, he consults for innumerable organizations and institutions worldwide, and has been publishing in the academic field since 1969. But it is his recent work with psilocybin that has attracted enormous attention from the psychedelic community. Having explored, in 2006, psilocybin's ability to produce spontaneous spiritual experiences, he is now going on to determine the extent to which the drug can produce lasting positive personality changes and how this might be applied to two fields of psychiatry that are notoriously difficult to treat: addictions and personality disorders. Pictured here, with David Luke, catching a morning coffee by the canal side, before delivering our respective talks at the International Conference on Psychedelic Research, Amsterdam, 2016.

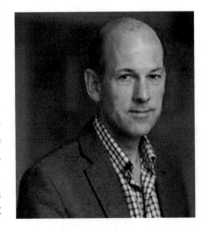

Rupert McShane is a British psychiatrist working clinically and academically at Oxford University He is carrying out a large study into ketamine as a treatment for depression[86]. It was a great pleasure having him come and speak to the delegates at Breaking Convention 2015.

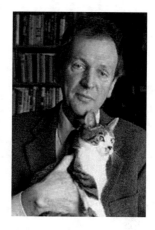

Rupert Sheldrake has risen to fame for his esoteric ideas that transcend mainstream scientific thinking. His theories challenge our understanding of the very fabric of the universe and the forces that hold it together. He also presents a healthy oppositional view about the dogma of modern scientific models[87]. Always a keen supporter of altered states of consciousness, he sees the value of psychedelics as tools for individuals' personal growth and development, and as agents of change for a scientific community that needs to broaden its horizons of nature's possibilities. And we've finally snared him for Breaking Convention in 2017.

Shlomi Raz is an important figure in emerging applied research. He founded the private company Eleusis in 2013 to discover and develop innovative, first-in-class therapies utilising serotonergic psychedelic compounds. Having come from a corporate city background, Shlomi has the skills and courage to take psychedelic research in new directions, with a bold vision of harnessing the therapeutic potential of psychedelic drugs for the collective benefit of humanity.

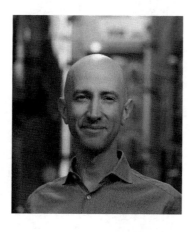

Stanislav Grof is a psychiatrist from Czechoslovakia who, following his immersion into psychedelic research in

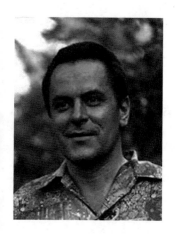

the 1950s, then moved to the USA where he carried out many years of pioneering research using LSD therapy at Spring Grove Hospital in Maryland; particularly as a tool to assist the existential process of dying[88,89,90]. He subsequently went on to develop a formal method for conducting psychotherapy in non-drug induced altered states of consciousness, the Breathwork technique, which has become an important grounding technique for many of the world's psychedelic therapists[91]. He writes wonderfully and continues to inspire many followers into the field.

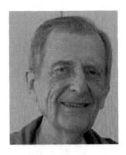

Stanley Krippner is an American psychologist and parapsychologist. He has been working in the psychedelic research field since the 60s and has written extensively on creativity[92], hypnosis, shamanism, altered states of consciousness, dream telepathy and parapsychological subjects.

Stephen Reid is a multitalented, media savvy activist who formed the UK's *Psychedelic Society* in 2014. Under his inspirational guidance local branches have sprung up in Edinburgh, Newcastle, Manchester, Liverpool, Leeds, Bristol and Brighton. The Society fosters a spirit of active participation with the goal of changing hearts and minds, debunking myths about psychedelics and tackling the long-term prohibitions that result in increased risks to psychedelic users and the public. He is pictured here talk-

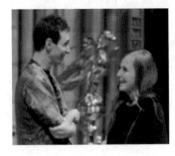

ing to Rita, the organiser of the Czech Republic's Beyond Psychedelics conference.

Stephen Szara is a psychiatrist and chemist from Hungary who pioneered the study of DMT in the 1950s[93]. He was one of the first scientists to pro-

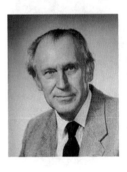

pose that the psychedelic state could teach us something useful about understanding neuroscience and further the field of psychotherapy. He is now an Emeritus Fellow of the American College of Neuropsychopharmacology and Collegium Internationale Neuro-Psychopharmacologicum, and a member of the Scientific Advisory Board of the Heffter Research Institute.

Susan Blackmore is a psychologist with a special interest in memetics (the study of memes) and has become widely known through her book *The Meme Machine*[96]. She is also a well-known broadcaster in the UK and never shies from supporting broad-minded and progressive research. She has a degree in parapsychology and has spoken out vociferously in support of psychedelic research.

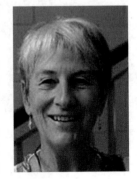

Teri Krebs is a psychedelic researcher from Norway, who together with her colleague, **Pal Johansen**, has contributed numerous papers to the

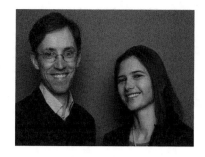

field in recent years. Their important large scale population-based epidemiological study demonstrated that recreational psychedelic use is associated with improved, not worsened lifetime mental health[97]. Teri and Pal also revisited the LSD studies for alcohol use disorder of the 1960s with a meta-analysis, demonstrating an overall positive effect size[98]. Teri (pictured her with Pal, two inspiriational people) has been an important has been an important influence on me; encouraging me in my presentations to use the word 'safety' instead of 'risks' when described psychedelics to the public. Her research has demonstrated that for most people these drugs are virtually harmless and bring many psychological and well-being benefits.

Thomas Roberts is a professor at the Department of Leadership, Educational Psychology and Foundations at Northern Illinois University, USA. He has had a long history studying the psychedelic drugs and their impact on the development of the human species. He has been teaching his students about this subject since the 1980s and is also author of the wonderfully futuristic and enthusiastic book *Psychedelic Horizons*[98] and co-editor of the two-volume *Psychedelic Medicine*[95].

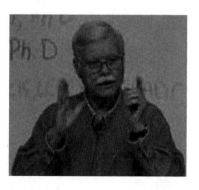

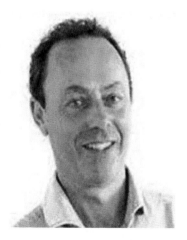

Tim Read is a psychiatrist from London, trained in Holotropic Breathwork and a superb supporter of psychedelic research and practice. Through his publishing house Muswell Hill Press[97] he has brought non-ordinary states of consciousness to the attention of millions with his fine collection of published works from many talented and particularly attractive authors.

Tim Williams is a consultant psychiatrist from Bristol, who has been a willing and experienced study doctor on many, if not

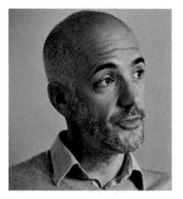

most, of the UK psychedelic studies of recent years. He has certainly dosed me on several occasions. As medical director of psychiatric services in Bristol his presence and experience has been invaluable when proposing psychedelic research in that town.

Torsten Passie is Assistant Professor for Consciousness Studies at Hannover Medical School

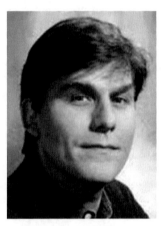

in Germany. For more than twenty years he has studied psychedelic drugs, altered states of consciousness and clinical shamanic practices. Torsten has worked with Hanscarl Leuner, a leading authority on psychedelic drugs and carried out research with cannabis, ketamine, nitrous oxide, and psilocybin. In 2011, he published a detailed account of the psychopharmacology of LSD[99,100].

Valerie Curran is Professor of Psychopharmacology at University College London,

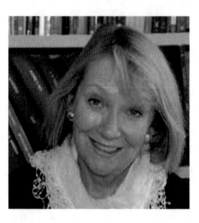

where she specialises in research that links our understanding of how drugs work at a neurotransmitter level with how they are producing subjective psychological and cognitive effects. During her career, she has carried out important work with cannabis, ketamine and MDMA[101]. As clinical lead in her local NHS Substance Misuse Service, she is keen to see that her research accurately reflects the risk and safety profiles of the psychedelic drugs. In this respect, she has contributed valuably to the evidence-based argument about the relative safety of MDMA-assisted psychotherapy.

William 'Bill' Richards is a psychologist who cut his psychedelic teeth in the 1960s and '70s working at the Maryland Psychiatric Institute alongside Walter Pahnke, Stan Grof and Richard Yensen. With a special interest

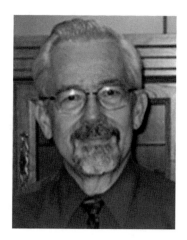

and expertise in the connections between the psychedelic state and mysticism he has been at the forefront of psychedelic research throughout his life; working with the team at Johns Hopkins University[102].

Together with the reams of important people not included in this list (I do apologise!), these people are continuing to contribute to the development of psychedelic research as a valid topic for mainstream scientific and social study in the 21st century and beyond. One thing all these people have in common is their ability to move seamlessly through the obscure world of today's psychedelic community while also being able to orientate themselves within the environment of modern research and media platforms. The capacity to do this is essential if we are to see these compounds returning to mainstream practice and study.

CHAPTER 9

The Psychedelic Renaissance Part Two: Contemporary Studies

Evidence-based practice!
When do we want it
After peer review!
— Banner held by anonymous protester at a 2011 Occupy March

When Did the Psychedelic Renaissance Begin?

The truth is psychedelic research never stopped entirely, but after LSD was made illegal it certainly drastically reduced in volume, and ceased being mainstream by the end of the 1960s. After this point, it was difficult to obtain a licence to research or work clinically with psychedelic drugs. Sandoz also stopped distributing its product and recalled all remaining stocks from people who had stockpiled *Delysid*, although, by then, many other places were synthesizing the drug. Czechoslovakia had a particularly good record for LSD manufacture. While these restrictions significantly reduced psychedelic research, not everyone gave up. Behind the Iron Curtain, beyond the restrictions of the Western World's struggle with the developing drug culture, LSD research continued — especially in Czechoslovakia up until 1974 in Sadska under Dr Milan Hausner[1]. leaving a rich legacy of psychedelic interest throughout that country[2].

In the UK, any psychiatrists who still had supplies of LSD could continue prescribing it if they wished; and this carried on into the 1970s, with the last recorded dose being given to a patient in private practice in 1976[9]. As noted, the next time a classical psychedelic was legally given to anyone in the UK was 33 years later, when David Nutt injected me with psilocybin[3].

MDMA emerged in the late seventies and was used legally by a small handful of therapists right up to 1985. When it was banned, there followed a further 25 years of persistent campaigning to get the next MDMA human clinical research published.

Superficially the 1970s and '80s do look a bit like the Dark Ages for psychedelic research. There was certainly a big comedown from the exuberance enjoyed in the fifties and sixties, but not all the lights were out. In 1971 Nixon launched The War On Drugs (though of course legislation to limit the range of legally sanctioned states of consciousness had actually been in place since the beginning of the century). Throughout the world psychedelics found themselves targeted by politicians. There were still some medical voices prepared to stand up for psychedelic research, but once LSD was banned most doctors were not happy to work outside the law. There were simply not enough medics prepared to stand up to the antipsychedelic stance forced upon the profession by paranoid governments[4].

In the 1970s it became a fashionable topic in psychiatric research to propose biological mechanisms for schizophrenia. The psychoanalytical and 'schizophrenogenic mother' theories of the 1950s were being rapidly eroded as the profession learned more about neurobiology[5]. With the prevailing social attack on psychedelics in the early 1970s, there was a flurry of research proposing links between drugs and schizophrenia and LSD was one of the first candidates explored. Despite the lack of similarities between the psychedelic state and schizophrenia that had been adequately dismissed by the psychedelic researchers of the 1960s, the suggestion that LSD could *cause* schizophrenia became hotly debated[6]. Whilst it is arguable that a person with pre-existing psychosis ought best to avoid psychedelics for fear of precipitating an acute episode, there were, at the time, many important objections against the suggestion that LSD causes schizophrenia; including the phenomenological distinctions and the lack of epidemiological correlations[7]. The overall rates of schizophrenia did not increase during the wide scale use of LSD nor decline as the drug became less popular in subsequent decades. As discussed earlier, schizophrenia has remained at a reasonably steady rate throughout the world, for generations, with a lifetime prevalence of around 1%. And as the 1970s progressed and more research emerged it became clear that other drugs, not the psychedelics, were more likely candidates as a primary cause for schizophrenia[8]. Most studies found higher associations between schizophrenia and the use of potent dopamine agonists such as cocaine and amphetamine, as opposed to the use of hallucinogens.

However, LSD and her cousins remained under the spotlight as drugs that cause harm. And throughout the 1970s, LSD became difficult to get hold of for legal medical uses. By then it did look as if it was all over for LSD as a mainstream treatment for mental illness. What a long, strange trip it had been.

So, although psychedelic research never completely went away, in the last 20 years we have seen an unprecedented growth of psychedelic interest *within the mainstream*, which is what this renaissance is all about.

How to Get a Drug to Market

For those not familiar with how a research team gets a drug approved as a clinical medicine, I will give a very brief description of the process[10].

Many clinical treatments in medicine first arise out of accidental anecdotal experience. Many others arise because a pharmaceutical company has specifically designed a new molecule with a target in mind. When a new chemical emerges in this way, there are pre-clinical studies that must be carried out to test whether the chemical is safe to be given to humans. *In vitro* tests involve adding concentrations of the chemical to isolated slices of tissues (heart, lungs, kidneys, brain, etc.) to determine the drug's toxicity. The new chemical will also be tested against animal models, which provides further information about safety and toxicity. This process of animal testing is highly controversial for many people outside the field of pharmacology and understandably often arouses a strong emotional response — especially amongst many in the psychedelic community. Nevertheless, it is doubtful LSD would have ever made it out of Hofmann's lab without such studies. (Whether someone else might have discovered LSD had Hofmann not, remains an interesting question).

The next part of the process of drug development is known as 'Phase I clinical studies' in which the drug is tested on healthy human volunteers; that is, people without the specific disorder the drug is intended to treat. The purpose of such tests is to gather information about appropriate safe doses and subjective effects of the new drug. Volunteers, often students at the university where the research is being carried out, are usually paid for their services. I have taken part in lots of such trials, though never paid, because I find them interesting. Once this part is over, one can begin the Phase II studies. These involve small-scale clinical trials in which the drug is given to handfuls of patients with the disorder one is testing. Between 10 to 40 people is usual.

Clinical studies must be rigorously designed to reduce as many aspects of bias as possible. The gold standard for drug development is the double-blind placebo controlled randomised study in which identically matched subjects are randomly assigned into a control group or an experimental group. Then one group gets the active drug and the other gets the placebo drug (they look identical). Neither the subjects nor the examiners who will be testing the subjects' outcomes know which group has been given which drug. In this way one hopes to demonstrate that any differences seen in outcomes between the two groups can be put down entirely to the physiological action of the drug and not due to any influences from either the test subjects or the experimenters.

After Phase II comes Phase III, in which the established best treatment regime with the new drug is rolled out to larger, multicentre groups for wide-scale testing on clinical patients. In this way, many hundreds of patients will receive treatment under a standardised protocol to ensure uniform results. From here the drug may then go out to market but under a very restricted license. Thousands of patients will get to use it in an open-label fashion (that is, they know what they are taking, rather than blindly) and their doctors will closely monitor their process and document any adverse effects to the drug company.

The timescale and costs of the process described above are extremely variable. It can take between 5 and 20 years to get a drug to market in this way. Today the average cost of getting a brand-new drug to market is around £75 million.

How This Research Method Relates to Psychedelic Drugs

The interesting thing about the psychedelic drugs is that we have literally tens of millions of cases of anecdotal uses of the drugs LSD, psilocybin, MDMA, ketamine, ibogaine, ayahuasca, cannabis and others over many decades — largely with safe and positive therapeutic effects. This is great, but because these 'clinical' uses have been occurring outside of the official clinical environment such cases are not enough for the regulatory authorities to immediately support these drugs becoming licensed medicines. And although people have been consuming psychedelic drugs for millennia and their toxicity profiles are low, we still must carry out all the pre-clinical studies described above. Only once the drugs are deemed safe for human consumption using the standardized tests, can the Phase I dosage studies on healthy volunteers take place. Then, if they are successful, the drug can go to Phase II and then Phase III studies.

One might have thought that the costs and timescales for getting psychedelic drugs to market ought to be quicker than for a newly invented chemical with no documented human use, but this is not the case. Although we may already know from anecdotal use it is relatively safe, this does not count as sufficient data for regulatory authorities. Furthermore, because the psychedelic drugs are all controlled or illegal drugs, one must have government approval to work with them, which means jumping through many legal and political loopholes and even putting up with unwanted media intrusions into one's research. The sum of the unbelievably harsh regulatory processes applied to this kind of research makes the process prohibitively lengthy and costly — as we have seen earlier with the hard road from MDMA being banned in 1985 to the publication of the first Phase II study in 2010. If MDMA, a drug which is not new, but rather one with a very well-known level of toxicity and a record of safety at dosages recommended for therapy, *does* finally get its license in 2021, as MAPS are planning, this mean it has taken at least 35 years to get to market.

Looking at the Contemporary Research for the Drugs

Below, we will look at each of the major psychedelic compounds in turn, outlining some of the published studies and discussing some of the future planned projects. It is a great pleasure to state that because of the rapidly expanding growth of this subject this section will be outdated even before it is published.

1. MDMA

Contemporary Clinical Research Completed

Most contemporary research with MDMA has centred on its role as an adjunct to trauma-focused psychotherapy for PTSD. I have described above in preceding chapters why MDMA is so perfectly suited for this kind of work. It is almost as if the drug were designed with this purpose in mind (though this is not actually the case). Having experienced first-hand the massive difficulties in helping stuck patients with repressed and intrusive memories of severe psychological trauma, my colleagues and I are absolutely committed to putting ourselves behind this research.

The Multidisciplinary Association for Psychedelic Studies (MAPS) lead the way in global MDMA-for-PTSD studies. In preparation for their forthcoming Phase III studies MAPS has amassed an impressive pool of data from Phase II studies in USA, Switzerland, Israel and Canada. The first study (now referred to as their 'flagship' study) was that carried out by Michael Mithoefer et al., and published in 2010[11].

In this initial study Michael Mithoefer, together with his co-therapist wife, the enigmatic Annie Mithoefer, provided MDMA-assisted psychotherapy for 20 patients with chronic PTSD, refractory to both psychotherapy and psychopharmacology. 12 patients received inactive placebo and eight received two or three sessions of MDMA (initial dose of 125mg, followed two hours later by a further booster of 62.5mg). Both groups received a course of preparatory and follow-up non-drug psychotherapy. Using the Clinician-Administered PTSD Scale (CAPS) as a primary outcome measure, Mithoefer demonstrated that at two and twelve-month follow-up 83% of the experimental group no longer met the criteria for PTSD, compared to just 25% of the patients in the placebo group. He also looked at neurocognitive and neurophysiological measures and showed that there were no drug-related serious adverse events, adverse neurocognitive effects or clinically significant blood pressure increases.

The Mithoefers' study set a high benchmark for others to follow. Since the publication of this initial study in 2010, the Mithoefers immediately began collecting long-term follow-up data. And in 2013 they published the results of the long-term follow-up study — having tracked the cohort of successfully treated patients with severe PTSD for up to four years after the initial single course of MDMA-assisted psychotherapy. The results showed that rates of remission were maintained; without having any further doses of MDMA since the original study, over 80% of the original cohort remain free from the diagnosis of PTSD[12].

When the incredibly positive results of the flagship pilot study were released in 2010 there were initially some critical responses; with some commentators finding fault with the impossibility of maintaining the blind control. Other critics attributed the positive results to the fact that the Mithoefers themselves were so inspirational and positive that such strongly significant results could never be reproducible in further studies. However, as we can see below, the MAPS armoury of positive MDMA-PTSD results now extends far beyond the magical reach of just Michael and Annie; a mantle I am certain they are happy to hand on to others in the field.

The MDMA/PTSD Switzerland Study by Oehen et al

As the world persisted seamlessly into 2013, and the pseudo-scientific elements of the psychedelic community came to terms with the realization that the ending of the Mayan calendar had absolutely no demonstrable effect on the planet, PTSD continued to be high on the agenda for psychedelic research. That year Peter Oehen published the results of his MAPS-sponsored Swiss MDMA Psychotherapy study for treatment-resistant PTSD. Together with co-therapist, Verena Widmer, Oehen's was a smaller study than Mithoefer's and although there was a definite trend in the direction of MDMA therapy being superior to placebo, at first sight the statistics failed to demonstrate a significant reduction in CAPS for the experimental subjects[13]. However, Henri Chabrol of Toulouse University looked at the data again using effect size as a measure. Chabrol concluded that Oehen had

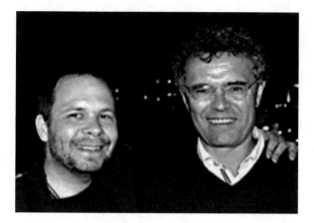

Picture 70: Few psychedelic therapists in recent times have had the experiential opportunities of (legal) therapy that Peter Oehen and his close colleagues received as part of the Swiss Psycholytic Society open training between 1988–1993. They have all gone on to do great things. Here is Peter in San Francisco in 2013.

been overly conservative and the results *were* indicative of MDMA psychotherapy providing substantial improvements for treatment resistant PTSD[14].

Recent MDMA Studies Terminated Early

Given the complexities of MDMA research in today's political climate, not all of those proposed have managed to get off the ground. The following studies illustrate the difficulties involved in clinical research with psychedelic compounds. The hurdles can sometimes feel insurmountable and the scale of problems faced are testament to the sheer determination of those researchers who initiate such work.

The Spanish MDMA for PTSD study was run by José Carlos Bouso in Madrid. It started in 1999, then, in 2002, after treating just six of 29 planned patients, the permission was revoked and the study was shut down because of political pressure.

An MDMA study run by John Halpern at Harvard University planned to explore the role for MDMA-assisted therapy to treat Anxiety Secondary to Advanced Stage Cancer. It began recruiting soon after its approval in 2004 and planned to treat twelve subjects. But only one subject completed the study and after the second subject dropped out the study was closed due to enrolment challenges.

Another MAPS-sponsored MDMA study that was initially planned, but has sadly floundered since 2011, is the one in Jordan. A team lead by

Nasser Shuriquie from Amman continue to await Jordanian approval to begin their project.

Similarly, in Australia a team lead by Stuart Saker and Fiona MacKenzie from Sydney got to the stage of working with MAPS to develop a protocol for their MDMA/PTSD study, which has since met with authoritarian resistance and failed to progress.

It is also worthy of note that Dr. Charles Grob's study of psilocybin therapy for end-stage cancer patients was originally planning to use MDMA, until the regulatory barriers to using MDMA were considered insurmountable, when Grob switched to psilocybin.

Further MDMA Studies Underway

Given the problems described above, at the time of writing this 2nd edition of this book we have had only two contemporary completed and published clinical studies for MDMA-assisted psychotherapy. But there are many new studies that are either still ongoing, completed or awaiting publication.

MDMA / PTSD in Veterans Study

Following the success of his pilot study, Mithoefer went on to study the role of MDMA-assisted psychotherapy specifically for treating military veterans, firefighters and police officers ("first responders") with service-related PTSD. This is a very important topic and a shrewd move on the part of the Mithoefers and MAPS. The non-evidence based politically biased wars in Iraq, Afghanistan, Syria and Yemen are taking their toll on the US and UK military personnel and nations at large. Governments are spending billions in disability payments for tens of thousands of sufferers of post-combat PTSD returning from warzones. It has become a medical, financial and political problem of growing proportions. The military is desperate for a way out, but the current treatments for PTSD are less than perfect and too many veterans are going untreated.

Some commentators within the psychedelic community object strongly to psychedelic researchers working with the military; citing that there ought to be no part for psychedelic research aimed at treating veterans of America's arrogant wars. But, thankfully, Doblin and Mithoefer — neither of them supporters of war themselves — do not see things this way. Rather, they accept that if the military is going to continue to do what it is doing, then someone must be there to pick up the casualties. And if MDMA can offer a ray of hope to such hapless sufferers then that is all well and good.

MDMA/PTSD U.S. Relapse Study

Michael Mithoefer has also revisited the original cohort that relapsed following their initial treatment with MDMA in his flagship pilot study. The idea is to explore whether some extra booster sessions with MDMA-assisted therapy can demonstrate that the positive effects of the treatment can be maintained, even for those people that relapsed. This study marks an important precedent. So far MDMA clinical research has been burdened by the need to show that MDMA therapy acts like a one-off magic bullet. By why should that be the case? After all, the current traditional treatments for PTSD involve taking *daily* SSRI drugs and carrying out multiple courses of trauma-focused psychotherapy. Who says, therefore, that in order to be considered efficacious, MDMA-therapy must work the first time if it is to be deemed a success? This study by Mithoefer, when published, may set the trend for repeated courses of MDMA-assisted therapy for those subjects whose severity of PTSD warrants such an approach.

International MDMA Research in the Pipeline

MAPS, Heffter and The Beckley Foundation are truly international. They are working with clinical teams all over the world, gathering and pooling their resources. The eventual goal of these organisations is to submit their data to regulatory authorities in support of seeing psychedelic compounds licensed as treatments for clinical medicine. Whilst Heffter has tended to concentrate solely on psilocybin in recent years, MAPS have focused primarily on MDMA.

Since the original Mithoefer Phase II MDMA-PTSD study there are now multiple ongoing MAPS-sponsored MDMA-PTSD studies.

These include one in Boulder, Colorado, USA, run by principal investigator Marcela Ot'alora. Also in the States is the Conjoint Therapy Study, in Charleston, South Carolina, in which Michael Mithoefer is working with Candice Monson and Julie Holland in a study exploring Cognitive-Behavioural Conjoint Therapy (CBCT) integrated with MDMA-assisted psychotherapy for the treatment of PTSD. In a departure from Mithoefer's previous study design, this study is being delivered for ten pairs of participants consisting of one person diagnosed with PTSD, and another who does not have a PTSD diagnosis but who is experiencing problems associated with their partner's PTSD. This study opens a whole new paradigm for MDMA research. Given its novelty, this study is not placebo-controlled but rather an open-label design — meaning all participants know they are given MDMA.

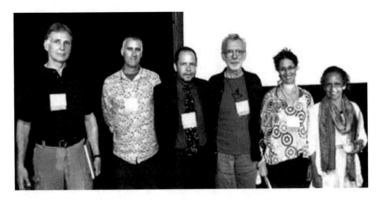

Picture 71: Speakers on the International MDMA Research symposium, at Psychedelic Science, Oakland, USA, 2013. Representing ongoing projects from Canada, Israel, USA, Australia and the UK. Featuring: Jim Grigsby, Martin Williams, Andrew Feldmar and Marcela Ot'alora.

In Vancouver, Canada, principle investigator Ingrid Pacey together with Andrew Feldmar is running another MAPS-sponsored MDMA-PTSD study. And in Beer Yaakov, Israel, another MDMA-PTSD study is being run by Principal Investigator Moshe Kotler.

Having submitted the pooled data of these studies, MAPS' plan is to eventually run a series of Phase III studies within the next few years, with a goal to see MDMA licensed by the FDA in America by 2021. If all goes to plan this form of PTSD treatment could be entering mainstream practice within the next 10 years. Now wouldn't that be amazing?

The Cardiff MDMA/PTSD Study: Its Development and Growth

For at least ten years, since first meeting Michael Mithoefer at the ENCP conference in Vienna, I have been talking to MAPS about a wish to develop a UK-based MDMA study. We have been through several different ideas before settling on our current approach. A big problem at first was finding a group of psychotherapists and psychologists willing to work on such a project. I never had any problems gathering the psychopharmacology support (having had David Nutt on board from the beginning), but the psychotherapy side was proving more challenging. Then I met Jonathan Bisson in 2009 when I was invited with Mithoefer and Grob to convene a panel on psychedelic therapy for the Royal College of Psychiatrists annual conference in Liverpool. Bisson, who is ex-services himself, is the lead of a large clinical research facility at Cardiff University, which specialises in cases of post-combat trauma. He sees hundreds of new cases every year and is an open-minded doctor with a passionate desire to try anything that could reliably work to improve the treatment rates for PTSD.

However, after several years of trying, we failed to find funding for our initial planned therapeutic study and it ran to ground. But now the Cardiff study is back up and running, with a jointly-funded quartet of financial backers, including MAPS, the Beckley Foundation and Anton Bilton of the Tyringham Research Institute. The current study design involves myself and Welsh psychiatrist, Mat Hoskins, assisted by co-therapist Chrissie Turner-Wilson. We plan to give patients with treatment-resistant PTSD either MDMA or placebo, and perform fMRI on them as we get them to recall their trauma histories.

The hypothesis is that on MDMA, compared to placebo, participants will show a reduced fear response, which through neuroimaging, we hope to demonstrate is associated with reduced amygdala and boosted pre-frontal cortex responses. The study will be carried out at the new CUBRIC-2 imaging centre in Cardiff and is sponsored by Cardiff University. It will add valuable data towards the raft of clinical studies underway; demonstrating the physiological substrate for MDMA-assisted psychotherapy's effects. Although this is, strictly speaking, not a therapeutic study (we will not be providing any formal psychotherapy for the participants), we hope to demonstrate that even a single dose of MDMA, delivered in facilitative setting by trained MDMA therapists, can have a positive effect on the

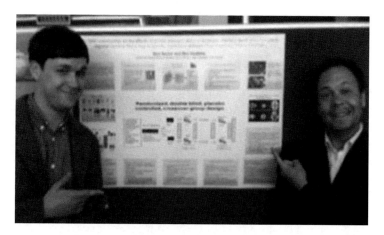

Picture 72: Mat Hoskins, psychiatrist from Cardiff University with a keen eye on the evitable role MDMA will play in the future of his profession. Here displaying our poster of our Cardiff plans at an event at Imperial College London to mark the press launch of Robin Carhart-Harris' LSD study results in 2016.

participants' PTSD symptoms. Indeed, this 'MDMA-*lite*' approach could even herald a new model for global MDMA therapy in the future. Demonstrating the clinical deliverability of MDMA in a standard NHS clinic, is, we feel, an essential component of MDMA research if we are to convince the regulatory authorities that it is not only experienced and inspirational experts like Mithoefer and Oehen that can make this sort of therapy effective.

Original Ideas for New MDMA Research

So far, I have mostly talked about MDMA therapy as an agent to manage PTSD, but that need not be the limit of its effectiveness as a clinical tool. Indeed, there are some other theoretical uses for MDMA described below, and some interesting pilot studies are now getting underway around the world.

MDMA for Depression

What about MDMA for depression? MDMA has a very clear effect on raising mood and improving feelings of wellbeing. After all, that is why 750,000 people *every weekend* in the UK take the drug recreationally. But what happens when depressed people take MDMA[15]? Because of the gap in our knowledge about therapeutic applications for MDMA, this question cannot yet be answered with confidence. The theoretical potential of using MDMA as a potent serotonin-enhancer to treat depression has been postulated by Riedlinger and Montagne in a chapter in Julie Holland's *Ecstasy* book[16]. But there is very little empirical clinical information regarding the effects of MDMA on depressed patients. There exist numerous anecdotal reports of the expected transient rise in mood during recreational use of MDMA by depressed people, but for a significant minority this is followed by a subsequent depressed mood and other associated unpleasant psychological and physiological 'hangover' effects. Because of these negative effects, there is little evidence — anecdotal or otherwise — of depressed people carrying out long-term self-medication with MDMA.

The existence of a hangover associated with MDMA is well documented by recreational users of Ecstasy. Among Ecstasy users, this hangover effect (sometimes called the 'mid-week blues' or 'Suicide Tuesday'), may last for between one and seven days, exacerbated by the adverse environmental circumstances in which recreational Ecstasy is often consumed (i.e., at night with consequent sleep deprivation, missing meals, excessive physical exertion and often being taken with other psychoactive drugs, including alcohol). No one has ever explored the MDMA mid-week blues in detail with a controlled clinical study, despite it being such a prevalent narrative amongst ravers. In our two forthcoming MDMA studies in Cardiff and Bristol we will be assessing mood, sleep distur-bance and suicidal measures for five-to-seven days post-MDMA in 40 patients. This might shed some light on the phenomenon. But a better study would be one that rigorously tests MDMA versus placebo in sub-jects who are variously exposed to lack of sleep versus being allowed to sleep, being allowed food versus being starved, after vigorous exercise versus relaxation, with cannabis and other drugs versus no other concomi-tant drugs; thereby mimicking all the various 'raving' experiences. *Then* we might get a better idea as to whether the mid-week post-MDMA blues truly exist or not. Sounds like a great study — but one fraught with ethical considerations.

There is certainly a place, however, for a trial that examines the pos-sible role for MDMA in treating depression. Recreationally, and in the cur-rent MDMA-assisted psychotherapy studies, subjects tend to use doses of 120mg plus. But it is not known what effect the drug may have if taken at much smaller dosages (say 10–25mg) for longer periods of time. Taken repeatedly at these lower doses, could sub-threshold MDMA microdosing have a gradual, beneficial effect on mood? One might expect the drug to have similar effects to the SSRI drugs, but because one need not wait for serotonin levels to build up slowly through inhibiting re-uptake of the neu-rotransmitter, one might propose the mood-enhancing effects of low-dose MDMA might be noticed much quicker than with an SSRI drug. And per-haps, if taken in such low doses, there might not be such a dramatic rebound serotonin depletion causing a significant hangover effect. The possibility of using MDMA to lift mood early and then transfer to an SSRI or other antidepressant to continue longer term might be considered. Be on the lookout to see if this sort of research emerges to explore whether MDMA could be developed as an antidepressant.

MDMA as an Alternative to ECT

One area where MDMA's rapid onset of action may be of use clinically is in circumstances where mood elevation is required quickly for emergency reasons and there is no time to wait for up to six weeks for the antidepres-sant effects of traditional drugs. In these situations, the current treatment is electro-convulsive therapy (ECT). In this scenario, could MDMA be used instead of ECT[15,16]?

ECT, like psychedelic therapy, is one of those great areas of psychia-try where there exist many erroneous preconceptions in the public that have the net result of withholding an effective, safe, cheap and relatively unobtrusive treatment from those patients who might otherwise benefit from it. The general public's understanding of ECT is appallingly bad. This is the case, at least, in the Western world. It is of note that in many non-Western countries they queue up for ECT, which they do not consider to be nearly as barbaric as we do in the West (perhaps because the 1976 film *One Flew Over the Cuckoo's Nest* was not seen so prolifically). Indeed, in India the general public consider the practice of taking daily doses of drugs as treatments for depression — as we are so prone to do here — to be far more invasive and unsavoury than a few quick and effective doses of electricity. So the idea that ECT is a bad thing can be seen as a cultural construct. This illustrates well that our opinions about psychiatric treatments are often based not on any particular evidence, but on where we live and what sort of propaganda we have been exposed to. All though I am sure some people within the profession of psychiatry would disagree with me, the vast majority of those with experience of working with severe mental illness will generally opt to choose ECT for resistant depression, as evidenced by a survey in which the majority of Indian psychiatrists themselves said it would be their first choice if they had severe depression[17].

In the West, we reserve ECT only for the most severe cases, those in which other treatments have failed or in which we need a rapid serotonin rush to kick-start someone out of the depths of severe — often catatonic — depression in which, by refusing food, the sufferer risks death by starvation. I have always been interested to know what would happen if you gave a high dose (say 150mg) of MDMA to a severely depressed catatonic patient. Who knows? My guess is that it would rapidly bounce them out of their catatonic state. If so, it could be life-saving.

So this is another study to look out for in coming years. Furthermore, because ECT is generally seen as such an unsavoury thing in the West then I believe a study that could be billed as 'the nail in the coffin for ECT' might get easily approved and supported.

MDMA for Social Anxiety in people with Autism

The idea of using MDMA to relieve anxiety associated with autism is currently being studied by Charles Grob and Alicia Danforth in a MAPS-sponsored randomised, double-blind, placebo-controlled exploratory **pilot study** in collaboration with the Los Angeles Biomedical Research Institute at Harbor-UCLA Medical Center and Stanford University[18,19].

Those with experience of autism — which certainly includes all child psychiatrists — will know that this is a spectrum of clinical disorders that

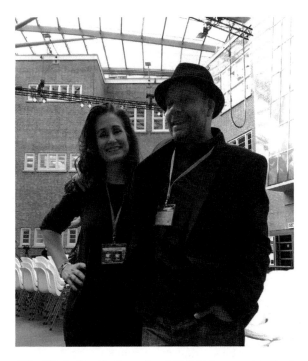

Picture 73: Alicia Danforth, using MDMA's capacity for boosting empathy to develop innovative approaches for treating social anxiety in adults with autism. Enjoying the Open Foundation's conference in Amsterdam in 2016.

share the common characteristics of restricted ranges of interest (obsessional behavioural or repetitive habits), impaired social functioning (characterised by a lack of understanding of social cues and rules), impaired communication, and abnormal use of language. At the more severe end of the spectrum sufferers may have learning difficulties and no development of speech and language at all. At the other end of the spectrum (sometimes called high-functioning autism or Asperger's Syndrome, although they are not quite the same thing), a person may have an abnormally high intelligence and very advanced language use but still suffer with social functioning difficulties and a tendency to be overly pedantic and inflexible.

One of the cardinal features of autism is a tendency for a sufferer to lack empathy. That is, they do not appear to recognise the emotional responses of others and may appear aloof and disinterested in other people's worlds. In this book, we have already described how MDMA has the effect of increasing levels of empathy in the user. Danforth and Grob's motivation to carry out such a study started came out of the observed anecdotal positive effects that autistic adults experience after taking recreational Ecstasy. Many demonstrate reduced empathy impairments during, and for some time after, the intoxication with the drug. This is certainly, therefore, an avenue worthy of further study. The current treatments for autism are largely either educational, social, functional or purely symptomatic — with the full range of psychiatric drugs used as and when they are needed. If MDMA can offer a way out of the 'locked in/locked out' aspect of social impairments secondary to autism, it would be greatly welcomed by those clinicians working with the condition.

Could MDMA-psychotherapy be Applied to Borderline Personality Disorder?

Aside from PTSD, as it appears in its 'simple' form (associated with discrete trauma such as post-combat-PTSD), a variation of the diagnosis is increasingly pervading psychiatry. It is now being applied in an expanded form as 'complex-PTSD', which refers to a history of trauma in which a person might not necessarily have had a single *life-threatening* traumatic episode, but might have suffered multiple episodes of non-life-threatening but equally frightening experiences of trauma — such as repetitive episodes of child sexual abuse. Such a history can lead to an emotionally unstable (for example, borderline) personality disorder (BPD), which is often very difficult to treat.

There are high rates of treatment resistance for BPD because the effects of repeated abuse render the sufferer highly prone to dissociative episodes in which they readily re-experience the frightening memories of their abuse. Whenever they attempt to 'go back there' in their thoughts, they dissociate, which may happen spontaneously at any time of the day, or in their nightmares. This makes undergoing trauma-focused psychotherapy (where the subject is *expected* to reflect upon their experience of abuse) extremely difficult. In such cases, an agent such as MDMA could be useful.

Clinically, I have seen many teenagers with emerging BPD. They so often present with a horrendous clinical picture of repetitive self-harm and suicide attempts. They have all the hallmark features of PTSD (hypervigilance, avoidance of cues that remind them of their abuse, flashbacks and nightmares), as well as drug and alcohol problems and a worrying tendency to seek out new abusive relationships that maintain them in the cycle of trauma. All of this develops as an attempt to mask the symptoms of PTSD. It is very difficult to treat these young people because they are so terrified of their memories of trauma that they go out of their way to avoid therapies aimed at encouraging them to discuss their past. Their sense of being stuck is painful to watch. I have known several tragic cases of teen-agers taking their life despite all their own hard work and good intentions, as well as the help and support of their families, their social workers and the committed psychiatric staff caring for them.

In the current MDMA PTSD studies, there have always been careful exclusion criteria to avoid enrolling patients with too many rigid border-line tendencies. This is understandable, as the last thing researchers need at this crucial early stage of modern psychedelic research is patients suf-fering episodes of high-profile self-harm or even completed suicide. Mithoefer and others have intentionally shied away from such risky patients and excluded them when writing their protocols, and who can blame them?

Ultimately, however, this is the group of patients I would like to help the most with MDMA-assisted psychotherapy. I think it could be just what is needed to allow these fragile and desperate people the kind of psycho-logical protection they need to allow them to break through their heavily fortified defences; it might enable them to stare their histories of abuse in the face, while feeling sufficiently bolstered by MDMA's effects to be able to do the trauma-focused work.

MDMA has unique properties to augment trauma-focused psycho-therapy. It acts like a life raft or a rubber ring. It can buffer the most intense and frightening aspects of the traumatic memories, yet it still allows the patient to experience enough of the pain to carry out real-time trauma-focused psychotherapy. This is a hugely valuable tool for patients who, up until now, have been unable to approach their past without being overwhelmed by negative affect and subsequently fleeing the ther-apy, back into their 'safe' world of self-harm, drug abuse and severe self-neglect.

This does not mean that trauma-focused therapy with MDMA is a walk in the park. Indeed, one of Mithoefer's patients told him: 'I don't know why they call this ecstasy!' Under MDMA-therapy, these trau-matised patients certainly do still experience the pain of their memo-ries. But the MDMA acts as cushion to make doing this work possible. As a psychiatrist who has seen too many young patients give up their fight against the past, I am very excited by the prospect of a clinical tool that can assist them to do this. In recent years, I have even likened the potentially paradigm-shifting effect that MDMA could hold for psychia-try as comparable to the impact the discovery of antibiotics had on gen-eral medicine one hundred years ago[20]. This was the theme of a TEDx talk I gave in Bristol in 2016. It fits well with the treatment-resistance of BPD and will be expanded upon in more detail in the final chapter of this book.

MDMA for Alcoholism

I am proud to be chief investigator, alongside my supervisor David Nutt, research associate Claire Durant, co-therapist Laurie Higbed and consultant psychiatrist Tim Williams in this ground-breaking UK study. The physical, mental and societal problems associated with alcohol misuse are pervasive and on the increase. The UK has a peculiarly harmful relationship with alcohol. Over half of adults in the UK drink above the maximum recommended weekly limits and a quarter are labelled as problem drinkers.

The burden of alcohol abuse in Britain in horrendous, with 8,000 deaths each year, one person in twelve dependent on alcohol, 20% of suicides and 65% of suicide attempts related to alcoholism, up to 1.3 million children adversely affected by family drinking, around 35% of accident and emergency attendance and ambulance costs alcohol related, and drink driving responsible for 17% of all road deaths[21].

In psychiatry, we have a large range of traditional treatments available, including many different pharmacological approaches and a raft of psychotherapies of varying efficacies. The current treatments for alcohol dependence are not great. A meta-analysis conducted ten years ago looked at 361 controlled studies and ranked treatment modalities[22]. Top of the list was the 'brief intervention approach', followed by 'motivational enhancement' and two different pharmacotherapies: GABA agonist treatment (e.g., acamprosate) and opiate antagonists (e.g., naltrexone). Those approaches that attempted to simply educate or shock fared the least effective at reducing rates of alcoholism.

So how good are acamprosate and naltrexone for treating alcoholism? A meta- analysis of 20 controlled trials involving 4,000 patients treated with acamprosate showed that at 12 months, abstinence rates were 27% for acamprosate compared to 13% for placebo, so basically not that great[23]. And a meta-analysis of 24 trials for naltrexone treatment only found significantly improved abstinence rates for the first 12 weeks and no differences between placebo and naltrexone at 12 months[24]. When acamprosate and naltrexone are combined, results are slightly better, with up to 73% abstinence after a 12-weeks treatment period compared to just 20% on placebo. But this rate of improvement had dropped to 66% at three-month follow-up and by 12 months combined treatment was no better than naltrexone alone[25].

None of these current treatments are particularly effective at providing a lasting treatment for alcohol dependence. Indeed, rates of relapse three-years post-treatment for alcohol dependence approach 90%. After 100 years of modern psychiatry this is not good enough.

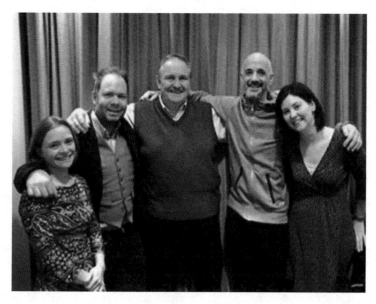

Picture 74: The Bristol-Imperial MDMA-Alcoholism (BIMA) Study
Team, Bristol 2015.
Left to right: Claire Durant, Ben Sessa, David Nutt, Tim Williams and
Laurie Higbed.

Successive UK governments have a transparently sinister relationship
with the UK drinks industry, which I liken to our equivalent of the US's
National Rifle Association, in which money and power trump evidence-
based data and influence political decision-making. Governments ignore
the calls for legislation to increase the price of alcohol and reduce its availability (which are the two most effective evidence-based to reduce the
harms of alcohol use) and we have seen in recent years a proliferation of
availability and normalization of heavy alcohol consumption.

Alcoholism is therefore an area of medicine that is well in need of an
innovative approach. Our Bristol-based study, sponsored by Imperial College London, will deliver an eight-week course of MDMA-Assisted therapy in a safe setting, after thorough screening of suitable patients, scrutiny
of physiological measures and intensive integrative follow-up. Using an
open-label design, with strict inclusion and exclusion criteria, we will
examine whether 20 patients who have been medically detoxed off alcohol
can use two sessions of MDMA-assisted Therapy to access, explore and
resolve ingrained negative psychological dynamics that maintain addictive
behaviours — most of which are underpinned by long-standing psychological trauma. The hope is this can provide an important opportunity for
patients with alcohol dependence to maintain abstinence and recovery.

But will MDMA Therapy for alcoholism even work? It does, after all, not provide the same level of 'spiritual / mystical' experience of the classical psychedelics. And all the other addictions studies with the classical compounds have emphasised that it is the depth of the induced subjective spiritual effects of the experience that best predicts maintained abstinence from substance use. But there *is* a slight subjective spiritual / mystical experience associated with MDMA use. True, it is less pronounced; with around 17% of MDMA first-time users reporting spiritual effects compared to around 80–90% of classical users[26,27]. However, Mithoefer described MDMA's capacity to "make yourself present in the moment", which is a core concept of mindfulness; and, crucially, the MDMA experience is generally more easily tolerated than the classical psychedelics, with less perceptually disturbing effects compared to LSD and psilocybin. Not all patients are able to tolerate the classical psychedelic experience, or even the idea of a treatment involving these experiences, and compliance is a critical part of addiction therapy. Therefore, MDMA offers, we anticipate, an alternative opportunity for enhanced psychotherapy for many patients.

To date there has been no previous study that applies the techniques of MDMA Therapy to the treatment of alcoholism. This landmark study will test the hypothesis that MDMA Therapy can be delivered safely and effectively in a clinical setting to patients with alcoholism; offering them a potential new approach to this devastating, chronic and relapsing condition. Watch this space.

Going Forward: Training MDMA Therapists for the Future

MAPS received official approval from the FDA on 29th November 2016 to go ahead with their Phase III studies. If we are truly to tackle the vast numbers of patients who could benefit from MDMA Therapy, and if we are going to see MDMA licensed for prescribed practice as soon as 2021, then we need a whole load of MDMA therapists and we need them fast! We organised a UK-based video training session together with MAPS for around 30 people in December 2014; all part of preparing the groundwork for the eventual European Phase III MDMA-PTSD studies.

People often ask me what are the qualifications for becoming an MDMA therapist and how can they become one. Whilst there are some well-formed opinions and structured approaches to answering this question— especially from the crew at MAPS who, rightly, have been spearheading the training for international MDMA therapists — the truth is that no one knows exactly. MDMA Therapy, in the mainstream, is new and there are no formal guidelines or prescribed training techniques.

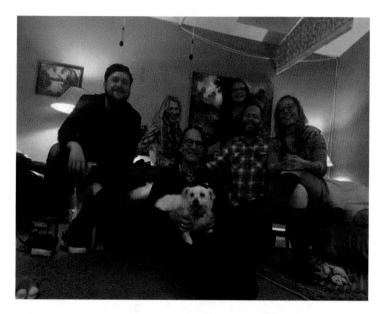

Picture 75: Training the Cardiff MDMA fMRI Team 2015: In
Charleston, South Carolina in 2015. Living with them for ten days
and receiving clinical-grade MDMA as part of our training was a most
memorable experience.
Left to right: Mat Hoskins, Chrissie Turner-Wilson, Michael & Annie
Mithoefer, Sarah Sadler and Flynn.

The MAPS system is good, and there are two teams — based in Boulder, Colorado, and Charleston, South Carolina, that are training the world's new generation of MDMA therapists. Training entails four basic stages: Firstly, read the MAPS manual on how to deliver MDMA therapy for PTSD, secondly, complete the MAPS online training modules, thirdly, undertake a week-long video training, in which one watches many hours of video footage of patients undergoing MDMA therapy and finally, undergo an MDMA and a placebo therapy session with trained guides. This is the model that those of us on the planned Cardiff and Bristol MDMA studies underwent. Only a small handful of people around the world have completed such training to date.

It is relatively easy to organize large scale video training groups, like the one above, but there is certainly a bottle-neck when it comes to getting the experiential training with MDMA. However, like any therapy, the real expertise comes with years of clinical expertise; or in the terminology of MDMA therapy, Flight Hours.

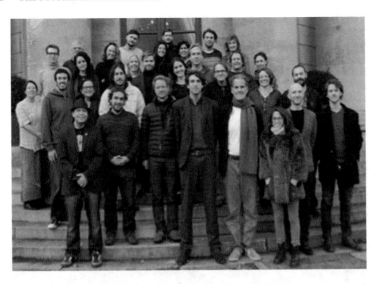

Picture 76: UK gathering of European MDMA Therapy research teams. At Tyringham Hall for a week of video training with Michael and Annie Mithoefer in December 2014. With Natalie Rodriguez, Iker Puente, Eduardo Schenberg, Maximilian von Heyden, Mendel Kaelen, Rick Doblin, Mat Hoskins, Amanda Feilding, Amy Emerson, Luke Williams, Robin Carhart-Harris, Felix Schuldt, Daniel Pinchbeck, Anton Bilton, Shlomi Raz, Katherine MacLean, Marc B.A, Anoushka Thomas, Rê Estevez, Manuela Maciel, Leor Roseman, Neiloufar Faamily, Natalie Lyla Ginsberg and Mendel Kaelen — among other new friends.

Transpersonal therapies such as Breathwork provide an important underpinning for any psychedelic therapist and training for these methods are readily available. Many practitioners have also had experience working in psychedelic emergency care, e.g. festival support services such as the Zendo Project[28] and Kosmicare[29]. And of course, many of the people interested in becoming MDMA therapists are already involved in psychological services. Having a clinical training is essential for at least one half of the MDMA therapy co-therapist pair and of course, when it comes to prescribing a medicine there must also be a doctor present to administer the drug — there is no way around that once we see this substance licensed.

But as we take this part of the clinical psychedelic renaissance forward I see no reason why MDMA therapists must be confined to being wholly psychiatrists, psychologists, nurses or psychotherapists. The key to progress is an understanding of non-ordinary states of consciousness and a willingness to be with and alongside people undergoing traumatic memory recall. There are many allied professions and complimentary therapy models that are good at that kind of work. In coming years, we will see a great many more people becoming trained to deliver MDMA therapy.

2. LSD

This next section on completed clinical studies with LSD is short. As it stands, at the time of writing the 2nd edition of this book there has been only one completed clinical study of LSD psychotherapy, and a couple of review papers discussing the role for LSD as an analgesic agent. This is despite an extensive history of LSD psychotherapy and many thousands of papers written during the 1950s and '60s describing its use — from Sandison, Grof, Leary, Osmond, Hoffer, Fadiman, Stolaroff and countless others.

There are several reasons why LSD has not been studied more extensively during the latest psychedelic renaissance, some of which are psychopharmacological but most of which are political. Many contemporary studies in which the researchers wanted to use a 'classical' psychedelic have opted for psilocybin rather than LSD. This may be because psilocybin is slightly easier to use than LSD; it is shorter acting, less cumbersome for a clinical study involving many patients and repeated sessions with the drug, and the high itself is generally a little less intense and perceptually distorting (though many would challenge this). But the main reason why researchers have opted for psilocybin is simply that LSD has such a widespread negative reputation in the eyes of the media, politicians, ethics boards and parents everywhere, which has a detrimental effect on obtaining a research license and funding. Many lay people, while perhaps familiar with magic mushrooms, have not heard of the drug psilocybin, which makes it an altogether easier proposition to use for a study in which researchers are keen to avoid unwanted media intrusions.

Basically, then, some 40 years since the dreaded 'psychedelic sixties' came to an end, those three little letters L.S.D. are still enough to strike fear into people's hearts and make research very difficult indeed.

Peter Gasser's LSD Study

Because of the reasons described above — and in homage to Albert Hofmann — when the Swiss psychotherapist Peter Gasser designed his clinical trial of psychedelic-drug assisted psychotherapy for the treatment of anxiety associated with end-stage cancer, he was determined not to take the easy route and choose psilocybin. He insisted on using LSD. Gasser was keen to get his study off the ground during Hoffman's lifetime, which he achieved. Hofmann died in 2008 after a lifetime dedicated to psychedelic research during which he saw his creation, LSD, initially hailed as a 'wonder drug' in the 1950s, turn into a 'problem child' in the 1960s, and then almost entirely disappear in modern medicine.

Gasser was granted permission to carry out his study in December 2007, prompting Hofmann to say: 'My wish has come true. I didn't think I'd live to find out that LSD had finally taken its place in medicine'.

Peter carried out a double-blind, randomized, active placebo-controlled pilot study to examine the safety and efficacy of LSD-assisted psychotherapy in 12 patients with anxiety associated with life-threatening diseases[31]. Treatment included drug-free psychotherapy sessions supplemented by two LSD-assisted psychotherapy sessions 2 to 3 weeks apart. The participants received either 200 μg of LSD or 20 μg of LSD, a sub-threshold dose in most people, as a control group. At the 2-month follow-up, anxiety was found to be reduced with no acute or chronic adverse effects persisting beyond 1 day after treatment or treatment-related serious adverse events.

Gasser then carried out a second, follow-up, qualitative study at 12 months, and showed that reductions in anxiety were sustained[30]. The implications of this study are enormous; not only in demonstrating the clinical efficacy of LSD as a potential treatment for anxiety, but also in terms of the political hurdles that had to be surmounted to see the project reach fruition. Albert would have been extremely proud.

LSD as an Analgesic for Treating Cluster Headaches

It has long been known anecdotally that the classical psychedelic drugs LSD and psilocybin, when used recreationally, have a positive analgesic effect at treating the severe pain associated with cluster headaches. This incredibly disabling condition has sometimes been referred to as 'suicide headaches' because the intensity of pain has been known to drive some sufferers to kill themselves.

Yet frequently, when people take small, sub-psychedelic doses of LSD or magic mushrooms, not only does their headache disappear during the intoxication, but also for many weeks or even months afterwards. The mechanism for how this works is not fully understood but it probably relates to the classical psychedelics' role as central vasoregulators. The anaesthetist Eric Kast discovered these analgesic effects of LSD in the 1960s. He carried out studies with the drug and found it to be more effective and better tolerated than traditional opiate-based analgesics[32].

In modern times, the idea to study cluster headache sufferers arose when, in 2004, the internet-based support group Clusterbusters approached

MAPS and asked them to evaluate the large numbers of anecdotal reports that the website was getting about the usefulness of recreational classical psychedelics for relieving cluster headache pain. A subsequent case review paper was published by the late Andrew Sewell, John Halpern and Harrison Pope in 2006[33].

Together with Matthias Kurst, Michael Bernateck and Torsten Passie at Medizinische Hoschule Hannover in Germany, John Halpern has also been in the process of developing a non-psychedelic analogue (2-Bromo-LSD, or 'BOL') to

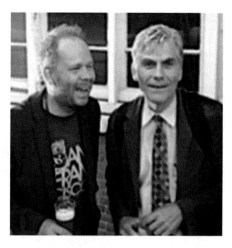

Picture 77: Torsten Passie. Veteran psychedelic researcher whose experience continues to inspire. Here in Amsterdam in 2016.

be used as an alternative to the hallucinogenic effects of LSD. They subsequently carried results of their internet survey of 53 patients with cluster headaches[34,35].

The implications for this work could be far-reaching and stretch well beyond psychiatry. Because it seems that the drugs exert their analgesic effects at such low doses and without the need for specialised psychedelic psychotherapy, this kind of psychopharmacology research could radically rewrite the textbooks as far as standard analgesia for general medicine goes.

A Re-Visiting of Psychedelic Creativity with LSD

As described in an earlier section of this book on creativity, the enigmatic Shlomi Raz of *Eleusis Benefit Corporation* has done much to push regulatory authorities further by running a small study in the UK administering LSD to healthy participants. Like Peter Gasser's Swiss study, Shlomi's study, which was a Phase 1 clinical study, stands as an important demonstration that human research with LSD can happen. The scientific world eagerly awaits the published results of the Eleusis team's research. As do I, as I was fortunate enough to be the study doctor for some of the Eleusis trials in London in 2016. Whatever the data shows, I can vouch for the fact that the participants certainly enjoyed their day being pampered by men and women in white coats whilst they consummated their brains with surrounding cosmic splendour from the 5th floor of a London hospital.

LSD Microdosing

Using sub-threshold (non-psychedelic) doses of classical tryptamine psychedelics has become flavour of the month in recent years within the psychedelic community. The internet is now awash with positive anecdotal stories of people (mainly in West Coast America, it seems) going to work on LSD doses of 5 to 20 mcg; having no obvious psychedelic effects but reporting back improved connectivity with their work colleagues, a greater clarity of thinking and an improved ability to focus and concentrate. This role of psychedelics as cognitive enhancers is certainly an area in need of more research. I am sure it will get this in coming years.

One researcher who thankfully just refuses to give up his work, is James Fadiman, who was involved in many of the ground-breaking studies of the 1960s. In recent years, he has turned his attention to microdosing and is bringing some promising results to the field.

One clinical application for cognitive enhancement is for dementia in the elderly. Most grandparents do not want to be burdened with daily psychedelic experiences (although I can think of some who wouldn't mind), but if it turns out that low dose LSD can improve their ailing cognitions, this could herald a huge leap forward for psychiatry. As we see our populations living longer to experience the gradual destruction of their brains, the race is on by pharmaceutical companies to develop more and more sophisticated cognitive enhancers. How ironic it would be, therefore, if it turns out LSD — a generic, non-patented substance — could be what they are reaching for in a few years.

And here steps in Shlomi Raz again. *Eleusis* have recently conducted a small pilot study testing different doses, from 5 to 25 mcg, of LSD in a group of older people. The micro-dosing study was intended to provide Eleusis with valuable safety/tolerability data as part of their programme to develop LSD and other compounds as disease modifying agents in Alzheimer's Disease. Results are, again, eagerly awaited.

LSD and Neuroscience Studies

And finally, before we leave LSD, we cannot overlook another mention of the work, described earlier, carried out by Robin Carhart-Harris, David Nutt, Amanda Feilding and the Beckley-Imperial research team at Imperial College London. In 2015 the team carried out an initial dose-response pilot study on healthy volunteers, followed by fMRI ASL and BOLD scans and Magnetoencephalography (*MEG*). In a similar way to the original Bristol-Imperial-Beckley psilocybin studies were carried out years earlier, subjects attended for two study days; one placebo and one intravenous LSD.

The results of this work, published in the distinguished *Proceedings of the National Academy of Sciences* (PNAS), were tremendously well

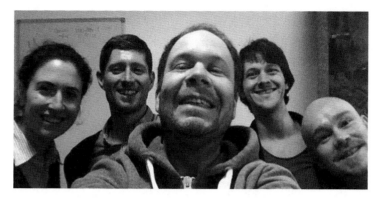

Picture 78: The Beckley-Imperial College LSD Pilot Study crew in 2015. With Neiloufar Family, Robin Carhart-Harris, Mendel Kaelen and Mark Bolstridge. A selfie at the end of a day's dosing from one of their intravenous LSD volunteer test subjects.

received. A glitzy press launch sponsored by the Beckley Foundation at the Royal Society in London in April 2016 was attended by psychedelic pioneers of old and new and caught the media's attention. Using LSD as a tool alongside multi-modal imaging techniques to investigate the neural correlates of consciousness, the study has advanced the understanding of neuroscience by decades. Results showed that LSD increases connectivity between multiple neural networks in the brain and modulates the brain's default mode by reducing blood flow to the posterior cingulate cortex and medial prefrontal cortex. Activity and connectivity between the occipital cortex (the visual centre) and other parts of the brain is greatly increased[36]. As Robin describes it:

"Normally our brain consists of independent networks that perform separate specialised functions, such as vision, movement and hearing - as well as more complex things like attention. However, under LSD the separateness of these networks breaks down and instead you see a more integrated or unified brain.

"Our results suggest that this effect underlies the profound altered state of consciousness that people often describe during an LSD experience. It is also related to what people sometimes call 'ego-dissolution', which means the normal sense of self is broken down and replaced by a sense of reconnection with themselves, others and the natural world. This experience is sometimes framed in a religious or spiritual way - and seems to be associated with improvements in well-being after the drug's effects have subsided."

LSD science is now well and truly back on track throughout the world. For the rest of the summer of 2016 and as we go into 2017 the media is full of one positive account of research or non-research use of psychedelics.

The work carried out by Feilding and Nutt's team is at the forefront of the psychedelic renaissance.

3. Psilocybin

In recent years, psilocybin has risen to the top of the list as the classical psychedelic substance with greatest potential for clinical research, for the reasons mentioned above. There have been several important studies looking specifically at the role for this drug in treating anxiety disorders and addictions, and some highly significant non-clinical studies have pushed forward our understanding of essential neuro-physiological processes and the nature of consciousness. And it looks like there is much more to come.

Psilocybin to Treat Obsessive Compulsive Disorder

It has long been known anecdotally that many sufferers with obsessive-compulsive disorder (OCD) frequently show a spontaneous remission of symptoms, sometimes lasting several weeks, when they take LSD or magic mushrooms. When MAPS sponsored this double-blind placebo-controlled pilot study by Francisco Moreno at the University of Arizona in 2006, it became the first piece of clinical psilocybin research since 1970. Moreno looked at nine patients with severe OCD, which had not responded to traditional treatments. Psilocybin was shown to substantially reduce OCD symptoms in several of the patients, one for several weeks after the treatment[37].

It is just early days in the research of this approach to OCD with psilocybin, but there is certainly more to come in this field in the future. Unremitting OCD is a very disabling and difficult to treat condition. Patients — and their psychiatrists — will welcome any new and innovative approach that is likely to contribute to the management of the disorder.

Psilocybin to Treat Anxiety Associated with End-stage Cancer

Charles Grob, Professor of Child and Adolescent Psychiatry at the Harbor-UCLA Medical Center, Torrance, California, started out with the proposal to use MDMA as the active agent, but Grob then switched to psilocybin because of the apparently insurmountable regulatory problems associated at that time with MDMA research.

There is a rich history of using psychedelics to assist patients with the existential issues associated with dying, with much of the work in this field being done by Stanislav Grof and Joan Halifax in the 1960s. Charlie Grob's study became the first psychedelic treatment with terminally ill patients

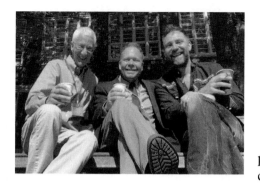 **Picture 79:** With Roland Griffiths and Dave Luke. Sitting in the morning sun drinking coffee by a canal in Amsterdam at the 2016 ICPR Conference; about to present our papers to an eager audience of young psychedelic enthusiasts. What could possibly go wrong now?

since the early 1970s. All the patients in the study had end-stage cancer and were experiencing unremitting anxiety. Using a double-blind placebo-controlled method, Grob demonstrated that psilocybin-assisted psychotherapy reduced psycho-spiritual anxiety, depression, and physical pain for these patients[38].

Of note, another psilocybin clinical study for sufferers of cancer is currently underway by Roland Griffiths' team at Johns Hopkins University. In this study 44 patients will be treated with psilocybin-assisted psychotherapy. It is like Grob's study, but Griffiths will be working with early-stage as well as late-stage cancer patients. Similar outcome measures will be employed, as Griffiths is hoping to show that psilocybin relieves the pain associated with cancer as well as improving quality of life, and helping patients to overcome the anxiety and existential crises associated with their diagnosis of cancer.

Psilocybin to Treat Depression

When Carhart-Harris and his Beckley-Imperial Research Programme (initially housed at Nutt's Bristol University Psychopharmacology Unit) started their studies using fMRI to explore the neurophysiological basis of psilocybin back in 2009, by injecting me with the stuff, no one knew exactly what they would find. It was a chance finding that psilocybin appeared to reduce neural activity in the anterior cingulate cortex (ACC) and the medial pre-frontal cortex (mPFC). It was known, however, that the ACC and the mPFC are areas that are *over*-active in depressed patients. This pointed the way to a new study exploring whether there may be a role for the drug as an antidepressant. Findings from their initial, open-label pilot study — in which 12 patients were given two doses of psilocybin 7 days apart — support the feasibility and safety of the proposed larger-scale double-blind placebo controlled study, with preliminary efficacy data suggesting an antidepressant effect[39]. The main study is underway right now and, just like those other studies whose promise for psychiatry could be profound, the consequences of this one, looking at depression — perhaps the single greatest clinical burden for humanity in the 21st century — could be colossal.

Psilocybin in the treatment of Addictions: Nicotine

In 2012 Matthew Johnson PhD, one of the team at Johns Hopkins who had worked with Roland Griffiths on the now-famous 2006 psilocybin mystical experiences studies, turned his hand to a psilocybin study for addictions. He started an open-label pilot study to determine the safety and feasibility of psilocybin as an adjunct to tobacco smoking cessation treatment. Smoking is by far and away the biggest killing drug humans have; taking around 120,000 lives each year in the UK.

As addictive pharmacological compounds go one must take one's hat off to nicotine. It is staggeringly addictive. One could say it is the perfect dangerous addictive drug: it has an immensely high dopamine-mediated affinity for the nucleus accumbens pleasure centre — meaning the compulsion to dose is intense (much higher than crack cocaine and heroin — I have heaps of patients who have successfully beaten heroin and crack addictions but cannot stop smoking). Each cigarette provides a mild but clearly noticeable stimulant effect that enhances cognitions, is alerting and boosts focus and concentration. Yet at the same time each cigarette also provides a subtle sense of relaxation and calmness. Indeed, smokers can control the extent to which the cigarette is a stimulant or a relaxant depending on hard they pull each drag; a remarkable system of idiosyncratic drug titration. Furthermore, nicotine is a very short-acting drug; to maintain a steady blood level of nicotine one would need to smoke a cigarette every four minutes. This means that smokers are constantly in a rollercoaster cycle of dose-withdraw-dose-withdraw all day long. The withdrawal syndrome itself is subtle but noticeably unpleasant; with irritability, poor focus and an intense craving to re-dose.

But above all, the 'best' thing about nicotine that makes it the perfect damaging drug is that the delivery method, cigarette smoking, is *spectacularly* bad for you. The alveoli of the lungs are arguably the most delicate and fragile tissue in the body. And the way people extract the drug nicotine (which itself is relatively harmless) from its bound state in the leaves of the Solanaceae (nightshade) family plant, Nicotiana *tabacum*, is by setting alight to the dried leaves and pulling that hot cauldron of burning smoke between the teeth, through the soft palette, down through the trachea and pumped into the furthest reaches of all the lobes of the lungs, in order that the nicotine molecules — alongside the another 6,000 chemicals, of which at least 400 are known to be highly toxic — can pass into the circulating blood of the alveoli and carry the nicotine to the brain for three seconds. You can see why it has caught on.

So Matt Johnson took 15 psychiatrically healthy nicotine-dependent smokers (10 males; mean age of 51 years), who were smoking on average 19 cigarettes per day for an average of 31 years and who had made an average of six previous lifetime attempts to quit their addiction. He administered a course of psilocybin-assisted psychotherapy using psilocybin doses between 20mg and 30mg, delivered as part of a structured 15-week smoking cessation treatment protocol. He used biomarkers to provide definitive proof of smoking behaviour as well as collecting self-report measures.

The results of Matt's pilot study showed that 12 of 15 participants (80%) showed seven-day point prevalence abstinence at 6-month follow-up. This substantially exceeds the recovery rates of all other current psychotherapeutic or pharmacological therapies for smoking cessation (which on average manage about 35% success rates) — by a very long way[40].

As with many other studies using psychedelics as tools for addictions (i.e. Osmond's LSD studies in the 1950s, Krupitsky's ketamine studies in the 1990s and Bogenshutz's psilocybin studies more recently), Johnson found that the patients who reported the most profound spiritual experiences had the greater rates of abstinence. Wow. It's true: God does hate fags.

Psilocybin in the treatment of Addictions: Alcohol

Using psychedelic-assisted psychotherapy to treat alcohol use disorder goes back to the very earliest history of psychedelics in medicine, with Osmond's use of LSD in the early 1950s. And since Teri Krebs' important 2012 meta-analysis that demonstrated the efficacy of those early LSD studies as viable treatments for alcoholism, psychiatry has been waiting for someone to recreate a modern psychedelic study with alcoholics[41].

Along comes New Mexico psychiatrist Michael Bogenshutz. Having first written an influential paper reviewing the history and potential mechanisms of classical psychedelics as treatments for addictions[42] he then went to on to do a study. Using psilocybin rather than LSD, for all the reasons described above, Bogenshutz carried out a single-group proof-of-concept study on 10 volunteers with alcohol dependence. They received two doses of oral psilocybin (0.3 mg/kg and 0.4 mg/kg — approximately 21–28 mg) separated by 4 weeks in combination with 12 weeks of outpatient psychosocial treatment including preparation, debriefing, and motivational enhancement therapy.

Results showed abstinence increased significantly following psilocybin administration ($p < 0.05$). The gains were largely maintained at follow-up to 36 weeks. There were no significant treatment-related adverse events. And, like all the other addictions studies, the intensity of positive, especially spiritual, effects in the first psilocybin session predicted decreases in craving and increases in abstinence[43].

Both Matthew Johnson and Michael Johnson have been very supportive in helping me set-up my own MDMA addiction study and I owe them a debt of gratitude. It was a great pleasure, therefore, when Matt and I wrote a jointly-authored editorial for the British Journal of Psychiatry about psychedelic therapies for addictions, which appeared in that 2015 journal with Sasha Shulgin on the cover[44].

Important Non-Clinical Contemporary Psilocybin Research

There have been lots of pre-clinical and neurophysiological studies conducted in recent years, many of which have come out of the laboratories of Franz Vollenweider and Dave Nichols, from projects overseen by the Heffter Research Institute on both sides of the Atlantic. Below are described some of these important non-clinical studies that are having profound effects on the way we view consciousness and spirituality. They will also have an important impact on the future of clinical research.

Psilocybin: The Spiritual Experience and Personality Change

I have already alluded to this piece of work throughout this book[45]. It was carried out by Roland Griffiths, Bill Richards et al. at Johns Hopkins

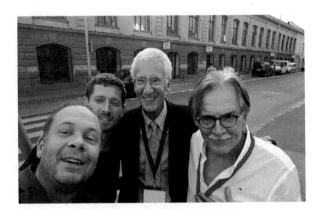

Picture 80: Carhart-Harris, Griffiths and Vollenweider; the brain teams of the psychedelic renaissance in Prague in 2016. As the renaissance broadens studies on clinical subjects are now becoming more prevalent.

School of Medicine and published in 2006. Some call it a recreation or re-visitation of the famous Good Friday Experiment by Walter Pahnke, but there were some significant differences.

Griffiths took a group of 30 healthy volunteers who had never taken a psychedelic drug before and gave them alternate sessions with either high-dose psilocybin (30mg orally) or an identical-looking placebo capsule of methylphenidate, which provided a light, stimulating effect to fool the user into thinking they had taken an active drug, but with no psychedelic effect. Sessions were spaced two-months apart and rating scales were used to test subjects' appreciation of drug effects and mystical experience at three stages: immediately after each session, at two months after the session and at fourteen months' follow-up. It was a double-blind study, with neither subjects nor examiners knowing whether each person had received the psilocybin or the placebo during each session. Sessions, which lasted an average of eight hours each, were carried out individually in a relaxed and supportive environment with minimal interventions from the investigators. Mainly, subjects usually chose to lie down and relax with eye-shades on, listening to music. They were encouraged to simply just 'go inside their heads'.

The results showed that 61% of the psilocybin group versus 13% of the control group reported a 'complete mystical experience'. Notably, one third of subjects also described the psilocybin experience as unpleasant and anxiety provoking at times. All the subjects taking high-dose psilocybin considered it a deeply profound experience, with one third describing it as 'the single most spiritually significant event of their lives' and two thirds saying it was 'among their five most meaningful and spiritually significant events'. These results were sustained: at fourteen months after the last session, the psilocybin group continued to attribute deep personal meaning to the experience. Roland Griffiths has gone on to publish further results as a spin-off from this initial study. More recent papers have described how the optimum dose for a mystical or spiritual experience is between 20 mg and 30 mg of psilocybin. Any less than this does not produce such a profound effect, whilst higher doses than this tend to be overly anxiety-provoking.

But perhaps the most interesting results to come out of this work by Griffiths and Richards are those that relate to the subtle but lasting personality changes that have occurred in the cohort of subjects who experienced high-dose psilocybin for the first time in his study. The investigators measured the long-term effects of the treatment on five broad domains of personality: neuroticism, extroversion, openness, agreeableness, and conscientiousness. Subjects frequently reported increases in their aesthetic appreciation, imagination, and creativity and there were lasting observable increases in the domain of openness following a high-dose psilocybin session[46].

The potential importance of these results is profound. It is the first time that science has demonstrated a phenomenon that is anecdotally obvious, namely, that a spiritually significant mystical experience predicts changes in behaviours, attitudes and values that are positive and long-lasting. The reason this has such great importance in psychiatry — and is of interest to me — is that it relates to my earlier comments about those patients with personality disorder who had no apparent hope of a way out of their condition. An adage in psychiatry, but one that is increasingly being challenged, is that 'once your (maladaptive or functional) personality has been formed nothing can change it'. Such a negative and fatalistic statement grates with every psychiatrist who has seen patients suffering because their ingrained personality appears to resist any attempts to relieve them of their suffering. If psilocybin can seriously lead to long-lasting positive personality change — which many would claim is the case, certainly anecdotally — this is an avenue worthy of much more exploration.

Psilocybin and the Beyond Within

The Heffter Research Institute's laboratories in Switzerland, run by Franz Vollenweider, have been responsible for some of the world-leading

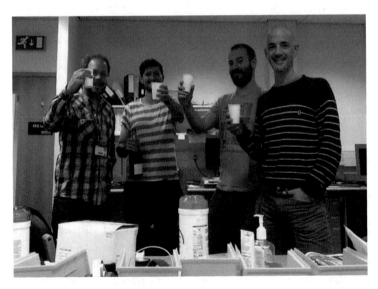

Picture 81: The Beckley-Imperial Psilocybin fMRI Team, Cardiff, UK, 2014. Drinking non-alcoholic fizz out of plastic cups after discharging the final participant. Robin Carhart-Harris, Luke Williams and Tim Williams.

neurophysiological studies with psilocybin in recent years. This work, with both humans and animals, has taught the scientific world a lot about the mechanisms of the 5-HT_{2A} receptor and the role it, and other mechanisms, play in the psychedelic experience and the neurophysiological basis for consciousness[47-55].

In the UK Robin Carhart-Harris and colleagues at the Beckle-Imperial Psychedelic Research Project have used functional Magnetic Resonance Imaging (fMRI) to look at the effects of psilocybin on healthy volunteers. While working with Robin in Bristol, I was privileged to help with, and co-author, the dose-response pilot study that preceded the actual imaging studies. In the pilot, with me as the first subject, we tested healthy volunteers on different doses of intravenous psilocybin while they lay inside a wooden mock fMRI scanner[56].

The basic rationale for Robin's first fMRI psilocybin project was to measure the functional activity in the medial prefrontal cortex after psilocybin[57]. Large decreases in activity and blood flow were observed, contrary to popular assumptions that under the influence of psychedelic drugs there is an increase in brain blood flow and activity. Because the medial prefrontal cortex is known to exert a top-down inhibitory control over limbic activity (the site of the brain that governs emotional experiences), it was postulated that a psilocybin-induced deactivation of the medial prefrontal cortex leads to a disinhibition of limbic activity and an associated increased emotional response.

Further psilocybin studies by Robin's team with fMRI measured the subjective psychological effects of psilocybin when a subject was experiencing recall of positive emotional memories[58]. Subsequent studies used Magnetoencephalography (MEG) and infused psilocybin. They found decreased frontoparietal connectivity consistent with the previous fMRI findings[53]. I must thank Robin again for the opportunity to enjoy some particularly colourful train journeys back to Bristol because of this work.

The reason these studies were so important for psychiatry is because they finally proved what had been known anecdotally for the last 60 years, since psychotherapists first began using LSD as a tool to enhance psychotherapy, namely, that *psychedelic drugs increase access to repressed emotional memories*[59]. The results became extremely helpful for future psychedelic psychotherapy studies. Robin had demonstrated graphically that this is how these drugs work[60].

Robin Carhart-Harris' psilocybin studies represented the most in-depth multi-imaging neuroscientific studies done thus far with a psychedelic drug. They wouldn't be matched until the same team went on and showed some even more impressive results in the following years; this time using LSD.

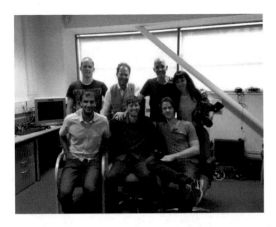

Picture 82: The Beckley-Imperial-Cardiff Magnetoencephalography (MEG) Psilocybin Crew in 2014. With Wouter, Suresh Muthukumaraswamy, Robin Carhart-Harris, Tim Williams, Mendel Kaelen and Georgina Cammalleri.

4. Dimethyltryptamine (DMT)

Since Rick Strassman's pioneering human DMT study of 1995 launched the new renaissance of psychedelic research, there have been very few other published human studies of its use[61]. One paper, however, by Daumann et al. in 2008, describes a study in which healthy human volunteers were given both DMT and ketamine under fMRI conditions[62]. This paper explores the potential role for DMT as a psychotomimetic to assist researchers developing psychopharmacological models for studying schizophrenia. (Funny how things come back into fashion isn't it?) The study suggests ketamine makes for a better psychotomimetic than DMT, because the former mimics both positive and negative symptoms of schizophrenia whereas the latter only models the positive symptoms.

Another important recent pre-clinical DMT study is by Fontanilla et al., published in the journal *Science* in 2009, which postulated that DMT binds to the sigma-1 receptor in the brain[63]. This is an important discovery because the sigma-1 receptor was previously considered an 'orphan receptor', as no endogenous chemical had been found that binds to it. In their biochemical, physiological, and behavioural experiments with mice, they suggest DMT is an endogenous agonist for the sigma-1 receptor. This opens the debate further made by McKenna, Strassman and others about endogenous DMT.

DMT's role as a neuroprotective agent, saving the brain from death in the context of hypoxic stress, is being hotly pursued by Ede Frecska and others[64].

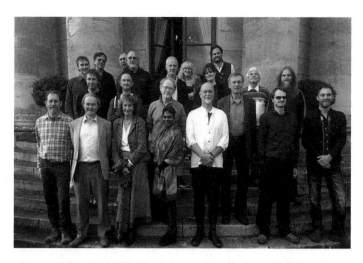

Picture 83: DMT Study Group at Tyringham Hall in 2015.
Left to Right: Erik Davis, Cosmo Feilding Mellen, Bernard Carr, Jeremy
Narby, Luis Eduardo Luna, Ede Frecska, Andrew Gallimore, Amanda
Feilding, Dennis McKenna, Santha Hancock, Graham Hancock, Jill
Purce, Dar Pan, Rory Spowers, Rupert Sheldrake, Peter Meyer, Graham
St John, Tony Wright and David Luke.

At Imperial College London we see 2017 begin with another ground-
breaking multi-imaging study — this time with DMT. A team lead by
Christopher Timmerman, and including Luke Williams and Robin Carhart-
Harris, will use concurrent fMRI and EEG to look at the neurophysiological actions of intravenous DMT. Carrying out EEG measurements whilst
someone is also in an fMRI scanner is a relatively new technique, and this
is certainly the first time it has been done with a psychedelic drug. Imperial's previous studies with psilocybin and LSD involved being injected
with the compound, going into the fMRI scanner then getting out of there
and going into a MEG scanner, whilst hoping that the drug effects were
still at their peak. By having participants (of which I was one!) wear an
EEG helmet whilst inside the fMRI scanner Chris hopes to demonstrate a
clearer picture of multiple imaging for this fascinating substance.

5. Ayahuasca

While human studies with *pure* DMT have been few and far between since
Strassman's study, a lot of contemporary research with DMT in the form
of ayahuasca is now taking place. Numerous scholars have been at looking at the anthropological and social aspects of ayahuasca in non-Western

cultures, how this relates to the stability of those populations and how it is increasingly emerging as a tool for self-exploration and healing in the West. For an excellent extensive review of many of the earlier studies with ayahuasca, see Dennis McKenna's review of research[65]. For further reading on the anthropological aspects of human development alongside ayahuasca it is always a pleasure to read Graham Hancock's book *Supernatural: Meetings with the Ancient Teachers of Mankind*[66].

The subject of ayahuasca — given just how much has been written and how quickly the subject is progressing — is enough to fill a textbook like this several times over. I cannot possibly do it justice and so I will not try to cover everything here. However, I can recommend other good books on the subject include Ralph Metzner's *Ayahuasca: Human Consciousness and the Spirits of Nature*[67] and *Sacred Vine of Spirits*[68]. Plus, the extremely informative book by Luis Eduardo Luna and Steven White (editors), *Ayahuasca Reader: Encounters with the Amazon's Sacred Vine*[69], which has recently been re-released in 2016 in an updated mammoth 2nd edition, containing a rich variety of new reflections about this entangled and enthralling subject.

In 2010 Joel Porfírio Pinto of the University of Sao Paulo published his thesis studying the fMRI, SPECT scans and neuropsychological changes in healthy volunteers given ayahuasca. SPECT showed activation of the frontal and temporal cortex and limbic areas. Cerebral blood flow decreased in a region of the right cerebellar hemisphere, and fMRI data showed decreased activation of areas involved in language processing. Pinto suggests ayahuasca could be useful for the study of the neurobiology of psychosis[70]. There are further series of pre-clinical and neurophysiological studies with ayahuasca that have been carried out by Jordi Riba in Spain. Details are given on the MAPS website.

In 2005 Charles Grob and Marlene Dobkin de Rios published a qualitative evaluation of Brazilian teenagers of the União do Vegetal Church who ritually use ayahuasca, and compared them to local matched non-users. Data showed that the ayahuasca-using teenagers appeared to be healthy, thoughtful, considerate and bonded to their families and religious peers, with no evidence of any harm caused by their use of the plant compounds[71].

Also in South America, there is currently a long-term evaluation being sponsored by MAPS of the very well established ayahuasca treatment program at the Takiwasi Center in Peru. The director of Takiwasi, Jacques Mabit, also wrote a good review of the history and ongoing efforts at the centre in the 2007 book *Hallucinogens and Health*[72].

Ayahuasca has a rich tradition in the treatment of addictions, with some renowned centres dedicated to treating substance misuse problems.

An open-label observational study investigated the safety and long-term effectiveness of ayahuasca treatment for individuals suffering from addiction and dependence. Combining Western psychotherapeutic techniques with South American shamanic healing practices, participants on a retreat in British Columbia, Canada received four days of group counselling consisting of psychosomatic techniques coupled with group sharing and dialogue and two expert-led ayahuasca ceremonies[73].

Participants showed reductions in their use of cannabis, alcohol and tobacco, with statistically significant reductions in cocaine use. There were also improvements in measures of hopefulness, empowerment, mindfulness and two measures of quality of life that were sustained at six-month follow-up.

Pharmacological Research with Ayahuasca

One individual who has done lots in recent years to advance formal human ayahuasca studies is Jordi Riba, a Spanish pharmacologist working at Sant Pau hospital in Barcelona. Jordi gained approval for the world's first pharmacology study of healthy volunteers under the influence of ayahuasca in 1998. The MAPS-sponsored study provided vital information about ayahuasca's pharmacokinetics and tolerability in humans, as well as collecting data about its neurophysiological and subjective effects. Using EEG, Jordi aimed to model the relationship between DMT plasma levels and changes observed in the brain's electrical activity[74]. Jordi has since gone on to publish more widely in the field[75,76].

In February 2016, I gave a positive recommendation to the *Journal of Psychopharmacology* for publication of an excellent systemic review of 28 peer-reviewed papers on ayahuasca up to 2015, written by Dos Santos et al[77]. The review analysed multiple published papers exploring the acute, subacute, and long-term effects of ayahuasca in terms of safety and toxicity and included published research on neuropsychological functioning and neuroimaging. The review described (and I quote some of the paper's abstract here) that ayahuasca administration was well tolerated, increased introspection and positive mood, altered visual perceptions, activated frontal and paralimbic regions and decreased default mode network activity. It also concluded that ayahuasca improved planning and inhibitory control improved working memory and showed anti-depressive and anti-addictive potentials. Long-term ayahuasca use was associated with increased cortical thickness of the anterior cingulate cortex and cortical thinning of the posterior cingulate cortex, which was inversely correlated to age of onset, intensity of prior ayahuasca use, and spirituality. Subacute and long-term ayahuasca use was not associated with increased psychopathology or cognitive deficits, instead being associated with enhanced mood and cognition, increased spirituality, and reduced impulsivity. In summary, ayahuasca is shown to have low toxicity and multiple potential benefits to the user. It did also conclude, however, that many of the studies lacked good methodological robustness and a lot more research is needed. I think we can all agree with that.

Future Studies with Ayahuasca

Jordi Riba's team in Barcelona are currently undergoing research, sponsored by the Beckley Foundation, investigating the role of glutamate transmission in ayahuasca's effects using MRI and spectroscopy, and has shown that ayahuasca facilitates aspects of mindfulness[78]. Another fascinating — and potentially epoch shattering — development with ayahuasca is the observation that it could play a role in neurogenesis; the growth of new nerve cells. A preliminary study suggests that harmine and

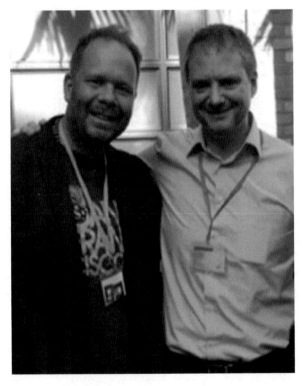

Picture 84: Jordi Riba, whose work in collaboration with the Beckley Foundation is trail-blazing advances in the field of neuro-regeneration. Here at the ICPR conference in Amsterdam in 2016.

tetrahydroharmine, alkaloids present in ayahuasca, increase the differentiation and maturation of stem cells into neurons[79].

Further studies in vivo could represent an important advance in the development of therapies to treat physical brain damage and stroke.

In the field of addictions, Brazilian psychiatrist, Luís Fernando Tófoli is currently putting together a study, like ours in Bristol with MDMA; treating post-detox alcoholics with a course of psychotherapy involving several sessions with ayahuasca. We have met and spoken about our shared difficulties in instigating such research and I wish him the best of luck with his project.

And finally, I wish to mention Benjamin Mudge, an Australian psychedelic researcher whose PhD I am currently supervising. He is carrying out a very ambitious project looking at whether ayahuasca ceremonies can have a positive effect on reducing symptoms for people with Bipolar 1 affective disorder. This is a brave move, as usually participants with any form of psychosis are excluded from psychedelic research studies. However, Mudge is responding to a raft of anecdotal reports that some people with Bipolar (and I stress, not everyone) who has had genuine and well-facilitated ayahuasca ceremonies do improve after drinking the ceremonial tea. Mudge's work looks set to broaden the horizons of how we look at psychedelics as potential treatments for psychosis. Exciting stuff.

6. Ketamine

Ketamine to Combat Addictions

So far, most contemporary psychiatric research with ketamine has focused on its capacity to treat addictions. In this regard, the work of Evgeny Krupitsky, the Clinical Director of Research for the Saint Petersburg Regional Center for Research in Addiction and Psychopharmacology, has set out the way. In the 1990s, he developed a model of ketamine-assisted psychotherapy to treat alcohol and opiate addictions.

Krupitsky and Grinenko compared 111 alcoholic patients treated with ketamine-assisted psychotherapy (KPT) with 100 alcoholic patients treated with conventional treatment[80]. 66% of those treated with ketamine-assisted psychotherapy (KPT) remained sober after one year, compared to 24% of the control group. I first met Evgeny at a conference in Vienna in 2007 when I was answering questions after a talk on psychedelic therapies. Someone in the audience asked me about ketamine and I answered that I was no expert on ketamine but recommended they get in touch with Dr. Krupitsky in St. Petersburg; the world authority on the subject. The questioner replied, "I am Evgeny Krupitsky!" We got on well and I subsequently invited him to speak at Breaking Convention 2011. Evgeny puts a lot of faith in the induction of a spiritual experience to explain his good results, which fits with the importance of the mystical experience to effect positive personality change.

Krupitsky further developed his technique and applied it to treating heroin addiction. He showed that one single session of KPT (compared to a placebo session) was enough to significantly promote improved abstinence from heroin for one year without any adverse reactions. He went on to study whether follow-up sessions, with two further monthly KPT sessions after discharge from hospital following this initial KPT session, improved long-term outcomes compared to those randomly allocated into a placebo group. At one-year follow-up there was a significantly higher rate of success in the multiple KPT group, with 50% of subjects remaining abstinent from heroin compared to just 22% in the single KPT group[81].

Krupitsky, although the most prolific, is not the only researcher to study the use of ketamine as a tool to improve addiction treatment. Another extraordinary study by Jovaisa et al. from Lithuania used low-dose ketamine, without combining it with psychotherapy, to demonstrate how the effects of the drug reduce the unpleasant withdrawal symptoms of heroin addiction[82].

Ketamine as a Psychotomimetic

As mentioned earlier, ketamine has been studied in recent years as a potential psychotomimetic to improve our understanding of schizophrenia, and assist in the development of new antipsychotics. To appreciate how this works, one must first understand that ketamine is an NMDA-antagonist (a glutamate receptor antagonist) and that it mimics both positive and negative symptoms of schizophrenia. This has led psychopharmacologists to search for an effective glutamate receptor agonist as a potential treatment for psychosis. Using this ketamine psychotomimetic hypothesis as a model in healthy human subjects, we can give ketamine, induce psychotic symptoms and then test potential antipsychotic drugs against these induced effects. The role that ketamine plays in this kind of research can significantly push forward our understanding of schizophrenia (just as LSD did in the 1950s). This was carried out for the first time successfully in a recent study by D'Souza et al[83].

Ketamine as an Antidepressant

Several recent contemporary publications suggest there may be a role for ketamine in the future of antidepressant developments. The first is a simple case series involving just two patients who coincidentally showed reductions in pre-existing depressive symptoms when being given injections of ketamine for a different condition (Complex Regional Pain Syndrome)[84]. In another study, which was randomised, double blind and placebo controlled, a single injection of ketamine significantly improved symptoms in depressed patients who had been taken off all their usual antidepressant medication for up to a week. The effect size was large and the ketamine treatment was well tolerated[85]. This study by Zarate opened up an interesting new line of research in treating depression. Most licensed antidepressants work by raising levels of the monoamines (particularly serotonin and noradrenaline), but ketamine, which exerts its effects by glutamate inhibition — perhaps via increased activity at AMPA receptors — is getting a lot of psychiatrists talking right now. The concept that depression could be managed by a monthly or fortnightly injection, rather than having to take daily antidepressant tablets, is revolutionary. It is not unlike dialysis for the brain. Furthermore, because — unlike LSD, psilocybin, MDMA and most other psychedelic drugs — ketamine is already a licensed drug (albeit not for psychiatric depression or other psychiatric disorders, but rather as an anaesthetic) doctors can prescribe it 'off label' with far greater ease and far fewer regulatory hurdles than those required for the other psychedelics. This means series of case studies can be built up over time to test its relative safety and efficacy.

One large, ongoing series of tests is coming from the UK from Rupert McShane, a consultant psychiatrist in Oxford. In his initial open-label study, which was carried out on patients with severe depression attending the ECT clinic in Oxford[86], he showed that ketamine infusions could be given safely to patients attending an NHS clinic. The effects on depression were moderately good, with 29% of patients responding to the treatment and in half of the sample, depression remitted completely. Patients did not experience any memory loss because of being given ketamine. Whilst these results, on face value, do not look particularly spectacular, one must bear in mind that these are severely depressed patients (who in many cases would otherwise be getting ECT). So, the remittance rates are not too bad at all. The project is still ongoing.

There has been a useful meta-analysis of published studies into ketamine for depression, covering the years up to 2014[87]. The review acknowledged that the "clinical evidence demonstrates rapid improvements in mood and suicidal thinking in most participants", but rightly pointed out that thus far, "study numbers have generally been small and many trials are unblinded and methodologically weak". The review went on to state that some studies suggest ketamine might also augment electroconvulsive therapy. The review reflected that one of the problems with ketamine is that the antidepressant effects are, "relatively temporary, disappearing after days to weeks". Nevertheless, the review concludes that the research is highlighting some: "exciting data providing new insights into neurobiological models of depression, and potentially opening up a new class of antidepressants."

And even more recently, we have seen two studies with ketamine conducted not on patients with severe unipolar depression, but on patients with bipolar depression. Early results suggest ketamine can improve mood and reduce and suicidality in this group[88,89].

It seems that there is still a long way to go before we will see ketamine challenging the long-held position that SSRIs have in mainstream psychiatry for treating affective disorders.

Ketamine as Treatment for other psychiatric conditions: Such as Obsessive-Compulsive Disorder?

Obsessive-compulsive disorder is a seriously disabling condition in approximately 0.5% of the population. First-line treatments are with cognitive behavioral therapy (CBT) and selective serotonin reuptake inhibitors (SSRIs). But there is a high treatment resistance and psychiatrists are increasingly looking for innovative options.

A single case study published in 2011 showed that a ketamine infusion rapidly reduced obsessive symptoms in a patient[90]. And whilst a subsequent open-label study failed to demonstrate significant improvements in OCD with ketamine[91] a small randomised cross-over study published in 2013 showed that 50% of patients with OCD responded positively to the drug[92]. Keep watching for ketamine in OCD.

And finally, before we leave ketamine completely, in a very exciting local development (the study is taking place at Exeter University, just down the M5 from where I work in Bristol), my friend Professor Celia Morgan, Professor of Psychopharmacology at the University of Exeter, is currently collaborating with researchers at University College London and Imperial College London to create a multi-site project in both the South West of England and London looking at ketamine as a treatment for alcoholism. Participants will receive a low-dose of ketamine by injection once a week for three weeks in conjunction with seven 90 minute sessions of psychological therapy. Ketamine certainly has a long way to go in psychiatry.

7. Ibogaine

Returning to the psychedelics' capacity for treating addictions, the drug ibogaine has long been known to combat addiction to alcohol, as evidenced by much lower rates of alcoholism in native ibogaine-using cultures. Alper et al. have highlighted several pre-clinical animal studies describing its effectiveness as an agent to combat addiction[93].

In an open-label (not placebo controlled) study by Alper, ibogaine was explored as a treatment for opiate dependence. Thirty-three patients with previous intravenous heroin addiction were given a single dose of ibogaine on stopping their opiate drugs. Twenty-five of them showed a resolution of the signs of opiate withdrawal within 24 hours, which was maintained for a total of 72 hours[94].

In recent years, ibogaine treatment clinics, both underground and licensed, have sprung up all over the world. MAPS is currently sponsoring research at ibogaine clinics in Mexico (with investigator Thomas Brown) and in New Zealand (with investigator Geoff Noller). These observational studies are gathering data about outcomes of long-running clinical programs. There are also treatment programs underway in Canada being evaluated by Leah Martin and Sandra Karpetas[95].

It is not only alcohol and opiates that are purported to benefit from ibogaine treatment; increasing reports about its efficacy at combating cocaine addiction and methamphetamine abuse are also emerging.

Whilst ibogaine therapies for addictions certainly hold a lot of promise, it is a substance with potential toxicity that needs to be borne in mind by clinicians. There have been some high-profile deaths in recent years of people undergoing underground ibogaine treatments — usually caused by cardiac arythmias[95,96]. However, note that with screening of high risk patients and careful monitoring these risks can be minimized in a clinical setting with screened patients. This toxicity need not be a barrier to its research and clinical use (all medical interventions carry some level of risks as well as benefits). But it does mean care and attention to appropriate screening and monitoring of use are essential.

For an excellent account of underground treatment with ibogaine for combatting opiate addiction I can highly recommend the films Iboga Nights and Detox or Die by film maker David Graham Scott[97,98].

Conclusion

As with all research, planning new projects using drugs that have a contentious history needs to be done cautiously to avoid the (often inaccurate) preconceptions about the relative usefulness and harm of these substances. However, common to all these drugs, there exists a rich wealth of anecdotal studies from 40 years ago that were abandoned prematurely before their full therapeutic potential was adequately reported or discounted. This area of psychedelic research is one that provides benefits for furthering our understanding of neuroscience and developing new treatments for our patients. If we are to strive to comprehend the brain in its entirety, these areas are worth revisiting with modern research methods. It is a pleasure to see this happening in so many places throughout the world today.

CHAPTER 10

Psychedelics Caught in the Crossfire of the War on Drugs

"LSD is a psychedelic drug which occasionally causes psychotic behavior in people *who have not taken it.*"—Timothy Leary

Crime Pays. War is a Money-spinner. But for Whom?

All wars generate propaganda. It is an effective weapon used on both sides of any debate and we hear a lot of claims about the relative dangers and safety issues in the so-called War on Drugs.

What an extraordinary notion, a war on drugs. It isn't even a war on drug users or drug dealers, but rather a war on the very concept of drugs themselves — well, some drugs, at least, but not alcohol or nicotine. Could we also wage a war on swearing or a war on nastiness?

Perhaps a more focused war on the *harmful use of drugs* is worth fighting. But increasing numbers of people in our society are now seeing that a prohibition against 998 out of 1,000 or more psychoactive substances is flawed on so many levels. Whether one approaches the problem from the point of view of health, finance, politics, international crime, class, religion or human rights, it is a war that looks increasingly unwinnable. And if it cannot be won, ought it be fought? And if it is worth fighting, then at what cost, how many resources should be put into it, and how many casualties and how much collateral damage are we prepared to accept?

Many people will say that not only cannot it not be won and ought not be fought, but that it is also a war whose core ideology is rooted in paternalism, religious restriction and even racism and not in the noble sentiments it pretends to uphold. At best, it undoubtedly supports a global crime scene of huge proportions and, at worst, may even *involve* shady government decisions and deals with criminal organisations.

Many people are happy to state that cannabis is the largest cash crop in the United States — more valuable than wheat — but totally unregulated. However, things are now changing and an exciting future lies ahead for America and, hopefully, the UK when it comes to cannabis laws. A system for legal medical cannabis operates in the majority of states in the US[1].

At the time of writing this, 29 out of the 50 U.S. states have a policy that allows for the legal use of medical cannabis. And both medical and recreational cannabis are recognized in 8 states (Alaska, California, Colorado, Maine, Massachusetts, Nevada, Oregon and Washington) and in the district of Columbia.

Tackling the idiocy of cannabis prohibition cannot come soon enough. Over the years, trillions of dollars have changed hands without a cent reaching the government purse. For the most part, the drugs industry has no registered companies, no CEOs, no managing directors, no line of responsibility or quality control in place. Instead, criminal gangs whose methods often involve violence and exploitation of vulnerable people shift money from the drug trade around the world.

On the other hand, there is also plenty of evidence that the illegal drugs industry supports many poor people and whole communities of peaceful folk who are otherwise unable to provide for themselves and their families. When the governments crack down on this cottage industry and attempt to crush the drugs trade, the sufferers are not the rich financiers but the end-game producers and users of the drugs. Meanwhile, the big-time suppliers simply drive off in their Mercedes to the next fertile ground for business.

We are told it is a supply-and-demand market perpetuated by the very war itself; it is a war waged against innocent people, ordinary citizens who have committed no other crime than that of having the creativity and enthusiasm to consider experiencing an alternative mental state to their waking consciousness. These innocents are immediately criminalized and forced to dabble in a risky underworld, fraternize with law-breakers and put their careers and livelihoods at risk.

Those calling for reform of the drug laws will say that the entire hopeless situation could be wiped out at a stroke of a pen by the lawmakers. The rug could be pulled from underneath those criminal gangs tomorrow by simply making all drugs legal and available to responsible adults who want them. Those in support of the war, on the other hand, claim such an action would lead to an increase in drug use and an increase in crime and health problems — though it is hard to imagine these issues being very much worse than they are presently. Those in support of legalisation will reply that such a vast sum of money currently goes into prosecuting people through the police, courts and prisons that the savings to be made there would more than adequately free-up funds to transform drug education and treatment services for any possible increase in use that might arise.

A dig at alcohol again: The alcohol lobby is very rich, very much favoured by governments and *very* against seeing other substances compared alongside the risks of booze. They have good reason to worry. Around £800 million is spent annually advertising alcohol in the UK[2]. It is notable that in 2009 the entire UK NHS budget for providing treatment services for alcohol dependency was the same as the cost of the first six seconds of a famous vodka brand's TV commercial. These are the sorts of economics those in favour of encouraging a debate about the evidence-based risks of different substances are up against.

I do not pretend to know enough about the politics and economics of the complex situation surrounding the drug laws to say for certain whose arguments are right in the debate. But as a clinical doctor — and, more critically, as a citizen who has lived through the War on Drugs all my life — I can say with great certainty that after 40 years of successive governments from all over the world fighting this campaign, what we still seem to have is a massive multi-substance drug problem anywhere one chooses to look. The prisons are full of offenders, trillions are spent on continuing the fight, and there is no shortage of new users, new suppliers and — from a clinical point of view — no end in sight of the casualties. Of course, proponents of the war will say these observations are more reason why we must keep fighting this war until we win.

There are some excellent organisations pushing tirelessly to encourage debate aimed at reform of the international drug laws[3]. In the UK, we have The Beckley Foundation[4], led by Amanda Feilding, who, alongside sponsoring all manner of consciousness research and psychedelic clinical drug studies, has used her influence in The House of Lords to work with policy makers throughout the world and keep the issue of drug law reforms on the political agenda. (The name of this chapter, incidentally, comes from an article I wrote with Amanda some years ago.)

Evidence-based Decriminalisation and Temple Balls

It is interesting to look at what has been going on in Amsterdam and more recently in Portugal, Uruguay, Canada, the Czech Republic and elsewhere, where legislators have made an evidence-based decision to apply levels of control that are deemed to be more in balance with the actual harms — or harmlessness — of the drugs. Statistics show that since decriminalising cannabis Holland has produced much lower rates of cocaine and heroin use

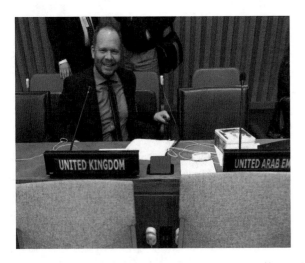

Picture 85: My experience at the United Nations in April was 2016 was disheartening and sobering (the conference part, at least, the trip itself, with Natalie Ginsberg from MAPS, was great). The UK, at present, is certainly down the more archaic end of the scale when it comes to the global nations' attitudes to drug policy reform.

and lower rates even of cannabis usage itself per capita than the UK — not to mention lower rates of organised crime, street violence, sexual assaults and teenage pregnancies[5]. Obviously, we cannot relate all these issues to the liberal Dutch approach to cannabis, but what we haven't seen in Holland is the whole country go to pot, as some people here might assume would happen if the UK adopted a similar approach.

When one is presenting lectures on the potential clinical benefits of psychedelic drugs, one frequently gets asked about and drawn into the question of the legalization of drugs for recreational purposes. Personally, I try to keep the two topics as separate as possible, as I see my role primarily as one to advocate for the use of the psychedelic drugs by doctors in a clinical setting. It is often difficult to keep the two issues apart, of course; as a scientist I find the errors, inefficiencies and sheer lack of evidence-base for the international drug laws so stark that they are almost impossible to ignore.

From a financial point of view, it would seem obvious that legalizing the production of cannabis for the hill farmers of Thailand or other poor communities in the world in Africa and Asia could transform countries like Malawi and Nepal, allowing local communities to finally provide the rest of the world with a unique and sought-after product that only they can make. Imagine that, Malawi Gold and Nepalese Temple Balls (both virtually harmless products, for those without a psychotic fragility) grown as a

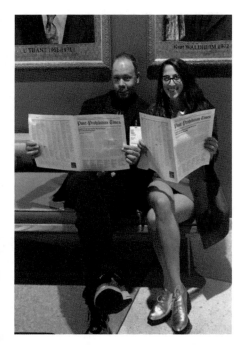

Picture 86: Representing MDMA Science at the United Nations, New York. With Natalie Ginsberg form MAPS, April 2016. Outside the UN building, activists dressed in 1930s attire were distributing copies of The Prohibition Times, dressed in 1930s attire. The UN were confiscating the pamphlets. We felt it was our civic duty to smuggle in and distribute a few copies.

legitimate cash crop and shipped all over the world to be used by non-law breaking responsible adults everywhere.

MDMA: Are We Throwing the Baby Out with the Bathwater?

But this chapter is not predominantly about the War On Drugs itself but, more specifically, on how it adversely effects medical psychedelic research. A subject I do know a lot about is MDMA and especially how it has been systematically demonised for 23 years in the popular and medical press, despite a wealth of evidence for its safe and therapeutic use. But while the politicians raved against the drug with a similar ferocity to the kids on the dance floors, the doctors and pharmacologists argued amongst themselves about the short, medium and long term dangers of MDMA. In the background, meanwhile, MDMA as a therapeutic tool was quietly becoming ancient history. Exactly as with LSD before it, the drug had now drifted so far from its clinical origin for this to become forgotten.

But have we missed something important when we allowed the political agenda to hijack MDMA from science and medicine? Has the politicians' single-minded demonization of all recreational drugs as 'Of No Medical Use' resulted in MDMA becoming an innocent bystander caught in the crossfire of the War on Drugs?

Those Evil Blacks and Mexican Drug Users

"There are 100,000 total marijuana smokers in the U.S., and most are Negroes, Hispanics, Filipinos and entertainers. Their Satanic music, jazz and swing result from marijuana use. This marijuana causes white women to seek sexual relations with Negroes, entertainers and any others."
- Harry Anslinger — Testimony to US Congress supporting Marihuana Tax Act, 1937.

MDMA is not the first such drug that has been treated in such an unscientific fashion. In 1937 cannabis was restricted by the Marijuana Tax Act[7] following a brutal racist campaign by Harry Anslinger and again in the 1951 by the Boggs Act[8] on the back of blatantly racist campaigns against Mexicans and black Americans, respectively. Indeed, even the name *marijuana* was propagated by the US government of the 1930s because it sounded sufficiently Hispanic to scare off the nice white folks from identifying with those nasty pot-smoking Mexicans. And in the 1950s, the campaign against cannabis was similarly transparently directed at encouraging the same nice white folk to avoid at all costs behaving anything like those crazy jazz-loving, sex-crazed blacks. In the UK, on the other hand, where there wasn't such a well-established large non-white community in the 1930s to align with the growing perceived problem of cannabis abuse, the plant has primarily been known simply as cannabis, the valuable source of that durable fabric hemp, and the origin of the word *canvas*. Perhaps this is something some politicians ought to bear in mind next time they are out canvassing support for the war on drugs. Or building walls.

The problem with restricting a drug's recreational use is that it also restricts researching the compound on humans for medical research. When politics pervades the field of medical research, it threatens to undermine the scientific goals of objectivity that are the cornerstones of practice in the search for evidence- based clinical excellence.[5] MDMA, like cannabis, LSD and psilocybin, could be a useful medical and research tool and all these drugs deserved to be explored in a dispassionate manner, without a political agenda influencing the scientific argument.

Just How Dangerous is MDMA?

Whenever a young person dies from a drug-related event involving Ecstasy, it tends to make the front page. But the number of column inches occupied by the perceived risks of MDMA is way out of proportion for the actual degree of physical harm that the drug presents and in stark contrast to those frequently occurring as a result of other drugs. Annually in the UK there are around 9,000 alcohol-related[9] and 80,000 tobacco-related deaths[10].

We have heard throughout this book how even the scientific studies exploring the relative harms and safety of MDMA have been misjudged, inaccurate and mislabelled (literally, at times) — all of which add up to a distorted view of the drug in both the scientific and popular opinions. It is difficult to accurately examine the large-scale risks of pure MDMA on human users because most people who take 'Ecstasy' (whatever that might consist of, in an uncontrolled market) use a host of other drugs too. One interesting study by John Halpern at Harvard looked at neurocognitive functioning in a population of Mormons in the USA who use MDMA *exclusively*, with no lifetime use of any other drugs including alcohol. The results of this study suggest subjects reporting 50 or fewer lifetime episodes of MDMA use displayed no neurocognitive differences approaching significance when compared to non-users[11].

How Frequently are Clinical Syndromes Attributed to Ecstasy Use?

There are no published studies suggesting psychiatric clinics and wards have become burdened by morbidity due to Ecstasy use, which suggests a low incidence of clinical neurotoxicity in human users. Data from a recent neuroimaging study at University College London suggests that MDMA use may not result in long-term damage to serotonin neurons when used recreationally by humans and, furthermore, that when even heavy users stop using the drug, within a year there are no demonstrable differences between their brains and brains of people who have never used the drug at all[12].

Other studies looking at the rates of depression and anxiety among Ecstasy users have demonstrated that, when higher levels of depression and anxiety are seen within a group of Ecstasy users, this can be related to pre-existing depression and anxiety as children and adolescents, before ever taking Ecstasy, emphasising the importance of taking temporal factors into consideration[13].

The data from retrospective studies measuring functioning in Ecstasy users is mixed and there remains a lack of firm conclusions about neurocognitive deficits and psychiatric morbidity. Nevertheless, the debate about the possible dangers of MDMA has had a lot of exposure in both the popular and scientific press in the last 20 years.

In 2012, just after the publication of the first edition of this book, Channel Four in the UK aired a program called *Drugs Live — Ecstasy*. The program, which received wide coverage and a lot of popular press, was made in conjunction with the Imperial College London study team and my colleagues David Nutt, Robin Carhart-Harris and Amanda Feilding were all involved. I was also consulted by the producers of the program who said they were keen to include segments about clinical research with MDMA for PTSD and I attended the screening, waiting anxiously in the studio audience to be approached to deliver the segment we had rehearsed. However, on the night things did not go as planned. The presenters never came to me.

Afterwards, in the Channel Four studios bar, I chatted to Jon Snow and the other presenters and they admitted, rather sadly it seemed, that the executive producers had found themselves bombarded with tweets and calls from the public complaining that the program was "too soft on drugs" and so the decision was made ad hoc to include more segments from the dissenting voices against MDMA and shy away from the likes of me. Channel Four has a tendency, apparently, to be somewhat obsessed with 'creating a 50/50 balance'.

So, we saw them pander to the subject of MDMA safety (which is in fact not a 50/50 but much more like a 95/5 issue) for the sake of their own reputational risk. It was deeply disappointing. Channel Four missed a trick there. It would have made much better copy and provided far more innovative and ground-breaking journalism, to talk about PTSD and the exciting contemporary clinical advances than to simply roll out the same old

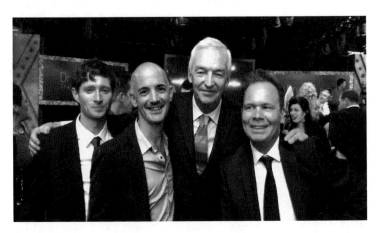

Picture 87: Robin Carhart-Harris, Tim Williams and Jon Snow on the set of Channel Four's Drugs Live: Ecstasy programme in 2012. A step in the right direction, but could they have been bolder and more progressive in their reporting of the benefits versus the risks of MDMA?

gurning ravers and out-dated (and frankly erroneous) stories about holes in the brains. On reflection, the program was nevertheless a small step forward. I just wish they'd been a bit more courageous.

Unscientific Attitudes Affecting Medical Research

The biggest travesty of all is when popular press media scares can impact on medical research for exploring a potential clinical role for MDMA as a therapeutic agent to treat mental illness. It is frustrating when scientific studies describing the dangers of taking Ecstasy recreationally refer to doses or patterns of use that are irrelevant to the clinical usage of MDMA for psychotherapy. A simple analogy would be to imagine doctors from the Royal College of Surgeons or Anaesthetists being denied access to prescribe, or even *research*, the opiate drugs for clinical use because of the existence of recreational heroin abuse. Opiates are vital components of these doctors' formulary, and while they are undeniably abused in society, they are also essential clinical tools when used safely by clinicians. MDMA (which is, incidentally, considerably less toxic than the opiates, when used either clinically or recreationally) may have the potential to be an equally important tool for psychiatry. All these questions make for an interesting proposal that there may be a much larger role for MDMA in clinical medicine than just as an adjunct to psychotherapy. However, with the current drug laws standing as they are, any researcher interested in this field still has significant barriers to overcome before proposing any such projects. Moreover, the controlled status of such compounds in most Western countries deters pharmaceutical companies from even exploring this arena, as they fear that any novel compound with action like MDMA would necessarily be subject to similar legal controls. These would probably hamper its being studied therapeutically and would limit its use and acceptability, even if it were to be shown to have efficacy and to be safer than MDMA in terms of abuse liability, hangover and neurotoxicity.

The Socio-political Agenda on Drugs has a Deleterious Effect on Medical Research

Clinicians, the police, pharmacologists and the public alike are increasingly questioning the current drug laws. David Nutt's major multidisciplinary review in *The Lancet* seriously challenged the current prohibition laws and declared the present system to be not based on scientific foundations[14]. But he was controversially sacked by the Labour government of the day for his opinions. He made some erudite — but clearly annoying for the authorities — comments. Outraged at the government disregarding the clear objective advice of experts in the field in favour of their preconceived political agenda he, in retrospect perhaps imprudently, overstepped the mark and openly criticised the government's policies. But he has lost no favour from the scientific community since that decision — far from it. Okay, so those supporting the Labour (and Conservative) policies of total prohibition may consider him a loose cannon and a maverick, but this is not at all tangible in the scientific community, where he remains as respected as ever — if not more so, for his courage.

Having split from the ACMD, Nutt formed a new committee in 2010 called the Independent Scientific Committee On Drugs (ISCD), which is not, as the name suggests 'a group of intoxicated independent scientists', but, rather, an attempt to gather and disseminate scientific research in an unbiased fashion without the influence of politicians putting their own spin on the data[15].This situation is bad for science and bad for patients and quite illogical. We must not let MDMA research be hijacked by politics, as has happened with LSD. MDMA is a medical tool, and it deserves to treated as such within the field of medicine.

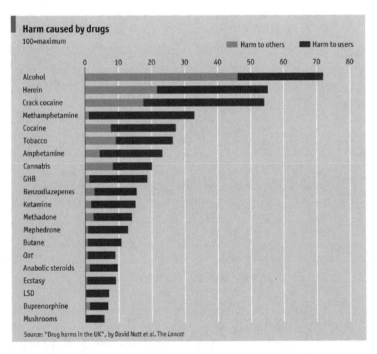

Picture 88: David Nutt's, now world famous, *Relative Drug Harms* graph, from the Lancet paper in 2010.

While it is clearly beyond the scope of this book to challenge such ingrained political dogmas as the international War On Drugs, what I can hope to do is encourage and support a technocratic approach to the drug laws, especially in regard to how they impact on psychiatric drug research.

It will take a brave politician to finally come off the fence and use the clear evidence wisely to review the archaic drug laws. But in reward for this bravery, that politician would be instantly popular and remembered historically for his or her good sense. That moment in history might still be some way off, although when the time comes it will come suddenly. The balance will tip with alarming speed once the politicians of the world realize they are freed from the senseless moral and twisted ethical constraints that keep the prohibition going. This is what political commentators call 'the seat belt effect' — that moment when, after years of intense resistance and debate, the arguments suddenly stop. It is now globally accepted by all that seat belts must be worn in cars, and we wonder now why there was ever a problem about it in the first place. Another good example of societal change that politicians feared could never happen is that of banning smoking in pubs. For decades, successive governments ignored the calls of the medical profession, saying it could never happen. Then it did. And no one complained. Much. The drugs debate could go the same way.

In the meantime we can hope that at least medical patients, if not the rest of the world's many safe and diligent users of psychedelic drugs, can be freed up to choose whichever mental states they wish to participate in, within the safety and privacy of their own minds.

The Concept of Harm Minimization

In 1998 the organisation DanceSafe was formed to provide information at raves and offer Ecstasy users a service for testing the quality of the pills they were taking to reduce casualties associated with low quality and adulterated substances[16]. But the concept of safe raving is much older than that. Since the sixties, festivals have included 'trip tents' where stressed-out users can go for psychological support or medical treatment. Currently, one such organisation is Kosmicare, which provides excellent support for ravers at festivals throughout Europe[17].

When I worked at the Glastonbury festival for six years in the medical tent as one of the resident psychiatrists, our main role was being with, and seeing people through, difficult drug experiences. Rarely were people in any significant physical harm — except for the ones who had drunk too much alcohol, who were always considered the riskiest. Those who had taken psychedelic drugs and were having a hard time because of their lack of attention to set and setting often presented as scared and lost in strange surroundings having become separated from their friends. All that was needed most of the time was a few hours chatting to our team and a cup of tea, and then they'd be on their way again. My friend Karin Silenzi de Stagni, the director and founder of Kosmicare UK, offers a more thorough approach to bewildered trippers, delivered by a skilled team of experienced psychonauts This is an important service for those who have become existentially separated from their buddies and/or their bodies.

In the late 1980s, when the concept of looking after ravers became established in the UK, there was outrage from right-wing groups. I remember talking to people at raves in the early 1990s that were campaigning for clubs to give out free drinking water and provide chill out rooms for overheated ravers. Critics argued that such measures were condoning Ecstasy use. But all these groups wanted to do was to save lives and reduce harm.

It is ironic that now, some 25 years later, the modern NHS has embraced the concept of harm minimization, rightly choosing it over total prohibition as the most appropriate and safe evidence-based approach to reducing the harms of casual drug use. Thankfully, those working with substance misuse disorders have been successful at convincing the authorities that people are going to continue to take drugs, whether the politicians like it or not, so measures that reduce the harm of such behaviours ought to be employed. A stark illustration of just how far harm minimization has come in the last 20 years can be found in the wealth of government leaflets and information available to today's drug users. I have seen NHS government-sanctioned cartoons aimed at children encouraging them to 'chase the dragon' rather than inject heroin, and I recently saw an interesting government leaflet on crack cocaine. It used a series of cartoons to advice the user to pay their rent and buy their week's groceries before going out and scoring their crack with their Job Seekers Allowance money. Then it recommended that, when coming to the last rock of the day, take time to savour and enjoy it, as there would be no more until tomorrow! It may sound crazy for those who would like to just say no to drugs, but the reality is this kind of advice does reduce harm and save lives and there is no evidence to suggest it makes people want to go out and start taking crack if they hadn't been inclined to do so in the first instance[18].

But there are still right-wing voices closing needle exchanges. David Nutt recently reiterated the call for pill testing in clubs but did not exactly get a lot of positive support from everyone. Harm minimization saves lives and people always have and always will take substances to alter their state of consciousness. It is the job of doctors and politicians to reduce harm, not try to deny or eradicate the urges of consenting adults who wish to indulge in what should be relatively harmless activities.

Demonization of Prohibition

It is interesting that the word *prohibition* is increasingly being used about the War on Drugs. The term *prohibition* is universally accepted as a political bad idea, a failed attempt to enforce an un-enforceable law against alcohol. It is widely recognised that the prohibition of the 1930s directly fuelled the development of the mafia-driven criminal networks. Perhaps we are seeing some positive steps towards enlightenment today about all illicit drugs? Personally I am sceptical, but it would not be before time if we were.

Perhaps one day we will look back on the War on Drugs and laugh in the same way as we do about the 1930s experiment. All those wasted years, money and lives. Current drug control laws ought to reflect the pharmacological and societal damage of respective drugs, but regulatory status is far from consistent with the actual harms — or potential benefits — of drugs[19]. The War On Drugs, waged by successive governments against all substances with abuse potential, threatens to strangle our advancement of knowledge about how these substances might be used safely and effectively to treat patients with unremitting mental illnesses. We do not seek to condone the recreational use of potentially dangerous compounds, but, rather, to view the subject with a scientific objectivity that the political agenda is often seen to be lacking. Such an approach is essential if we are to provide the most effective and targeted social policies around prohibition and, crucially, the best evidenced treatments for our patients.

The Misuse of Drugs Act — How Useful Is It?

In the UK the system of classification we use to categorize drugs that have been arbitrarily prohibited is called the Misuse of Drugs Act 1971 (MDA 1971). (http://www.legislation.gov.uk/ukpga/1971/38/contents) The Act sets out the legal penalties that apply to the crimes of either possession, or intent to supply, the various substances deemed too dangerous to be used. Alcohol — that intoxicating substance that produces an aggressive confusional state and is implicated as a causative factor in most domestic violence, sexual assault, road traffic accidents and completed suicide cases — as well as killing 15,000 people per year because of its profound toxicity on the human brain and body — is not included in the Act. The death rates from all the other drugs put together amounts to approximately 4,000 deaths per year — around 3,000 of which are deaths from prescribed drugs.

The MDA 1971 is over 45 years old. It was written in another time and place which now has no relevance to today's culture or society. It is, in my opinion, one of the most striking examples of pseudoscience in the British legal constitution. The Act separates the various classified drugs into different classes, see table below.

Having read this far through this book, reader, you will know that this ranking of drugs with this system bears little or no relation to the actual harms — or benefits — of the drugs. That is putting it mildly. In fact, from what we know about the actual rates of morbidity and mortality of the drugs that present as clinical problems to drug services, the table above has *no empirical validity whatsoever*. The classes, and the allocation of the drugs to them, are meaningless. They are based on peculiar arbitrary definitions that do not relate to the drugs' effects, addiction risks, social, physical or psychological harms.

The fact that psilocybin, LSD, MDMA and DMT are in Class A undermines the entire system of drug prohibition in the UK; or at least it ought

Class	Drugs in class	Potential penalties	
		For Possession	For Intent to Supply
A	Heroin, Cocaine (including crack) MDMA Methamphetamine, LSD, DMT Psilocybin (in the form of mushrooms)	Up to 7 years in prison	Up to Life in prison
B	Amphetamine, Cannabis Codeine, Ketamine, Methoxetamine Methylphenidate. (Any class B drug that is prepared for injections becomes a class A substance)	Up to 5 years in prison	Up to 14 years in prison
C	GHB Diazepam and most and other benzodiazepines. Anabolic steroids.	Up to 2 years in prison	Up to 14 years in prison

Picture 89: The arbitrary pseudoscience of the Misuse of Drugs Act. Compounds in each group have little relevance to their actual risks to recreational users or their potential benefits to medicine.

to. The addiction and toxicity risks from these drugs is virtually zero. As David Nutt said, the MDA is not fit for purpose and therefore sends the wrong message about drugs.

I would go further to say the MDA causes significant harm. People need not die from *any* of these drugs (yes, including methamphetamine, heroin and cocaine). All the drugs in that table can be used safely with the correct care and scrutiny — and most of them *are* used safely daily as clinical tools within hospitals all over the world. The reason we see people dying from their illicit use is not simply because of an inherent toxicity factor of the drug; but rather a combination of the drug effects, unknown ingredients (precisely what and how much), and the way they are used. And it is these last factors, uncertain substances and unsafe practices, that arise as a direct result of the drugs' prohibited status.

When drugs of variable quality, with an unknown and impure dose, are bought and used in clandestine circumstances, harms will occur. Imagine if you bought a bottle of alcohol and you did not know what strength it was, you drank it quickly in secret, you refused to get help when you started becoming ill and, if you found yourself becoming addicted over time, you avoided approaching care services because of fear of prosecution. That scenario is how prohibition causes drug harms. It encourages unsafe use. It does not deter use; in fact, data shows that prohibition increases use amongst certain groups.

I hate drug misuse and drug deaths. I hate knife misuse and knife deaths. I hate hang glider misuse and hang glider deaths.

But all these activities *can* be done safely and can provide people with positive experiences that they deserve to have. If we made knives or hang gliding illegal they would not be eradicated. But they would become a lot more dangerous and the harms and deaths associated with their use would increase. As we have established, drug addiction results from complex psycho-social factors; not just the drugs themselves. Banning all drugs to solve drug addiction is like amputating your legs to save money on shoes. It is dangerous, disabling and will, of course, cost you a lot more money.

So why do we do this with drugs? Successive governments of the last 45 years who blindly support the MDA 1971 narrative of total prohibition based on a deeply flawed, non-evidence based document with no calls for audit or review have blood on their hands for the cause of preventable drug harms.

Prohibition turns drug use into drug abuse.
Drugs don't kill people. Prohibition does.

Why Does This Issue Matter?

There are dangers associated with inaccurately reporting an exaggerated risk of drug use in the scientific and popular press. It may provoke a public health scare resulting in disproportionate use of resources and money, which could be better directed elsewhere and it risks directing attention and education away from more effective harm-minimization programs. But perhaps the most important side effect of inaccurate reporting is the damage it inflicts to research exploring potential positive therapeutic benefits of the drug.

No attempt is being made to condone recreational drug use or suggest that MDMA or any other illegal substance is an entirely safe drug; after all, there is no such thing. There are valid concerns that MDMA, for instance, can induce low mood as its effects wear off, that it can induce pre-existing anxiety and depression in susceptible individuals, that it produces unwanted acute side-effects such as spasmodic contractions of the jaw muscles and that in very rare cases of uncontrolled recreational use it can cause an idiosyncratic adverse reaction that may even be fatal. But for all drugs, whether used recreationally or prescribed, the public deserve to be given a realistic risk-benefit ratio and accurate reporting of relative risks as they apply to them.

A lot of water has passed under the bridge since Ecstasy emerged as a potential problem in 1988 and since then an abundance of studies has neither confirmed irreversible neurotoxicity in humans, nor an associated rise in clinical morbidity, from the use of MDMA.

Recreational Drug Use for Psycho-spiritual Growth

Before this current renaissance got underway, Albert Hofmann famously said that next time psychedelic drugs enjoy a resurgence in society 'the medical doctors must not be allowed to run the show'. Earlier, I made the statement that as a clinical doctor campaigning for the medical use of psychedelic drugs (as opposed to commenting on the recreational use of drugs), I must not allow myself to be dragged into the debate about whether non-clinical populations ought to be able to use the psychedelics. I am nevertheless now going to contradict myself. This is because I do believe there are some circumstances in which healthy, non-clinical members of society can use these currently illegal drugs safely. Drugs such as LSD, DMT, psilocybin, cannabis and MDMA *can* be used carefully, with adequate preparation, by an individual in order to enrich their life. These substances can provide valuable insights and opportunities for reflection, especially about important personal existential issues, and questions regarding their relationships with others.

I therefore support those lobbies of safe users who choose to push for legalisation of drugs to be used judiciously for such positive uses.

Hofmann hoped that one day his discovery, LSD, might become available legally, to be used in clinics where people can safely connect with one another and with nature in a facilitative environment. In effect, such places do already exist legitimately in the form of those recognised religious organisations that use substances, such as the Santo Daime and União do Vegetal Church's use of ayahuasca, the West African use of ibogaine and the Native American Church's use of peyote.

But why not imagine a day where psychedelics can be used lawfully in a Western context? American writer and psychedelic researcher Thomas Roberts has done just this and presents wonderful talks about his vision for a one-billion-dollar company, Community Psychedelic Centers International, which will provide education, training and opportunities for psychedelic voyages on the high street from registered premises[20]. His book *Psychedelic Horizons* is a marvellous piece of writing that avoids the clichéd backstory of psychedelic history and looks firmly towards the future[21].

The psychedelic journey is a deeply personal and profoundly important experience. To deny a healthy and functioning person such a unique existential experience is bordering on a restriction of fundamental human rights. And while these substances are not, in any shape or form, a panacea to cure all ills, there is good anecdotal evidence — from millions of users worldwide — that through the intentional (in the sense of 'with a mission') use of such drugs one can not only transform for the better one's personal life, but that this can have a positive effect on one's immediate environment by providing a space for community reflection. These are not formally tested suppositions, because of the ban on such widespread use of these drugs, but this is a potentially valuable area of study that deserves its place in the future of psychedelic research.

In Conclusion

There are many people battling for governments all over the world to look with sense at their drug laws for all kinds of reasons: from those wishing for medical research to progress unhindered by irritating regulatory processes, to those simply wanting the aesthetic freedom to choose to alter their mental state in whatever way they see fit within the safe confines of their own home.

But a major problem with the fight against the War On Drugs is that there are wildly different methodological arguments being used on either side of the debate. On the one side, there are the likes of David Nutt and the Beckley Foundation producing reams of accurate objective data supporting an end to prohibition. On the other side, are governments whose agenda

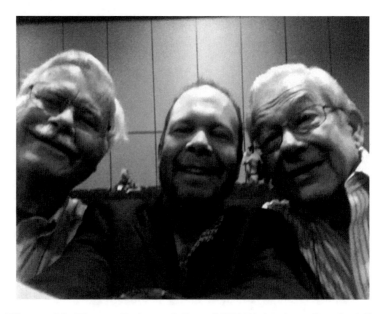

Picture 90: Thomas Roberts, left, and Bill Richards, at Psychedelic
Science, in Oakland, California in 2013.

is influenced by the powerful drinks industry, and a right-wing media
fuelled not by science but by a conservative sentimental approach. Being
seen to be 'soft on drugs' is regarded as a definite vote loser. But just
because the general masses fear a position that offers radical changes to the
current system does not mean the current position is right. One despairs
sometimes and wonders just how much more scientific or sociological data
will it take before the blinkered politicians take notice.

The world watches and waits the developments unfurling in America
regarding changes to cannabis laws. The hope being, that once enough
states exercise their rights to provide legal regulated markets for recreational cannabis use, the federal government will be forced to change the
law. Then, one hopes, a trickle-down effect reaches Europe and the UK. I
will not hold my breath or dust off my Peter Tosh records just yet.

Clearly, as Thomas Roberts says, rather than sitting back and waiting
for our esteemed leaders to become enlightened with a natural urge to
embrace transpersonal issues, the answer instead is to meet the business
people and the politicians (they are the same group) head on, with the kind
of argument they can understand: votes and money. If the culture can be
shifted towards an accurate assessment of the risks, then the public will
support whatever brave politician dares to put their head above the parapet
and propose a reform of the drug laws. And as soon as the politicians

realize that in doing so there is an awful lot of money to be made — and saved — by providing drugs to those who want them, and treatment for those that need it, then the seeds of change will be sown very quickly indeed. Until then we will just have to wait. The current situation certainly gives a lot of people a career. One thing is for sure, there is no way I would be writing this book if I had chosen to study the research of non-psychoactive, politically benign heart tablets.

Conclusion - Back to the Future

Psychiatry Needs Psychedelics, and Psychedelics Need Psychiatry

Without researching these drugs for medical therapy, psychiatry is turning its back on a group of compounds that could have great potential. Without the validation of the medical profession, the psychedelic drugs will remain archaic vestiges of the past, maligned as recreational drugs of abuse and subject to continued negative opinion. Similarly, the people who use them — even for psycho-spiritual purposes — will remain maligned and rejected by society.

These two disparate groups — psychiatrists and recreational psychedelic drug users — are united by their shared recognition of the healing potential of these compounds. Progression for both groups will come from professionals working together adapting to fit a conservative paradigm. This way they can provide the public with important treatments and raise the profile of expanded consciousness in mainstream society. Psychedelic drugs have had a consistent presence in Britain since the 1960s, as both a hedonistic recreational pursuit and as part of a creative subculture, while their clinical use has regrettably fallen from the medical curriculum for the last forty years. But recently, we have seen a re-emergence of these compounds in medicine. They have re-entered the mainstream with impressive force, pushing them to the forefront of contemporary brain research.

The three Breaking Convention Conferences held in the UK since 2011, and the more recent emergence of the UK Psychedelic Society, with local branches now springing up in every major British city, represent an important conduit to mainstream culture.

However, what about the hippies? The interplay between psychiatry and psychedelia has been part of the necessary developmental trajectory for our culture and we can now see a new way — a renaissance as some are calling it — initiating a reformation of the relationship between the people using these drugs, their society, science and greater spiritual consciousness. This is the future. We are going back to it.

Prehistoric and Recent Psychotherapy with Psychedelics

As we have seen in this book, the ancient use of hallucinogens for the augmentation of psychotherapy is well documented by scholars of anthropology. All cultures through history have used sacramental plants and fungi to assist individuals and communities access repressed memories. The role of shamans, with their combined roles of physicians, psychotherapists and priests, and the nature of their relationship with their patients, is not dissimilar to that of the today's psychotherapists.

The rediscovery of the healing aspects of psychedelics between the 1940s and 1970s provided psychiatrists with new tools to replace their primarily psychoanalytical methods and cruel, imprecise physical treatments such as insulin coma therapy, psychosurgery and un-anesthetised ECT. But after Hofmann's *Delysid* leaked from the medical clinics into popular culture a global interest in recreational psychedelic use lead to authoritarian clampdown.

Now, after some forty years of repressive actions of successive governments to effectively halt all psychedelic research (while the recreational use of every other drug has increased tenfold), we are seeing a growth of contemporary psychedelic research. New clinical and neurophysiological studies are being published every week. The expansive growth of our

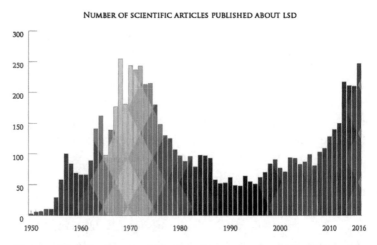

NUMBER OF SCIENTIFIC ARTICLES PUBLISHED ABOUT LSD

Picture 91: The Psychedelic Renaissance – a wonderful graphic (courtesy of The Beckley Foundation) demonstrating that the current published output is rivalling that of the first heydays of psychedelic research. With far more to come in the next decade.

understanding of the physiological processes behind the subjective psychological effects of psychedelic drugs is informed hugely by modern imaging techniques. This provides an envious perspective from which to re-visit studies of the 1950s and 1960s. Back then, we had to simply take it for granted that these substances 'increased access to repressed emotional memories'. Now we can demonstrate this graphically with cutting edge neuroimaging, which adds kudos to the field and courts greater interest from those mainstream-funding organisations that previously considered psychedelic research to be a thing of the archaic past.

The Problem with Psychiatry

But despite advances in neuroscience, psychiatry remains the Cinderella of the medical profession. Chronically underfunded, clinical and research psychiatry remains decades behind our general medical cousins in our understanding of the body's most challenging organ. This is not surprising given the brain's complexity. There are some hundred-billion neurons in the human brain connected to one another by up to ten-thousand dendrites per neuron. A single cubic millimetre of grey matter contains over three kilometres of axons. These are staggering statistics that make the liver, kidney and heart seem crude and simple by comparison.

However, we do not have to go far back in medical history to find an age when physicians were equally baffled by the physical body. 150 years ago doctors voluminously categorised the diseases they saw and mapped their progressions through populations but had little idea about the pathophysiological nature of the common fatal disorders and, crucially, they could not see a way to actually treat them. However, just around the corner was a critical advance, the antibiotics, and once discovered the face of mortality statistics were changed forever.

Today the psychiatric profession is in a similar position to those 19th century doctors. Perhaps it is time for us to ask: *Where is our psychiatric antibiotic?* Mainstream psychiatric research is not adequately challenging this status quo. And the pharmaceutical industry thrives on drug treatments that require a daily dose of their expensive product, to be taken indefinitely and with a transparent realization that it will never actually 'cure' them of their problem. Of course, as doctors we support the pharmaceutical industry and prescribe their drugs — we must — they are all we have. It would be unethical *not* to mask the symptoms of psychiatric disorder for our patients. We know the drugs we give are often not resolving their problems. And here is where we return to the intriguing therapeutic potential of psychedelic therapies.

Why Psychedelic Medicine Works

Psychedelics are the perfect drugs to assist psychotherapy. They are short-acting so can be administered for a single session of therapy. They have no significant dependency issues. They are completely non-toxic at doses proposed for therapy (and are considerably safer than many of the medications we currently use in psychiatry). They are shown to reduce depression. They raise arousal to enhance motivation for therapy, increase feelings of closeness between the patient and therapist, increase relaxation and reduce hypervigilance. They stimulate new ways of thinking to explore entrenched problems. And drugs such as MDMA can *reduce the fear of recalling traumatic memories* so the patient can focus on their trauma without being overwhelmed by negative feelings. When the pharmacological effects of psychedelic drugs are combined with effective and expertly guided psychotherapy, they can offer a new way of looking at old psychiatric problems and could just be the Holy Grail, the penicillin just around the corner for psychiatry.

Using the guided psychedelic experience as medicine, we can tentatively allow ourselves to use a forbidden word, a word that as medical students on our first psychiatric placement we are conditioned never to utter. It is the word *cure*. With psychedelic drug therapy, we *can* turn back time, return to face miserable childhood memories, back to the child's bedroom where that horrific abuse occurred and, psychologically at least, *rewrite history* for that patient. Under the influence of drugs such as MDMA, LSD, ketamine, ibogaine, ayahuasca and psilocybin — used with care and supervision — these patients can explore and repackage the sensory aspects of their traumatic recollections and *put that memory away* in the compartmentalized area of their past where it belongs. The memory will always be there; the psychedelic drugs do not simply nullify or blunt out history (we leave that to the toxic effects of the traditional prescribed psychotropics, and drugs like heroin and alcohol), but psychedelics can help patients re-label their past experiences and become masters of their minds, not remain slaves to the random emergence of unwanted memories that blight their waking and sleeping lives. This unique and powerful role of the psychedelic drugs is tailor-made for disorders based around anxiety. And these disorders are not rare. Anxiety, including PTSD and OCD, are the scourge of modern psychiatry, the smallpox and gangrene of our modern age.

But above these clinically useful effects of the psychedelic drugs there is something else — a mysterious, apparently *spiritual* element that defies our current medical language. The existential component of the psychedelic experience is undeniable and is why these compounds are so useful for improving the resolution of end-of-life anxiety. But the subject of psychedelic spirituality, while wholeheartedly embraced by the recreational users of these drugs, sits uncomfortably with most medical doctors. It was this spiritual element — and the hippies love of it — that blew the opportunity for medical psychedelic research in the past. This time round we must be more cautious.

The Problem with the Recreational Use of Psychedelics

When LSD was banned in the mid-sixties, medical research was severely limited worldwide. Illegalization had a paradoxical effect on restricting popular use, subsequently producing the massive 1960s drug culture. Young people embraced psychedelics and cannabis, popularly accepted as a rite of passage, a de rigour ticket to the swirling maelstrom of anti-authoritarianism left-wing protest and the rejection of the older generation. LSD became labelled as a drug to enhance creativity and was highly influential in colouring new approaches to multiple disciplines from art, music and architecture to fashion, product design, TV and film production and even cooking.

Inevitably, this revolution irked those in authority whose grip on power was threatened by a group of people whose *raison d'être* was to encourage freedom of thought beyond the preceding necessarily restricted modes of expression. Doctors, when banned from research with the drug except under very constrained circumstances, were forced to distance themselves from psychedelics and instead had to toe the party line. What had started as a legitimate and effective new line of psychiatric research was now driven underground. This was disheartening for those clinicians who had seen how useful psychedelic therapy was for patients where traditional methods had failed. Most gave up their research with psychedelics and returned to mainstream medicine, embracing the growing arsenal of new symptom-masking psychotropic chemicals flooding the market, fuelled by pharmaceutical corporations eager to cash in on the physical approach to treating mental disorders, which, ironically, was begun in part by the interest in LSD fifteen years earlier. Later, some of the early medical psychedelic pioneers turned their attention to the then-still-legal drug MDMA, and developed systems for its use in psychotherapy; until it too was banned in the 1980s and, following a broadly similar path to LSD, created the nineties rave generation.

Having lost the medical profession as allies, the late-sixties hippies were now free to become the mouthpiece of the psychedelic revolution. Building their churches and laboratories in the free festivals and communal living, they propagated their philosophy and re-wrote the political codes and boundaries of the New Age, combining the utopian dream of sham political organisation alongside the contradictory banner of boundary-free living, as informed by the ego-less freedom of the internal hallucinatory world. And when mainstream pop society came down from the 1960s and turned back to the grindstone of consumer-driven modern living, those brave pioneers still willing to fly the freak flag, as it were, became increasingly maligned. Their message of internal freedom fell on deaf ears for most clean-living (alcohol soaked) people.

The drugs themselves had moved on. The beautiful people of Haight-Ashbury had morphed into a homeless army of amphetamine and heroin addled ghosts. What had started out as a legitimate protest to an unwinnable foreign war in Vietnam now looked to many like senseless disturbance of the peace. The message was drugs are bad. Drugs ruin lives. Drugs are used only by directionless scroungers. Without the considered approach from the medical profession adding a level of evidence-based caution to the use of psychedelics as medicines, the hippies' message was lost. Gone were the academics preaching a careful methodological approach. All that was left was 'getting kicks'.

Of course, there always have been some pockets of well-organised users advocating a considered method of using psychedelic drugs as healing agents, but these were few and far between. The subsequent developing cocaine trade further restricted any honourable or noble message of the dying hippies and LSD was lost in the mire. The 1960s didn't work. Society had concluded that the hippies' drugs merely caused an 'acute confusional state' and did little to further our understanding of the complex re-evaluation of our social values. The 'normal' people had already decided that it was exactly these drugs that had caused society's problems in the first place.

Doctors, politicians and the other grey-suited 'men of wisdom' have always struggled with groups of long-haired soothsayers whose sentences end with the word 'man'. Glastonbury's stone circle and Burning Man — wonderful, beautiful, creative, life-affirming, progressive and spiritually awakened social melting pot experiments that they are — do not sit well within the austere chambers of the Royal Medical Colleges, Westminster or the US Senate. In these places the hair is neatly trimmed and the shirts well-pressed. It is arguable that such stolid attitudes need to be challenged — and, indeed, many before and since Leary have tried waving their placards and demanding for the last 50 years their cognitive liberty — the right to be high — but none have been successful.

Doctors and indeed politicians need randomised double-blind placebo controlled clinical studies, not reports of anecdotal drug experiences, no matter how convincing they may seem to the saucer-eyed users. Until recently, the medical profession had no choice but to reject the hippies and join forces with the politicians. They did their bit for the War on Drugs by churning out studies highlighting the dangers of wanton recreational use of substances. Forced to appraise individuals' mental breakdowns in the context of their drug use, they categorised illegal drugs as agents that solely cause harm. By the time we saw Ecstasy step up to take LSD's place of 'killer drug' in the early nineties, neurocognitive deficits and brain damage were the phrases of the day. Doctors and neuroscientists wrote voraciously, applying endless erroneous assumptions about doses and patterns of use of recreational Ecstasy users, forgetting that one man's cognitive impairment was another man's party. The medical profession, proudly contributing to the entrenched position of the system, pitched itself against the ravers in the same manner as they had long become accustomed to attacking the hippies. By the end of the 20th century the War on Drugs had stepped up a gear and The Man was clearly winning.

The Problem with the Medical Use of Psychedelics

But medicine does not have all the answers. Randomised controlled trials (RCTs), although the gold standard of research, the benchmark for all new treatments, are highly artificial phenomena. Psychedelic psychotherapy has never sat comfortably with RCTs. How do you design a reliable psychotherapy placebo? And how do you double-blind an experience as intensely *known* as high-dose LSD? But this is not the major hurdle to psychedelic research. And despite what some psychedelic conspiracy theorists might like to think, nor is the hurdle restrictions from fearful governments choosing to block psychedelic research because of a bias against such developments. No, the major impediment to psychedelic research is simple: it is money. The main challenge for the future lies in convincing a profession funded by the pharmaceutical industry to spend millions on researching and developing a therapy that could end up challenging the need for antidepressants.

Who normally pays for (non-psychedelic) psychotherapy? The couch makers? Large-scale randomised, controlled trials of psychotherapy are difficult to design and expensive to run. They are few and far between. It would be nice to imagine the pharmaceutical companies have patients' best interests at heart, that they wish to nobly pursue a programme that aims to wipe out mental disorder altogether, but control, not cure, is their agenda. And without the financial support of multi-million companies encouraging the media (and therefore the public) to look at psychedelics, the press is free to propagate whatever message it wants. Money dictates medical research. Doctors and researchers do not want to bite the hand that feeds them, no matter how subtly that food is supplied.

The delay by the medical profession to develop a consistent evidence-based approach to the relative harms and safety of recreational drugs with coincidental therapeutic potential has been continually hampered by a negative media profile. Psychedelic drugs are not *entirely* safe — no drug or indeed any medical intervention is — but, statistically, they are *very very* safe. And now, over a quarter of a century since 1988's Summer of Love, we are starting to get a balanced opinion in the press. Only a few lone voices from non-clinical opponents with limited experience of the plight of patients continue to be fearful of MDMA. The popular press is beginning to appreciate that psychedelic therapy bears little resemblance to unrestrained recreational use. The popular belief that 'All Recreational Drugs Kill' is no longer a valid argument against the low to moderate infrequent doses of psychedelics applied as medical treatments. Within mainstream media, at least, the tide is starting to turn for the better.

But we certainly didn't get here through the efforts of the ravers or the hippies. Most of their mental twittering of the last forty years has been ignored by mainstream society. It was only through the more recent and considered change in direction of hard-nosed scientists that we are seeing this so-called renaissance. Sadly, it took watering down the mystical-spiritual elements of psychedelics for today's researchers to have got their work underway. Even Roland Griffith's tremendous piece of scientific art, which is a point in case, uses a necessarily conservative language with which to disseminate his important message to his doubting medical colleagues. And all of us working in psychedelic research know that it is essential to downplay the more 'cosmic' components of our work to get funding and publication. It is only through developing a language of conservative banality that we are where we are today.

This is not a satisfactory position. Why should doctors not use words like *bliss* and *enlightenment*? Psychiatry is overly restricted and restrictive in describing mental states only in a language of pathology. The medical model is insufficient to accurately portray what it is to soar angelic on psychedelic drugs. By avoiding descriptions of the psychedelic experience in its glorious entirety, because of impositions from the bodies that fund the research, we risk missing the transpersonal and not eking from these drugs the full extent of their offering. By taking a polarised swing to the extreme of the hippies' standpoint, the medical profession may be missing the wood for the trees and developing substandard therapy paradigms that fail to incorporate the essential healing elements of the naturalistic psychedelic experience. The hippies, of course, have no qualms about including as much cosmic language as they can muster.

While a legitimate mainstream licence to practice for MDMA psycho-therapy for PTSD might now be only a few years away, it is hard to imag-ine that doctors will be embracing the full cross-cultural practice of in-the-field South American ayahuasca in dreary NHS clinics any time soon. It seems the little white pills will be given out long before Western doctors become comfortable prescribing night-long sessions with painted-faced shamans.

Does this matter? Yes it does. Psychedelic psychotherapy, if it is to be effective, must embrace the full healing element of the experience; a watered down capsulated version will not suffice. Furthermore, by con-forming to such restrictions the medical profession risks further polarising these drugs into those that are acceptable and those that are not. We would continue to operate on an uneven playing field. All healing substances used by all healers ought to have an equal footing in medicine. Doctors still have something to learn from the hippies.

Nightmare Scenarios for Commercial Psychedelics?

As the future unfolds and we see the increasing popular appeal of psyche-delics emerge, it might be only a matter of time before some unscrupulous entrepreneur recognizes the wider implications for commercial sectors of society. One could easily imagine the executive board at Google, Shell, Starbucks and Amazon sitting down to a shared LSD session, delivered legally for a high price by a team of commercial psychedelic guides. The potential creativity-boosting elements of the psychedelic experience could be utilized as tool for increasing product sales. For some this might seem like the antithesis of the peace, love and simplicity message of hippie sen-timent that heralded the initial birth of psychedelic culture. However, this is now the 21st century, Trumpism prevails, and from this point onwards anything is possible.

Resolution of These Problems

We need to introduce these drugs gently. By working within the necessarily restricting guidelines of mainstream methodological practice, we can hope to avoid giving our influential press-writers any excuse to align the overly hedonistic recreational use of non-psychedelic, more destructive drugs with the sober intentions of the medical psychedelic community. Boring, I know, but essential. Like it or not, we need to appeal to the sensibilities of the herd. Such a move does not, I believe, represent either selling out or buying into a Western system of capitalism, as I am often told by my more radical hippie friends. Rather, it is shrewd, creative and necessary. I for one refuse to sit by and watch another 50 years of senseless prohibition stagnate mine and my patients' development simply because I am too proud to put on a tie and speak to the men in suits.

But it's not just conservatives who need convincing. There are still many doubters of the healing effects of psychedelic drugs within the medical profession itself. We must get these people on our side now alongside persuading the public. Doctors must infiltrate their medical journals with case studies, book reviews and well-designed studies so cynics can understand that the psychedelic projects of recent years are some of the most eloquent, most cutting-edge neuroscientific studies around. The recent projects have had to be of the highest quality, with critics intensely vigilant and ready to strike at the first hint of methodological limitation. This approach includes the urgent need to tackle cringe-worthy pseudoscience being blurted from some corners of the psychedelic community. It is embarrassing to listen to the rigidity and small-mindedness of some such armchair commentators — who vociferously accuse the medical profession of being 'stuck in their ways', whilst rigidly propagating their erroneous claims about physiological mechanisms for psychedelics. The pineal gland delusion (the incorrect idea that it produces DMT) is, in my opinion, one such example of this folly.

Some scholars even suggest we need a new name for the psychedelic compounds (sorry Aldous and Humphrey). *Psycholytic, entheogen* or *entactogen* are all viable alternatives to the negative baggage accrued by *psychedelic*. Whilst others, in their turn, feel passionately we must promote the term 'psychedelic'; as the homosexual community embraced the word 'queer', making it their own and extinguishing stigmatisation of its use. What is for certain is that these substances are not mere recreational drugs, they are medical agents, pharmacological compounds designed in the main part in laboratories by and for the medical profession. That is where they started and that is where they deserve to return. We owe that much to the population of patients with intractable mental health disorders who may benefit from their effects.

Having been woefully absent from our education since the 1970s, the psychedelic drugs need to be bought back in to mainstream university teaching as viable medicines to treat a range of mental disorders. Negative attitudes to novel approaches often develop at medical school and then persist throughout the profession. Scholars must use creative techniques to bring psychedelic culture to the attention of new generations of psychiatrists. In 2015 the Royal College of Psychiatrists published a CPD-Online teaching module of psychedelic medicine. This is the first-time psychedelics have been formally recognised on a mainstream medical teaching program, providing an opportunity for trainee doctors to realize that clinical psychedelic medicine is a serious career choice.

We must simultaneously overcome the dispassionate attitude of the existing medical model and embrace the mental states of bliss, enlightenment and spiritual emergence experienced by many people. That they are difficult to comprehend and describe with our current medical language does not mean they do not exist, any more than suggesting the mental state of *love* doesn't exist, just because we find it difficult to describe with psychiatric language. The states of bliss and enlightenment have been the prime possession of the world's religions for too long. But why should they own them? These are *mental states*, with the same empirical validity as depression, anxiety and agitation — all perfectly recognised by psychiatrists. It is time for psychiatrists to wrestle these words back from religions and embrace them within the sphere of medicine.

The economics of psychedelic medicine are also convincing once understood. Effective psychotherapy augmented by psychedelics is a cost-effective way of treating otherwise unremitting mental illnesses. If, as the emerging evidence suggests, a few focused drug-assisted sessions with MDMA or psilocybin can truly eliminate the symptoms of chronic mental disorders *for good*, then this means the patient need not continue with lengthy and expensive pharmacological treatments, and the immense financial and personal burden of psychiatric disease on the community can be reduced. Doctors, politicians and the general public alike will embrace any new approach that can effectively demonstrate such a phenomenon. Psychedelic therapy clinics could become commonplace in our communities. In the future, psychedelic drugs need not be confined only to clinical populations but could be made available to much larger groups of healthy people. They could use these substances under appropriate supervision in licensed premises for their own personal psycho-spiritual growth and development. Why not?

Summary of this Book and Orientation for Future Direction

In conclusion, what the global psychedelic community needs more than ever is neither simply more hippies or more doctors shouting for the cause. Rather, we require some good PR. We need to learn from the struggles of other minority groups and use savvy media influences to get the message across. Why, when the safety and efficacy of psychedelics is so well established do most people in the public still fear these compounds so much?

We need to forget trying to change our pseudo-apocalyptical world and the course of human history with psychedelics as they did in the 1960s. Such arrogance is beyond reason in the 21st century when society is far too varied for such a restricted viewpoint. Everything possible must be done to avoid the past promises of chemical utopia. Indeed, an unfortunate but necessary truth is that professionals working in this field must remain as boring and staid as possible — as well as inspirational and enthusiastic — to get the message across.

But at the same time we could do with an 'outing' of psychedelic use; normal, non-stereotypical, everyday people standing up and saying: "Yes, I take LSD / MDMA / ayahuasca. So what? These compounds are safe and non-addictive, and a lot better for me than alcohol." This normalisation approach is what pushed forward the gay liberation cause in the 1990s, far more effectively than the more radical street protests and aggressive confrontations with authority seen in the 1970s and 80s. The Psychedelic Society in the UK is running such a campaign and I wish it luck.

To finish, and by way of a disclaimer, I do not say these dull and conservative things because I lack imagination or fail to appreciate the fun, wonder and spirituality of the psychedelic experience. On the contrary, I welcome and embrace it. But I firmly believe that those of us who see the benefits of psychedelic drugs have a much better chance of infiltrating our message into mainstream consciousness if we adopt a cautious approach. And the net result is that this way we may eventually get psychedelic psychotherapy culture and freedom in through the back door.

Then we will have a revolution, man.

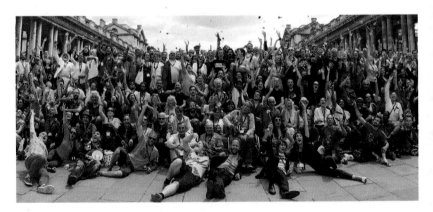

Picture 92: Breaking Convention, 2015, at Greenwich University, London.

Acknowledgments

It has been a great pleasure re-visiting this text to provide an updated version for the 2017 second edition. So many new studies, research projects, conferences, festivals, gatherings and internet groups have sprung up since the first edition of *The Psychedelic Renaissance* in 2012. And I have made many new friends in this ever-growing world wide web of psychedelic researchers and commentators.

Thank you to Mark Chaloner and that long-time inspirer of the less tangible, Tim Read, at Muswell Hill Press for their support and for giving me the opportunity to express in words with virtually unchecked passion what I have carried around in my head for so long.

I am grateful to Keiron Le Grice for reviewing the manuscript for the first edition of this book (2012) and providing not only prose-perfect editing, and feedback based on a knowledge of the subject, but also providing me with appropriate boundaries and helping me keep my feet on the ground while allowing my head to remain in the clouds. And for the 2nd edition (2017) thanks especially to Nikki Wyrd for your sensible injection of prose, wisdom and magick into the spidery fluffiness that I dare call writing.

Thank you, thank you to Robin Carhart-Harris, Dennis McKenna, Dave Nutt, Rick Doblin, Michael Mithoefer, Ralph Metzner and Amanda Feilding for blessing my humble work with your words of experience and kindness. Your years of inspirational encouragement have helped me to keep going and ignore the harbingers of doom with their comments of 'career suicide'. Broader shoulders are impossible to find. I will stand on them to peep over the wall into the garden of delights.

Cheers, man, to Spanny Dangle for the superb artwork and the years of tea and sympathy. Those of us who have known and loved you the longest and closest are convinced your best is yet to come. Whatever, stick around; I certainly intend to.

But most of all thank you to my perspicacious and pulchritudinous wife, Sarah, for enduring this process and believing in me, even if not always believing me.

Look! It's finished — I'm back — again!

B.S.J.S. February 2017

Notes/Reference List

Introduction

1. The song 'The Half Remarkable Question', by The Incredible String Band from the album Wee Tam and The Big Huge. This band's music is an excellent place to start for anyone interested in what the psychedelic experience sounds like.
2. Timothy Leary offers these words on his album of speech and psychedelic music from 1967, Turn On Tune In Drop Out.
3. McKenna, Terence (1982) Food of the Gods. London: Bantam.
4. http://www.legislation.gov.uk/ukpga/2016/2/contents

Chapter 1: A Personal Reflection

1. Strassman, Rick (1995) *DMT: The Spirit Molecule*. New York: Park Street Press.
2. www.maps.org
3. Sandison, R. and Sessa, B. (2008) 'An Interview with Dr Ronald Sandison – LSD Pioneer in UK Psychiatry'. *Multidisciplinary Association for Psychedelic Studies Bulletin*. Autumn Volume, 2008.
4. www.beckleyfoundation.org
5. Sessa, B. (2005) 'Can psychedelics have a role in psychiatry again?' *British Journal of Psychiatry 186*: 457–458.
6. Sessa, B. (2006) 'Psychosis, Psychedelics and the Transpersonal Journey': Proceedings of the Royal College of Psychiatrists Spirituality and Psychiatry Special Interest Group Programme for Friday 31st March, 2006.
7. Nutt, David J. et al (2007) 'The Development of a rational scale to assess the harm of drugs of potential misuse'. *The Lancet*, vol. 369: 1047–1053.
8. Home Office (2009) 'MDMA ('ecstasy'): A review of its harms and classification under the Misuse of Drugs Act 1971.' http://www.erowid.org/chemicals/mdma/mdma_info13.pdf

9. Nutt, D.J. (2009) Equasy – An overlooked addiction with implications for the current debate on drug harms. Journal of Psychopharmacology 23(1) (2009) 3–5

10. http://www.bbc.co.uk/blogs/thereporters/markeaston/2009/10/nutt_gets_the_sack.html

11. Carhart-Harris, Robin L.; Williams, Tim M.; Sessa, Ben, et al (2010). 'The administration of psilocybin to healthy, hallucinogen-experienced volunteers in a mock-functional magnetic resonance imaging environment: a preliminary investigation of tolerability'. *Journal of Psychopharmacology.*

12. https://www.youtube.com/watch?v=LBTr2JEyfXU

13. http://www.psychiatrycpd.co.uk/learningmodules/psychedelicdrug-therapyinps.aspx

14. Alexander, B.K., Coambs, R.B., and Hadaway, P.F. (1978). "The effect of housing and gender on morphine self-administration in rats," *Psychopharmacology*, Vol 58, 175–179

15. Freud, Sigmund (1940) 'An excerpt from *An Outline of Psychoanalysis*. London, Hogarth Press.

Chapter 2: The Experience and the Drugs

1. Sessa, B. (2014) One Man's Cognitive Impairment is Another Man's Party: Legalisation, Legislation and The Fair Trade Cannabis Company. *PsyPress UK.* Summer 2014

2. Adams, Douglas (1979) *The Hitchhikers Guide to the Galaxy.* London: Pan Books.

3. Leary, Timothy (1968) *High Priest.* New York: The New American Library Inc.

4. Lesh, Phil (2005) *Searching for the Sound: My Life with the Grateful Dead.* New York: Little, Brown and Company.

5. Pahnke, Walter N. (1966) 'Drugs and Mysticism'. *The International Journal of Parapsychology*, vol. VIII (no. 2), Spring 1966; 295–313.

6. Griffiths, Roland R., Richards, W. A., McCann, U., Jesse, R. (2006) 'Psilocybin can occasion mystical-type experiences having substantial and sustained personal meaning and spiritual significance.' *Psychopharmacology* (Berl) 187: 268–283.

7. Leary, Timothy (1968) *High Priest.* New York: The New American Library Inc.

8. McKenna, Terence (1982) *Food of the Gods.* London: Bantam Press.

9. Bill Richards, B. and Pahnke, W (1966) 'Implications of LSD and Experimental Mysticism'. *Journal of Religion and Health*, Vol. 5, 1966, 175–208.

10. The Jimi Hendrix Experience. From the album *Are You Experienced*? London: Track Records. By way of a footnote, apparently as a child Jimi had an imaginary friend whom he called 'Sessa'. Weird, I know. Especially as my youngest son is called Jimi.

11. Leary, Timothy, Ralph Metzner, and Richard Alpert (1963/1992). *The Psychedelic Experience: A Manual Based on the Tibetan Book of the Dead*. New York: Citadel Press.

12. Hofmann, Albert. (1979/2005) *LSD My Problem Child: Reflections on Sacred Drugs, Mysticism, and Science*. Sarasota: MAPS.

13. From the song 'Museum' by Donovan Leitch on his 1967 album *Mellow Yellow*. Produced by Mickie Most. Epic Records.

14. See www.erowid.org, www.bluelight.org, and www.shroomwithaview. org for examples of such drug forums. Well worth a browse.

15. Shulgin, Alexander and Shulgin, Anne. (1991) *PIHKAL: Phenethylamines I Have Known And Loved – A Chemical Love Story*. Berkley: Transform Press.

16. Shulgin, Alexander. and Shulgin, Anne. (1997) *TIHKAL: Tryptamines I Have Known And Loved – A Chemical Love Story*. Berkley: Transform Press.

17. Strassman, Rick. (1995) *DMT: The Spirit Molecule*.

18. Szabo, A., Kovacs, A., I., Riba, J., Frecska, E. (2016) The Endogenous Hallucinogen and Trace Amine N,N-Dimethyltryptamine (DMT) Displays Potent Protective Effects against Hypoxia via Sigma-1 Receptor Activation in Human Primary iPSC-Derived Cortical Neurons and Microglia- Like Immune Cells. Frontiers in Neuroscience 10(35)

19. Passie, Torsten, Halpern John H, Stichtenoth DO, Emrich HM, Hintzen A (2008). 'The Pharmacology of Lysergic Acid Diethylamide: a Review'. *CNS Neuroscience and Therapeutics* 14 (4): 295–314.

20. Bergson, H.; *Mind-energy (L'Énergie spirituelle, 1919)*. McMillan 1920. – a collection of essays and lectures.

21. Huxley, Aldous. (1954) *The Doors of Perception*. London: Chatto and Windus.

22. Carhart-Harris, Robin et al (2012) 'Psilocybin augments subjective and neural responses to autobiographical memory cues: An fMRI study with implications for psychedelic-assisted psychotherapy'. *British Journal of Psychiatry*. IN PRINT for 2012.

23. Roberts, A. (2014) Reservoir Drugs: The Enduring Myth of LSD in the Water Supply. PsyPress Journal. Vol 2.

24. Tendler, S. and May, D (1984) *Brotherhood of Eternal Love*. London: Harper Collins.

25. Fielding, Leaf. (2011) *To Live Outside the Law: Caught by Operation Julie, Britain's Biggest Drugs Bust*. London: Serpents Tail.

26. To see one of the world's largest collection of Blotter Art check out my friend Monkey's website at www.blotterart.co.uk. Monkey has consistently donated the blank (undipped!) perforated blotter paper from which we print our delegates' name badges for our Breaking Convention conferences. He also auctioned off some rare sheets signed by Tim Leary and gave the proceeds to the conference.

27. Fantegrossi W. E., Woods, J.H., and Winmge, G. (2004) 'Transient reinforc- ing effects of phenylisopropylamine and indoealkylamine hallucinogens in rhesus monkeys'. *Behavioural Pharmacology* 15:149–157.

28. Alexander, B.K., Coambs, R.B., and Hadaway, P.F. (1978). "The effect of housing and gender on morphine self-administration in rats," *Psychopharmacology*, Vol 58, 175–179).

29. Dishotsky, N. I., et al (1971). 'LSD and genetic damage'. *Science* 172 (3982): 431–40.

30. http://www.rcpsych.ac.uk/pdf/RCPsych%20ADD2015%20Programme%20at%2021April2015.pdf

31. Grof, Stan and Grof, Christina (eds.) (1989). *Spiritual Emergency: When Personal Transformation Becomes a Crisis.* Los Angeles: Tarcher.

32. Stamets, Paul (1996) *Psilocybin Mushrooms of the World: An Identification Guide.* New York: Ten Speed Press.

33. Griffiths, Roland R., Richards, W. A., McCann, U., Jesse, R. (2006) 'Psilocybin can occasion mystical-type experiences having substantial and sustained personal meaning and spiritual significance.' *Psychopharmacology* (Berl) 187: 268–283.

34. Carhart-Harris RL, Bolstridge M, Rucker J, et al. Psilocybin with psychological support for treatment-resistant depression: an open-label feasibility study. Lancet Psychiatry 2016; published online May 17. http://dx.doi.org/10.1016/S2215-0366(16)30065-7.

35. Bogenschutz MP, Forcehimes AA, Pommy JA, Wilcox CE, Barbosa PC, Strassman RJ. (2015) Psilocybin-assisted treatment for alcohol dependence: a proof-of-concept study. *J Psychopharmacol.* 2015 Mar;29(3):289–99

36. Strassman, Rick (2001) *DMT: The Spirit Molecule.* New York: Park Street Press.

37. Huxley, Aldous (1954) *The Doors of Perception.* London: Chatto and Windus.

38. Monte AP, Waldman SR, Marona-Lewicka D, et al. (September 1997). "Dihydrobenzofuran analogues of hallucinogens. 4. Mescaline derivatives". *J. Med. Chem.* **40** (19): 2997–3008.

39. Halpern, John H., Sherwood AR, Hudson, J. I., Yurgelun-Todd, D., Pope H. G. Jr. (2005) 'Psychological and cognitive effects of long-term peyote use among Native Americans'. *Biol Psychi.* 58(8):624–631.

40. Holland, J.(Editor) Metzner, Ralph; Adamson, Sophia (2001) *Ecstasy : the complete guide ; a comprehensive look at the risks and benefits of MDMA*. Rochester, Vt: Park Street Press. p. 182
41. Nichols, D. (1986). "Differences Between the Mechanism of Action of MDMA, MBDB, and the Classic Hallucinogens. Identification of a New Therapeutic Class: Entactogens". *J. Psychoactive Drugs*. **18** (4): 305–13
42. Sessa, Ben (2011) 'Can MDMA enhance Trauma-focused psychotherapy?' *Progress in Neurology and Psychiatry.* Volume 15, Issue 6, 4–7.
43. Sessa, B. (2017) Can MDMA Therapy Be Used to Treat Alcoholism? *Journal of Psychedelic Studies.* IN PRESS.
44. Sessa, B. (2016) MDMA and PTSD treatment: PTSD: From novel pathophysiology to innovative therapeutics. Neurosci Lett. 2016 Jul 6. pii: S0304-3940(16)30490-6. doi: 10.1016/j.neulet.2016.07.004
45. Cole, Jon et al (2002) 'The content of ecstasy tablets: implications for the study of their long-term effects.' *Addiction*. Volume 97, Issue 12, pages 1531–1536
46. Sessa, B. (2015) *The Ecstatic History of MDMA: From Raving Highs to Saving Lives*. From *Neurotransmissions: The Book of Proceedings from the 2013 Breaking Convention Conference*. (Editors: King, D, Luke, D, Sessa, B, Adams, C. and Tollan, A.) Strange Attractor Press, London.
47. Sessa, Ben (2007) Is there a role for MDMA Psychotherapy in the UK?' *Journal of Psychopharmacology*. Vol 21; 220–221
48. Schifano Francisco, Corkery J., Deluca P., Oyefeso A., Ghodse A. H. (2006) 'Ecstasy (MDMA, MDA, MDEA, MBDB) consumption, seizures, related offences, prices, dosage levels and deaths in the UK (1994–2003).' *Journal of Psychopharmacology* 20(3): 456–463
49. Schifano Francisco, Oyefeso A., Webb L., Pollard M., Corkery J., Ghodse A. H. (2003) 'Review of deaths related to taking ecstasy, England and Wales, 1997–2000.' *BMJ* 326: 80–81 NimmoS.M., KennedyB.W., TullettW.M., BlythA.S., DougallJ.R. (1993) 'Drug-induced hyperthermia'. *Anaesthesia* 48: 892–895
50. Malberg J. E., Seiden L. S. (1998) 'Small changes in ambient temperature causes large changes in 3,4-methylenedioxymethamphetamine (MDMA)- induced serotonin neurotoxicity and core body temperature in the rat.' *J. Neuroscience* 18: 5086–5094
51. Wolff K., Tsapakis E. M., Winstock A. R., Hartley D., Holt D., Forsling M. L., Aitchison K. J. (2006) 'Vasopressin and oxytocin secretion in response to the consumption of ecstasy in a clubbing population'. *Journal of Psychopharmacology* 20(3): 400–410

52. Sessa, Ben, Nutt, David (2007) 'MDMA, politics and medical research: Have we thrown the baby out with the bathwater?' *J Psychopharmacol* 21: 787–791.

53. Sessa, Ben and Nutt, David (2008) 'Reply to letter by Green, Marsden and Fone (2007) about Sessa and Nutt's editorial (MDMA: baby with the bath water) in the November 2007 Journal.' *Journal of Psychopharmacology,* Vol. 22, No. 4, 457–458

54. Selvaraj, S. et al (2009) 'Brain Serotonin transporter binding in former users of MDMA ('ecstasy').' *British Journal of Psychiatry.* 194: 355-359

55. Doblin R1, Greer G, Holland J, Jerome L, Mithoefer MC, Sessa B. (2014) A reconsideration and response to Parrott AC (2013) "Human psychobiology of MDMA or 'Ecstasy': an overview of 25 years of empirical research". Hum Psychopharmacol. 2014 Mar;29(2):105-8.

56. O'Shea, E., Orio, L., Escobedo, I., Sanchez, V., Camarero, J., Green, A. R., et al. (2006) 'MDMA-induced neurotoxicity: long-term effects on 5- HT biosynthesis and the influence of ambient temperature.' *Br J Pharmacol* 148: 778–785.

57. Hatzidimitriou, G., McCann, U. D., Ricaurte, George (1999) 'Altered Sero- tonin Innervation Patterns in the Forebrain of Monkeys Treated with (6)3, 4-Methylenedioxymethamphetamine 7 Years Previously: Factors Influ- encing Abnormal Recovery.' *J Neurosci* 19: 5096–5107.

58. Sabol, K. E., Lew, R., Richards, J. B., Vosmer, G. L., Seiden, L. S. (1996) 'Methylenedioxymethamphetamine-Induced Serotonin Deficits Are Followed by Partial Recovery Over a 52 Week Period. Part I: Synaptosomal Uptake and Tissue Concentrations.' *J Pharmacol Exp Ther* 276: 846–854.

59. Ricaurte, George et al (1985) 'Hallucinogenic amphetamine selectively destroys brain serotonin nerve terminals.' *Science,* 229, 986–988.

60. Stolaroff, Myron (2004) *The Secret Chief Revealed.* Sarasota: MAPS.

61. Greer, George R., Tolbert, R. (1986) 'Subjective reports of the effects of MDMA in a clinical setting.' *Journal of Psychoactive Drugs* 18(4): 319–327

62. Greer, George., Tolbert, R. (1990) 'The therapeutic use of MDMA.' In Peroutka, S. J. (ed.), *Ecstasy: the Clinical, Pharmacological and Neurotoxicological Effects of the Drug MDMA.* Kluwer: Holland

63. Bergman, S. (1999) 'Ketamine: review of its pharmacology and its use in pediatric anesthesia.' *Anesth Prog.* 46(1): 10–20.

64. Jansen, Karl. (2004) *Ketamine: Dreams and Realities.* Sarasota: MAPS.

65. Lilly John. (1973) *The Center of the Cyclone* (2nd ed.). London: Bantam Books.

66. Kohrs, R; Durieux, ME (November 1998). "Ketamine: Teaching an old drug new tricks". *Anesthesia & Analgesia.* 87 (5): 1186–93

67. Frohlich J, Van Horn JD. (2014) Reviewing the ketamine model for schizophrenia. J Psychopharmacol. 2014 Apr;28(4):287-302.

68. Wong, J. J., O'Daly, O., Mehta, M. A., Young, A. H., & Stone, J. M. (2016). Ketamine modulates subgenual cingulate connectivity with the memory-related neural circuit—a mechanism of relevance to resistant depression?.*PeerJ, 4*, e1710.

69. Pal, H.R., Berry, H., Kumar, R. &, Ray, R. (2002) Ketamine Dependence. Anaesth Intensive Care. 2002 Jun;30(3):382–4.

70. Middela, S; Pearce, I (January 2011). "Ketamine-induced vesicopathy: A literature review". *International Journal of Clinical Practice.* 65 (1): 27–30).

71. Moore, Marcia. (1978) *Journeys into the Bright World.* Rockport: Para Research Inc.

72. Morris, H.; Wallach, J. (2014). "From PCP to MXE: a comprehensive review of the non-medical use of dissociative drugs". *Drug Testing and Analysis* 6: 614–632.

73. Diamond PR, Farmery AD, Atkinson S, Haldar J, Williams N, Cowen PJ, et al. Ketamine infusions for treatment resistant depression: a series of 28 patients treated weekly or twice weekly in an ECT clinic. J Psychopharmacol 2014; 28: 536–44.

74. Shulgin, Alexander. and Shulgin, Anne. (1991) *'PIHKAL: Phenethylamines I Have Known And Loved – A Chemical Love Story.'* Berkley: Transform Press.

75. Moya, P.R.; Berg, K.A.; Gutiérrez-Hernandez, M.A., Sáez-Briones, P., Reyes- Parada, M., Cassels, B. K., Clarke, W. P. (2007). 'Functional selectivity of hallucinogenic phenethylamine and phenylisopropylamine derivatives at human 5-hydroxytryptamine (5-HT)2A and 5-HT2C receptors'. *The Journal of pharmacology and experimental therapeutics* 321 (3): 1054–61.

76. Ambrose,J. B., Bennett, H. D., Lee, H. S., Josephson, S. A. (May 2010). 'Cerebral vasculopathy after 4-bromo-2,5-dimethoxyphenethylamine ingestion'. *The Neurologist* 16 (3): 199–202.

77. Stolaroff, Myron (1994) *Thanatos to Eros – Thirty-Five years of psychedelic exploration.* Berlin: VWB

78. Stolaroff, Myron. (2004 / 1997) The Secret Chief Revealed: Conversations with a pioneer of the underground psychedelic therapy movement. Sarasota: MAPS.

79. Sessa, B and Meckel Fischer, F. (2015) Underground LSD, MDMA and 2-CB-assisted Individual and Group Psychotherapy in Zurich: Outcomes, Implications and Commentary. *Journal of Psychopharma-*

cology / Journal of Independent Scientific Committee on Drugs. March 2015. Vol1.

80. Fantegrossi, W. E., Harrington A. W,.Eckler, J. R., Arshad, S., Rabin, R.A., Winter, J. C., Coop, A., Rice, K. C., Woods, J. H.(September 2005). 'Hallucinogen-like actions of 2,5-dimethoxy-4-(n)-propyl-thiophenethylamine (2C-T-7) in mice and rats.' *Psychopharmacology (Berlin)* 181 (3): 496–503.

81. Theobald, D. S., Staack, R., Puetz, M., Mauer, H. H. (September 2005). 'New designer drug 2,5-dimethoxy-4-ethylthiophenethylamine (2C-T-2): studies on its metabolism and toxicological detection in rat urine using gas chromatography/mass spectrometry'. *J Mass Spectrom.* 2008 Mar ;43(3):305-16.

Chapter 3: Early Pioneers

1. Sessa, B. (2015) The History of Psychedelics in Medicine – Chapters One and Two in The Psychedelic Policy Quagmire: Health, Law, Freedom, and Society (Psychology, Religion, and Spirituality) Editors: Ellens, Harold and Roberts, Thomas. Published by Preager, USA.

2. Mitchell, S. Weir, (1896) 'The Effects of Anhelonium Lewinii (the Mescal Button)," Brit. Med. J. 2:1625-1629.

3. Ellis, Havelock (1897) 'The phenomena of mescal intoxication'. The Lancet, Volume 149, Issue 3849, Pages 1540 - 1542

4. Lewin, Louis. (1894) 'Über Anhalonium Lewinii und andere Cacteen' — On Anhalonium lewinii and other cacti.' *Archiv für Experimentelle Pathologie und Pharmakologie*. 24: 401-411

5. Stoll, Werner A. (1947) 'Lysergsäure-diäthyl-amid, ein Phantastikum aus der Mutterkorngruppe.' *Schweiz Arch Neut.* 60: 279.

6. Heffter, Arthur, C.W. (1898). 'Ueber Pellote - Beiträge zur chemischen und pharma- kologischen Kenntniss der Cacteen Zweite Mittheilung'. *Naunyn-Schmiede- berg's Archives of Pharmacology* 40 (5–6): 385–429

7. Roberts, Andy (2008) *Albion Dreaming: A popular history of LSD in Britain*. London: Marshall Cavendish.

8. Of note, there is another derivative of lysergic acid with psychedelic properties called *AL-LAD*, or 6-allyl-6-nor-LSD, which was described by Shulgin in TiHKAL. It is shorter-acting than LSD and was only very recently made illegal).

9. Piper, Alan (2013). "Leo Perutz And The Mystery Of St Peter's Snow". Time And Mind: The Journal Of Archaeology, Consciousness And Culture 6 (2): 175–198

10. Hofmann, Albert. (2005) 'LSD: Problem Child and Wonder Drug.' Sarasota: MAPS.

11. Stoll, W. A. "LSD, ein Phantastikum aus der Mutterkorngruppe." Schweizer Archiv für Neurologie und Psychiatrie 60 (1947): 279. 2.
12. Sandison, Ronald. and Sessa, Ben. (2008) 'An Interview with Dr Ronald Sandison – LSD Pioneer in UK Psychiatry.' *Multidisciplinary Association for Psychedelic Studies Bulletin.* (Autumn Volume, 2008).
13. Sandison, Ronald. A., Spencer, A. M., Whitelaw, J. D. (1954) 'The therapeutic value of LSD in mental illness.' *J Ment Sci.* 1954 Apr;100(419):491-507.
14. http://www.youtube.com/watch?v=Hd4rgyZzseY
15. Busch, A. K., Johnson, W. C. (1950) 'L.S.D. 25 as an aid in psychotherapy'. *Dis. Nerv. System.* 1950 August;11:241
16. Osmond, Humphrey and Smythies, John. (1952) 'Schizophrenia: A new approach.' *The British Journal of Psychiatry.* 98: 309-315
17. Ludwig, A. (1970) 'LSD treatment in alcoholism.' In Gamage, J. R. & Zerkin, E. L. *Hallucinogenic Drug Research.* Beloit, Wisconsin: Stash Press.
18. Krebs, T.S and Johansen, P.O. (2012) Lysergic acid diethylamide (LSD) for alcoholism: a meta-analysis of randomized controlled trials. Journal of Psychopharmacology, 9 March 2012 DOI:10.1177/0269881112439253
19. Krupitsky, Evgeny. M. (1995) 'Ketamine psychedelic therapy (KPT) of alcoholism and neurosis.' In: H. Leuner (Ed.) *Yearbook of the European College for the Study of Consciousness.* Berlin: Verlag Fur Wissenschaft und Bildung.
20. Alcoholics Anonymous (1984), *"Pass it on": the story of Bill Wilson and how the A.A. message reached the world.* New York: Alcoholics Anonymous World Services, Inc.
21. Huxley, Aldous. (1954) *The Doors of Perception.* London: Chatto and Windus.
22. By way of a footnote regarding this famous poem, in 2015 I had my first excursion away from scientific writing into the world of contemporary fiction, with the publication of, '*To Fathom Hell or Soar Angelic*', a story imagining the development of psychedelic medicine in the UK. (Sessa, B. (2015) To Fathom Hell of Soar Angelic. Published by Psychedelic Press, UK.)
23. Lee, M. A. and Shalin, B. (1992) *Acid Dreams. The complete social history of LSD: The CIA, the sixties and beyond.* New York: Grove Press.
24. Huxley, Aldous. (1962) *Island.* New York: Harper and Brothers.
25. Huxley, Aldous. edited by Michael Horowitz and Cynthia Palmer (1999) *Moksha: Aldous Huxley's Classic Writings on Psychedelics and the Visionary Experience.* Vermont: Park Street Press.

26. Grof, Stanislav (2001). *LSD Psychotherapy* (3rd ed.). Sarasota: MAPS.
27. Eyerman, J (2013) "A Clinical Report of Holotropic Breathwork in 11,000 Psychiatric Inpatients in a Community Hospital Setting" MAPS Bulletin Special Edition, 2013 23(1): 24-27
28. Greenfield, Robert. (2006) *Timothy Leary. A Biography.* Boston: Houghton Mifflin Harcourt
29. Leary, Timothy. (1957). *Interpersonal diagnosis of personality.* New York: Ronald Press.
30. Leary, Timothy. & Metzner, Ralph. (1968). 'Use of psychedelic drugs in prisoner rehabilitation.' *British Journal of Social Psychiatry* Vol. 2: 27–51.
31. Doblin, Rick. (1998) 'Dr. Leary's Concord Prison Experiment: a 34-year follow-up study.' *J Psychoactive Drugs.* 1998 Oct-Dec;30(4):419–26.
32. Hollingshead, Michael (1973) *The Man Who Turned On the World.* New York: Abelard-Schuman Publ. (also Blond & Briggs, Ltd.)
33. Leary, Timothy (1968) *High Priest.*(Second Edition, 1995). Berkeley: Ronin Press.
34. Pahnke, Walter N. (1969) 'Psychedelic drugs and mystical experience.' *Int Psychiatry Clin* 5: 149–162.
35. Doblin, Rick. (1991) 'The Good Friday Experiment – A twenty-five year follow-up and methodological critique.' *Journal of Transpersonal Psychology* Vol. 23 (1): 1–28.
36. Zaehner, R.C. (1972) *Drugs, Mysticism and Make Believe.* London: Collins.
37. Meher Baba (1966) *God in a Pill? On L.S.D. and The High Roads.* Walnut Creek: Sufism Reoriented, Inc.
38. Masters, Robert. L. and Houston, Jean. (1966). *The Varieties of Psychedelic Experience.* Vermont: Park Street Press.
39. Downing, Joseph J., and Wygant, William, Jr. (1964) 'Psychedelic experience and religious belief.' In R. Blum and Associates, editors. *Utopiates: The Use and Users of LSD-25.* New York: Atherton. Pp. 187–198.
40. Clark, W. H. (1974) 'Hallucinogen drug controversy'. In: Radouco-Thomas, S., Villeneuve, A., Radouco-Thomas, C. (eds) *Pharmacology, Toxicology, and Abuse of Psychomimetics (Hallucinogens).* Quebec: Les Presses de l'Universite' Laval: 411–418.
41. Sandison, Ronald. to Sessa, Ben. (2007) Personal communication.
42. Ling TM, Buckman J (1963) The Treatment of Anxiety with Lysergic Acid and Methylphenidate. Practitioner 191: 201–204
43. Kast, Eric (1967). 'Attenuation of anticipation: a therapeutic use of lysergic acid diethylamide' *Psychiat. Quart.* 41 (4): 646–57.
44. Grinspoon, Lester. and Bakalar, J. (1979) *Psychedelic Drugs Reconsidered.* New York: The Lindesmith Center.

45. Malleson, Nicolas. (1971) 'Acute Adverse Reactions to LSD in clinical and experimental use in the United Kingdom.' *Br J Psychiatry.* 1971 Feb;118(543):229–30.

46. Krebs TS & Johansen P-Ø (2013) Psychedelics and Mental Health: A Population Study. PLoS ONE 8(8): e63972. doi:10.1371/journal.pone.0063972.)

47. Laing, Adrian (1997) *R.D. Laing: A Biography.* London: Harper Collins.

48. In 1993, aged twenty-one, I first read Laing's *The Divided Self* (1960), whilst taking a year out from medicine to complete a psychology degree. He wrote it when he was a junior doctor himself, aged just 23. Fueled with anti-psychiatry sentiments, I devoured the book with admiration and envy. Such precise dissection of the rot and junk that littered psychiatry at the time blew me and my anti-authority student colleagues away.

49. Leary, Timothy. (1980) *The Politics of Ecstasy.* Berkley: Ronin Publishing.

50. Zeal, Paul. (2010) Personal communication – and this video we did: https://www.youtube.com/watch?v=K_b4bUHk8gs

51. Kyaga, S. et al (2011) 'Creativity and mental disorder: family study of 300,000 people with severe mental disorder.' *British Journal of Psychiatry* November 2011 199:373-379

Chapter 4: The Prehistory and Ancient History of Hallucinogens

1. Hawking, S. There is no God. There is no Fate. From Discovery Channel Curiosity S01E01.

2. McKenna, Terence (1982) Food of the Gods. London: Bantam Press.

3. Gould, Steven Jay 1997) *Evolution: The Pleasures of Pluralism.* The New York Review of Books, June 26, 1997, pp. 47–52.

4. Ramachandran, V.S. (2011) *The Tell-Tale Brain.* William Heinemann, London.

5. Sessa, Ben. (2012) '*The Tell-Tale Brain* by V.S. Ramachandran. Book review.' For the Journal of Neuropsychoanalysis. Vol 14, No.1. 2012.

6. Danforth, A.L., Struble, C.M., Yazar-Klosinski, B. and Grob, C.S. (2016) MDMA-assisted therapy: A new treatment model for social anxiety in autistic adults. Progress in Neuro-Psychopharmacology and Biological Psychiatry. Volume 64, 4 January 2016, Pages 237–249

7. Freedman, A.M. et al (1962) 'Autistic Schizophrenic Children. An Experiment in the Use of D-lysergic acid diethylamide (LSD-25).' *Archives of General Psychiatry,* 1962; 6 (203–213)

8. Simmons, J. et al (1966) 'Modification of Autistic Behavior with LSD-25.' *American Journal of Psychiatry,* May 1966, pp. 1201–1211

9. Mogar, R. E., Aldrich, R. W. (1969) 'The use of psychedelic agents with autistic schizophrenic children.' *Behav Neuropsychiatry* 1: 44–50.

10. Another interesting, and sad, association between psychedelics and elephants is that of the case in 1962 of a shady CIA government official, Dr. Louis Jolyon 'Jolly' West. Jolly injected an elephant, Tusko, the pride of Oklahoma Zoo, with 300mg of LSD, a wildly misjudged dose, using a dart rifle. Tusko experienced an unremitting seizure. Dr. West subsequently administered massive quantities of phenobarbitone and chlorpromazine and Tusko died an hour and a half later – most likely as a result of the heavy sedatives, not the LSD. A more accurate dose, given interspecies scaling and the size of an elephant's brain, would have been more like one milligram. Rumour has it that West, who was part of the CIA's MK-ULTRA programme, was high on his own supply at the time. This and other fascinating stories of psychedelic history can be found in: Lee, M. A., and Shalin, B. (1992) *Acid Dreams. The Complete Social History of LSD: The CIA, the Sixties and Beyond.* New York: Grove Press.

11. Eliade, Mercia (1951) *Le Chamanisme et les techniques archaïques de l'extase*, 1951 - *Shamanism: Archaic Techniques of Ecstasy.* Princeton: Princeton University Press.

12. Kehoe, Alice (2000) *Shamans and Religion: An Anthropological Exploration in Critical Thinking. Long* Grove: Waveland Press.

13. Harner, Michael, (1980) *The Way of the Shaman: A Guide to Power and Healing.* New York: Harper & Row.

14. Contemporary Western society does not always recognise the role of shamanic approaches to spirituality. In the UK BBC Radio 4, which likes to represent as wide a range of religions as possible on their morning 'Thought for the Day' slot, has so far never had a sermon about entheogenic spirituality. Perhaps one day this will change?

15. Schultes, Richard Evans; and Albert Hofmann (1980). *The Botany and Chemistry of Hallucinogens* (2nd ed. ed.). Springfield, Ill.: Thomas.

16. Hofmann, Albert., Wasson, G.R., Ruck, C. and Staples, B. (1998) *The Road to Eleusis: Unveiling the Secret of the Mysteries.* New Castle, PA: Hermes Press.

17. Ruck, Carl. P. and Webster, P. (2006) 'Symposium: The Mythology and Chemistry of the Eleusinian Mysteries.' *Proceedings of the 2006 World Psychedelic Forum conference: LSD.* Basel, Switzerland.

18. Forte, Robert (Editor) (1997) *Entheogens and the Future of Religion.* San Francisco: Council on Spiritual Practices.

19. Allegro, J. M., Irvin, J. R., Ruck, Carl P. (1970) *The Sacred Mushroom and The Cross: A study of the nature and origins of Christianity within*

the fertility cults of the ancient Near East. London: Hodder & Stoughton Ltd

20. Nemu, D. (2014) *Science Revealed.* Psychedelic Press, UK.
21. Nemu, D. (2014) *Neuro-Apocalypse.* Psychedelic Press, UK.
22. Heinrich, Clark (2002) *Magic Mushrooms in Religion and Alchemy,* Park Street Press, New York
23. Strassman, R. (2014) DMT and the Soul of Prophecy: A New Science of Spiritual Revelation in the Hebrew Bible. Park Street Press, New York, USA).
24. Merkur, Dan. (2000) The mystery of manna: the psychedelic sacrament of the Bible, Vermont: Inner Traditions / Bear and Co.
25. Deep Purple, (1968) 'Mandrake Root.' From the album *Shades of Deep Purple.* Produced by Derek Lawrence. Parlophone Records, UK.
26. Caporael, L. (1976). 'Ergotism: The Satan loosed in Salem?' *Science, 192* (4234), 21-26
27. Albarelli Jr., H.P. (2009) A Terrible Mistake: The Murder of Frank Olson and the CIA's Secret Cold War Experiments. Trine Day, Bigtownville, CO, USA).
28. Hagenbach, D. and Werthmüller, L. (2001) Mystic Chemist – The Life of Albert Hofmann and His Discovery of LSD. Pages 84-87. Synergetic Press, Santa Fe, New Mexico, USA).
29. Szasz, Thamas. (1961) T*he Myth of Mental Illness.* New York: Harper and Row.
30. Foucault, Michel. (1964) *Madness and Civilisation.* New York: Pantheon Books.
31. Goffman, Irvin. (1961) *Asylums: Essays on the Social Situation of Mental Patients and Other Inmates.* New York: Anchor Books.
32. https://www.theguardian.com/commentisfree/2016/sep/08/fabric-closure-drugs-policy-london-nightclub-dance
33. Henderson, Bobby (2005). "Open Letter To Kansas School Board". Available at: http://www.venganza.org/about/open-letter/
34. Why shouldn't the Gong Mythology be an equally valid explanation of spiritual truth as does Christianity? It goes briefly as follows: Once upon a time there was a planet called Planet Gong, from which came small green men, the Pot Head Pixies, with propellers on their heads. They fly in teapots by a process known as 'glidding'. On Planet Gong there is an Angel's Egg, guarded by the 32 Octave Doctors. The mystery of Planet Gong is revealed to an ordinary hapless human called Zero the Hero, who, after drinking a special tea, falls asleep and is taken to Gong by the passing Captain Capricorn. Zero realises he is specially chosen prophet, assigned to save planet Earth from the ignorant human race. But during a crucial point in his mission he chooses

to fraternise with the celestial groupies at a great cosmic party rather than build a temple, thereby failing to complete his task. But all is not lost. After he is dead, in his spiritual form in 2032, he manages to unite the hopeless souls of Earth in order that they can transcend this life, enter a new enlightened form of consciousness and save the planet. The most important aspect of the Gong story, which is the brainchild of the wonderfully psychedelic visionary Daevid Allen, is its sound empirical validity. A fine collection of albums from the band Gong are disseminated all over the world and regularly worshipped by many captive followers. The Gong story is no less magical or unbelievable than the Christian message of Jesus' relation to God. Albums by Gong well worth a listen to illustrate the famous Gong Mythology include: *Flying Teapot* (1973), *Angel's Egg* (1973) and *You* (1974). All on Virgin Records.

35. https://www.theguardian.com/music/2015/mar/13/daevid-allen
36. http://www.telegraph.co.uk/obituaries/2016/08/29/gilli-smyth-space-whisperer--obituary/
37. James, William. (1902) *The Varieties of Religious Experience*. London: Long- mans, Green and Co.
38. Masters, Robert L. and Houston, Jean. (1966). The Varieties of Psychedelic Experience. Vermont: Park Street Press.
39. Dawkins, R. (2006). *The God delusion*. Boston: Houghton Mifflin Co.

Chapter 5: Hippie Heydays and the Birth of Ecstasy

1. Withnail and I. (1987) Directed by Bruce Robinson.
2. Bateson, G. (1972). Double bind, 1969. Steps to an ecology of the mind: A revolutionary approach to man's understanding of himself, 271-278. Chicago: University of Chicago Press
3. Morgan, B. (2006) *I Celebrate Myself: The Somewhat Private Life of Allen Ginsberg*. London: Viking / Penguin.
4. Leary, Timothy. (1968) *High Priest*. New York: The New American Library Inc.
5. Lee, M. A. and Shalin, B. (1992) *Acid Dreams. The complete social history of LSD: The CIA, the sixties and beyond*. New York: Grove Press.
6. Stevens, Jay. (1987) *Storming Heaven: LSD and the American Dream*. New York: Grove Press.
7. Tendler, S. and May, D (1984) *Brotherhood of Eternal Love*. London: Harper Collins.
8. Kesey, Ken. (1962) *One Flew Over The Cuckoo's Nest*. New York: Viking Press.

9. Kerouac, Jack. (1957) *On The Road.* New York: Viking Press.
10. Wolfe, Tom. (1968) *The Electric Kool-Aid Acid Test.* New York: Farrar, Strous and Giroux.
11. Kripal, J. J. and Shuck, G. W. (2005) *On the Edge of the Future: Esalen and the Evolution of American Culture.* Bloomington: Indiana University Press.
12. Castaneda, Carlos. (1968) *The Teachings of Don Juan: A Yaqui Way of Knowledge.* Berkley: University of California Press.
13. Fikes, Jay Courtney (1996) Carlos Castaneda, Academic Opportunism and the Psychedelic Sixties. Millennia Press.
14. Greenfield, Robert. (2006) Timothy Leary. A Biography. Boston: Houghton Mifflin Harcourt
15. Going back to my early 90s DJ roots, from 2008 to 2012 I presented a monthly radio show on local Somerset radio. The show, called, *'Dr. Ben's Psychedelic Love-In presents 'In The Psychiatrist's Flares') was assisted by* lysergic colleagues Chris S. and Rupert M.. It provided an excellent excuse to spend my hours trawling through record shops. Remember them?
16. Perry, Charles. (2005) The Haight-Ashbury. New York: Wenner Books.
17. Jarnow, J. (2016) *Heads.* Da Capo Press, Boston, USA.
18. Kaelen, M., Barrett, F.S., Roseman, L., Lorenz, R., Family, N., Bolstridge, M., Curran, H.V., Feilding, A., Nutt, D.J., Carhart-Harris, R.L. (2015). LSD enhances the emotional response to music. Psychopharmacology (Berl.) 23, 3607–3614.
19. http://www.youtube.com/watch?v=aTgrioOyWEo
20. Miles, Barry. (2005) Hippie. London: Cassell Illustrated /Octopus Publishing Ltd.
21. Roberts, A. (2016) Acid Drops. Psychedelic Press, St. Ives, UK.
22. Neville, Richard. (2012) Hippie Hippie Shake. New York: Overlook TP.
23. Fielding, Leaf. (2011) To Live Outside The Law. London: Serpents Tail.
24. Bentley, S. (2016) Undercover: Operation Julie - The Inside Story. CreateSpace Independent Publishing Platform, London.
25. Sessa, B. (2015) The Ecstatic History of MDMA: From Raving Highs to Saving Lives. Accepted for publication in the Breaking Convention Book of Proceedings from the 2013 Conference. Strange Attractor Press, London.
26. Iversen, L. (2006) Speed, Ecstasy and Ritalin - The Science of Amphetamines. Chapter Four: Amphetamines as Performance Enhancers, Page 77-78. Oxford University Press, Oxford.
27. Shulgin, Alexander and Shulgin, Anne. (1991) 'PIHKAL: Phenethylamines I Have Known And Loved – A Chemical Love Story.' Berkley: Transform Press.

28. Eisner, Bruce. (1989) *Ecstasy: The MDMA Story.* Berkley: Ronin Publishing.

29. In 2000, whilst travelling around India alone for six months I came across the Osho ashram in Pune. Completely unaware of what sort of place it was, I took the obligatory AIDS test and stayed for six weeks, sharing my love, as one was encouraged to do. It was beautiful. I spent most of my time lying at the bottom of the swimming pool holding my breath and counting in Hindi; it was too hot to be anywhere else.

30. Colin, M. (1997) *Altered State: The Story of Ecstasy Culture and Acid House.* London: Serpents Tail.

31. I truly regret not making it out London for the Castlemorton event in my 2nd year of medical school. I did make it to the Criminal Justice Bill march and the Reclaim the Streets parties of the mid-nineties; raving alongside lines of policemen in scenes reminiscent of the sixties anti-Vietnam marches — or at least that's what we liked to think. At the time London was awash with impromptu raves in warehouses and squats. Pirate FM radio transmitted vinyl mixed rave from the roof of my tower block in Archway. I gather now they just upload playlists onto the internet, sigh.

32. My friends and I were in the BBC studio audience the night The Shamen played 'Ebenezer Goode' on Top of the Pops. From what I remember…

33. http://www.maps.org/research/mdma/studies/mp1/

34. As one of my patients once said to me when describing the bind he was in with his family, "It's a Catch 24." "You mean Catch 22?" I replied. "Oh, no, doc. It's way worse than that."

35. Grob, C.S., Poland, R.E., Chang, L. and Ernst, T. (1996) Psychobiologic effects of 3,4-methylenedioxymethamphetamine in humans: methodological considerations and preliminary observations. Behavioural Brain Research 73: 103-107.

36. Doblin, Rick. (2004) 'Exaggerating MDMA's Risks to Justify A Prohibitionist Policy.' Published on MAPS website: http://www.maps.org/mdma/rd011604. html

37. Sessa, Ben (2005) 'Can psychedelics have a role in psychiatry again?' *British Journal of Psychiatry186*: 457–459

38. Sessa, B. and Nutt, DJ (2015) Making a Medicine Out of MDMA. *British Journal of Psychiatry. 2015 Jan;206*(1): 4-6.

39. Sessa, B. and Johnson, M. (2015) Is There a Role for Psychedelics in the Treatment of Drug Dependency? *British Journal of Psychiatry,* 206 (1) 1–3

40. Sessa, B. and Grey, A. (2015) Painting of Dr Alexandra and Ann Shulgin by Alex Grey, with Commentary from Sessa and Grey – On the

cover of the *British Journal of Psychiatry.* January Vol. 206, No. 1. 2015).

Chapter 6: Psychedelic Creativity

1. Sessa, Ben. (2008) 'Is it time to revisit the role of psychedelic drugs in enhancing human creativity?' *J Psychopharmacology*; 22; 821
2. Carhart-Harris, Robin L.; Muthukumaraswamy, Suresh; Roseman, Leor; Kaelen, Mendel; Droog, Wouter; Murphy, Kevin; Tagliazucchi, Enzo; Schenberg, Eduardo E.; Nest, Timothy. "Neural correlates of the LSD experience revealed by multimodal neuroimaging". *Proceedings of the National Academy of Sciences.* vol. 113 no. 17; 4853–4858
3. Heilman, K. M., Nadeau, S. E., Beversdorf, D. O. (2003) Creative innovation: possible brain mechanisms.' *Neurocase* 9: 369–379
4. Zinkhan, G. (1993) 'Creativity in Advertising.' *Journal of Advertising* 22, 2: 1-3.
5. Ede Frecska, Vivien Magyar, Csaba E. Moré, and Luis E. Luna (2011) 'Enhancement of Creative Expression and Entoptic Phenomena as After-Effects of Repeated Ayahuasca Administration.' Submitted to *Journal of Psychopharmacology.* May 2011. Under peer review.
6. Luke, David (2010) Rock art or Rorsarch: Is there more to entopics than meets the eye? Time and Mind: *The Journal of Archaeology, Consciousness and Culture.* Volume 3—Issue 1, pp. 9–28
7. Thomas de Quincey, ed. Grevel Lindop. *Confessions of an English Opium-Eater and Other Writings.* New York: Oxford University Press, 1998.
8. Coleridge, ST (1816) *Kubla Khan.* New Ed edition (2004) Reading, UK: Two Rivers Press.
9. Dumas, A (1844) *The Count of Monte Cristo.* Penguin Classics (2003). London: Penguin.
10. Tennyson, AL (1832) *The Lotus Eaters.* New Ed edition (2000) Oxford, UK: Oxford University Press.
11. Artaud, A (1937) *The Peyote Dance.* (1976) New York: Farrar, Straus and Giroux.
12. Michaux, H (1956) Miserable Miracle. San Francisco: City Lights Books (1963).
13. Sessa, B. and Grey, A. (2015) Painting of Dr Alexandra and Ann Shulgin by Alex Grey, with Commentary from Sessa and Grey – On the cover of the *British Journal of Psychiatry.* January Vol. 206, No. 1. 2015).
14. Chamberline, Dean, and Sessa, Ben and (2007) 'Pictures in psychiatry: Albert Hofmann.' *British J Psychiatry* 190: 1-a2-1.

15. Dobkin de Rios, M, Janiger, Oscar (2003) LSD, *Spirituality and the Creative Process*. Vermont: Park Street Press.
16. Krippner, Stanley (1972) 'Mescaline psilocybin and creative artists.' In: Tart, Charles T., (ed), *Altered States of Consciousness*. New Jersey, USA: John Wiley and Sons.
17. Barron, Frank (1965) 'The Creative Process and the Psychedelic Experience.' *Explorations Magazine*. Berkley, California, June–July.
18. McGlothlin, WH, Cohen, S, McGlothlin, MS (1967) 'Long lasting effects of LSD on normals.' *Arch Gen Psychiatry* 17: 521–532.
19. Harman, W. W., McKim, R. H., Mogar, R. E., Fadiman, James, Stolaroff, Myron J. (1966) 'Psychedelic agents in creative problem solving: a pilot study.' *Psychol Rep* 19: 211–227.
20. Izumi, Kiyo. "LSD and Architectural Design." *Psychedelics: The Uses and Implications of Hallucinogenic Drugs*. Eds. Bernard Aaronson and Humphry Osmond. Garden City, NY: Anchor Books, 1970. 381-97.
21. Stafford, P.G., Golightly, B.H. (1967) *LSD – the problem-solving psychedelic*, chapter VII. London: Tandom Books, pp. 207–209.
22. Roberts, A. (2015) Francis Crick, DNA & LSD. Psychedelic Press U.K., 2015, Volume 2).
23. Markoff, J. (2006) *What the Dormouse Said: How the Sixties Counter- culture Shaped the Personal Computer Industry*. New York, USA: Penguin Group.
24. Kleps, Art (1967) 'Creative Problem Solving' in *LSD: The problem-solving psychedelic*, chapter III. by Stafford, PG, Golightly, BH (eds),. Award Books: New York p. 46.

Chapter 7: Modern Non-Western Uses of Natural Plant and Fungi Psychedelics

1. Pinchbeck, Daniel (2017) How Soon is Now? Watkins Publishing, London.
2. Gilk, Paul (2009). "*Green Politics is Eutopian*". Cambridge, UK: The Lutterworth Press.
3. Evans Schultes, Hofmann, Albert and Ratsch, Christian (1998) *Plants of the Gods*. New York: Healing Arts Press.
4. Wasson, R. Gordon (1957) 'Seeking the Magic Mushroom.' *Life magazine*, May 13, 1957
5. Maria Sabina quoted (in translation) in Halifax, J. (1979) Shamanic Voices: A Survey of Visionary Narratives, New York: E.P. Dutton. Pp 203-205. Taken from the tremendous book edited by Robert Forte, *Entheogens and the Future of Religion*. San Francisco: Council on Spiritual Practices.

6. Arthur, James (2003) *Mushrooms and Mankind: The Impact of Mushrooms on Human Consciousness and Religion.* San Diego, CA: The Book Tree.

7. Samorini, G. (2000) *Animals and Psychedelics.* Park Street Press, Rochester, Vermont.

8. Letcher, Andy. (2007) *Shroom: A Cultural History of the Magic Mushroom.* London: Ecco.

9. Letcher, Andy. (2011) Personal communication.

10. Gottlieb, Adam. (1977) *Peyote and other psychoactive cacti.* Berkley: Ronin Publishing.

11. Halpern John H., Sherwood AR, Hudson JI, Yurgelun-Todd D, Pope HG Jr. (2005) 'Psychological and cognitive effects of long-term peyote use among Native Americans.' *Biol Psychi.* 58(8):624-631.

12. Hagan, William T. (1995) *Quanah Parker, Comanche Chief.* University of Oklahoma, pg. 57.

13. Alper, K. and Cordell, G. (2001) *Ibogaine, Volume 56: Proceedings from the First International Conference (The Alkaloids).* Waltham, MA: Academic Press.

14. Scott, David Graham (2004) https://vimeo.com/25291673

15. Scott, David Graham (2014) https://vimeo.com/130630278

16. Ball, M. (2007) Sage Spirit: Salvia Divinorum and the Entheogenic Experience. Oregon: Kyandara Publishing

17. Metzner, Ralph. (2005) *Sacred Vine of Spirits: Ayahuasca.* Vermont: Park Street Press.

18. Burroughs, William S. (1963) *The Yage Letters.* San Francisco: City Lights.

19. McKenna, T. (1993) *True Hallucinations.* San Francisco: Harper.

20. McKenna, D. (2012) *Brotherhood of the Screaming Abyss: My Life with Terence McKenna.* North Star Press of St. Cloud. Clearwater, MN, USA.

21. http://www.guardian.co.uk/politics/2011/sep/05/psychedelic-therapy-war-on-drugs

22. Ludlow, F. H. (1857) *The Hasheesh Eater.* Fitz Hugh Ludlow Memorial Library Edition (1975) Level Press, San Francisco, USA.

23. Grinspoon, L. & Bakalar, J.B. (1993) *Marijuana: The Forbidden Medicine.* Yale University Press. New Haven and London.

24. Holland, Julie (Editor) (2010) The Pot Book: A Complete Guide to Cannabis: Its Role in Medicine, Politics, Science, and Culture. Sarasota: MAPS.

25. Holland, J. (Editor) (2001) *Ecstasy: The Complete Guide : A Comprehensive Look at the Risks and Benefits of MDMA.* Park Street Press. New York.

26. Rolles, S. & Murkin, G. (2013) *How to Regulate Cannabis: A Practical Guide*. Transform Drug Policy Foundation. www.tdpf.org.uk

27. Harris, B. (2015) *The Secrets of Medicinal Marijuana: A Guide for patients and those who care for them*. Muse House Press, USA.

28. Mechoulam, R.; M. Peters, Murillo-Rodriguez (21 Aug 2007). 'Cannabidiol - recent advances'. *Chemistry & Biodiversity* 4 (8): 1678–1692.

29. Melville, Nancy A. (14 Aug 2013), *Seizure Disorders Enter Medical Marijuana Debate, Medscape Medical News.*, retrieved 2014-01-14

30. Esther M. Blessing, Maria M. Steenkamp, Jorge Manzanares, Charles R. Marmar (2015) Cannabidiol as a Potential Treatment for Anxiety Disorders. Neurotherapeutics. 2015 October; 12(4): 825–836

31. Leweke FM, Mueller JK, Lange B, Rohleder C (2016). "Therapeutic Potential of Cannabinoids in Psychosis". *Biol. Psychiatry* 79 (7): 604–12

32. Hallak, E.C., Filho, S., Freitas-Ferrari, M.C., McGuire, P., Zuardi, A.... Fábio, L.S. (2011) Neural basis of anxiolytic effects of cannabidiol (CBD) in generalized social anxiety disorder: a preliminary report. Journal of Psychopharmacology 2011 25: 121-130

33. Bennett, C. (2010) *Cannabis and the Soma Solution*. Trine Day LLC. Waterville, OR, USA.

34. White, Timothy (2006) *Catch A Fire: The life of Bob Marley*. London: Omnibus Press.

35. https://www.theguardian.com/world/2015/feb/25/jamaica-decriminalises-marijuana).

36. Shrivastava, A., Johnston, M., & Tsuang, M. (2011). Cannabis use and cognitive dysfunction. *Indian Journal of Psychiatry, 53*(3), 187–191.

37. Tait, R. J., Mackinnon, A. and Christensen, H. (2011), Cannabis use and cognitive function: 8-year trajectory in a young adult cohort. Addiction, 106: 2195–2203.

38. Semple DM[1], McIntosh AM, Lawrie SM. (2005) Cannabis as a risk factor for psychosis: systematic review. J Psychopharmacol. 2005 Mar;19(2):187-194

39. Sharpley MS, Hutchinson G, Murray RM, McKenzie K. (2001) Understanding the excess of psychosis among the African-Caribbean population in England: review of current hypotheses. Br J Psychiatry2001;178(suppl 40):60–68

40. Harrison PJ, Owen MJ; Owen (February 2003). "Genes for schizophrenia? Recent findings and their pathophysiological implications". *Lancet*. 361 (9355): 417–9

41. Power, RA et al (2015) Genetic predisposition to schizophrenia associated with increased use of cannabis. Mol Psychiatry. 2014 Nov; 19(11): 1201–1204.)

42. Wang, Linda (June 28, 2010). "C&EN Talks With John W. Huffman". *Chemical & Engineering News*. **88** (26): 43.).
43. Papanti, D., Schifano, F., Botteon, G., et al (2013) "Spiceophrenia": a systematic overview of "Spice"-related psychopathological issues and a case report. *Human Psychopharmacology Clinical and Experimental* 28(4):379-89).
44. New psychoactive substances (NPS) in prisons A toolkit for prison staff (2015) PHE publications gateway number: 2015534)
45. Stafford, Peter. (1993) *Psychedelics Encyclopedia*. New York: Ronin Publishing.
46. Evans Schultes, Hofmann and Ratsch (1998) *Plants of the Gods*. New York: Healing Arts Press.

Chapter 8: The Psychedelic Renaissance Part One: Movers and Shakers

1. www.maps.org/psychedelicreview/
2. www.maps.org
3. www.heffter.org
4. www.beckleyfoundation.org
5. www.csp.org
6. www.gaiamedia.org
7. Hagenbach, D. and Werthmueller, L. (2013) *Mystic Chemist: The Life of Albert Hofmann and His Discovery of LSD*. Synergetic Press, Santa Fe, USA
8. www.horizonsnyc.org
9. www.breakingconvention.org - Breaking Convention has given me many happy memories in the last seven years. Despite taking a year off between gatherings, the work load is immense. Endless emails and Skype meetings (I counted over 10,000 messages in all) between members of the executive crew and furious last minute scrabbling for money to put together the necessary material. It is all worth it for a magical weekend coming-together of UK and international psychedelic communities. I knew we had got it right when, in 2011, veteran psychedelic researcher Roland Griffiths came up to me in the bustle of the opening party and said, 'Hey man, this is a great vibe. It reminds me of the Berkley campus in 1965!
10. The wider Breaking Convention crew now extends to Adam Malone (entertainments), Andy Roberts (merchandising and archive), Stuart Griggs and Maria Pap (art curators), Mark Lewis (IT and tech), Julian Vayne and Nikki Wyrd (front of house and volunteering), Rob Dickins (Psypress liaison), Stephen Reid (press and media),

Hattie Wells (speaker liaison), Cara Lavan and Luca (video directors), Ali Beiner and Ashleigh Murphy (sponsorship) and Sarah Watson and Will Rowlandson (workshop organisers). A more professional and enthusing crew one would be hard pushed to find.

11. www.stichtingopen.nl
12. www.erowid.org
13. www.bluelight.ru
14. www.psychedelicsociety.org.uk.
15. www. psypressuk.com
16. www.octobergallery.co.uk
17. www.ukcpsychedelics.co.uk
18. www.beyondpsychedelics.cz
19. www.neurosoup.com
20. Sessa, Ben. (2008) 'Self-medication of LSD and MDMA to treat mental disorders: A case series' in The *Neurosoup Yearly Review 2008*. *Neurosoup Trust*.
21. www.realitysandwich.com
22. www.ssdp.org
23. www.londoncannabisclub.com/feed-the-birds-campaign-2
24. www.muswellhillpress.co.uk
25. www.tyringhaminiative.com
26. Forgive me for omitting anyone from this alphabetically listed section. If you are not on this list, it does not diminish your importance but rather illustrates my ignorance and certainly reflects my greater knowledge of European, especially British, over American professionals.
27. Danforth, A.L., Struble, C.M., Yazar-Klosinski, B. and Grob, C.S. (2016) MDMA-assisted therapy: A new treatment model for social anxiety in autistic adults. Progress in Neuro-Psychopharmacology and Biological Psychiatry. Volume 64, 4 January 2016, Pages 237–249
28. Sewell RA, Halpern JH, Pope HG Jr. (2006) 'Response of cluster headache to psilocybin and LSD.' *Neurology* 27;66: 1920-1922.
29. Letcher, Andy. (2007) *Shroom: A Cultural History of the Magic Mushroom*. London: Ecco.
30. Roberts, Andy. (2008) *Albion Dreaming: A popular history of LSD in Britain*. London: Marshall Cavendish.
31. Roberts, A. (2016) Acid Drops. Psychedelic Press, St. Ives, UK.
32. Morgan, C.J. and Curran, H.V. (2012) Ketamine Use: A Review. Addiction. 107; 27-38
33. See Charlie's multiple publications here: www.heffter.org
34. Rätsch, C. (2005) *The Encyclopedia of Psychoactive Plants: Ethnopharmacology and Its Applications*. Park Street Press, Vermont.

35. *Heinrich, Clark (2002)Magic Mushrooms in Religion and Alchemy*, Park Street Press, New York
36. Pinchbeck, Daniel (2002) Breaking Open the Head: A Psychedelic Journey into the Heart of Contemporary Shamanism. Broadway Books, New York.
37. Pinchbeck, Daniel (2006) 2012: The Return of Quetzalcoatl. Jeremy P. Tacher/Penguin. New York.
38. Pinchbeck, Daniel (2017) How Soon is Now? Watkins Publishing, London.
39. Scott, David Graham (2004) https://vimeo.com/25291673
40. Scott, David Graham (2014) https://vimeo.com/130630278
41. See Dave Luke's multiple publications here: www.gre.ac.uk/eduhea/ study/pswc/staff/dr-david-luke
42. See Dave Nichols' multiple publications here: www.heffter.org
43. See Dave Nutt's multiple publications here: www.imperial.ac.uk/ people/d.nutt
44. www.synergeticpress.com
45. McKenna, D. & McKenna, T. (1994) The Invisible Landscape: Mind, Hallucinogens & the I Ching. HarperOne, San Francisco, USA.
46. www.dancesafe.org
47. Krupitsky EM, Grinenko AY (1997). 'Ketamine psychedelic therapy (KPT): a review of the results of ten years of research'. *Journal of Psychoactive Drugs* 29 (2): 165–83
48. See Franz's multiple publications here: www.researchgate.net/profile/ Franz_Vollenweider/publications
49. Frischer, Friederike (2015) Therapy With Substance. Muswell Hill Press, London).
50. Sessa, B and Meckel Fischer, F. (2015) Underground LSD, MDMA and 2-CB-assisted Individual and Group Psychotherapy in Zurich: Outcomes, Implications and Commentary. *Journal of Psychopharmacology / Journal of Independent Scientific Committee on Drugs*. March 2015. Vol1.
51. See George's multiple publications here: www.heffter.org
52. Ricaurte George A, Yuan J, Hatzidimitriou G, Cord BJ, McCann UD (2003B) 'Retraction.' *Science 301: 1429.*
53. www.grahamhancock.com
54. Bouso JC, Palhano-Fontes F, Rodríguez-Fornells A, Ribeiro S, Sanches R, Crippa JA, Hallak JE, de Araujo DB, Riba J. Long-term use of psychedelic drugs is associated with differences in brain structure and personality in humans. European Neuropsychopharmacology, Volume 25, Issue 4, 483 – 492
55. Vayne, J. & Wyrd, N. (2012) The Book of Baphomet. Mandrake, Oxford, UK.

56. Holland, Julie (2010) *Weekends at Belleview.* New York: Random House, Inc.
57. Holland, Julie (Editor) (2001) *Ecstasy: The Complete Guide : A Comprehensive Look at the Risks and Benefits of MDMA.* New York: Park Street Press.
58. Holland, Julie (Editor) (2010) The Pot Book: A Complete Guide to Cannabis: Its Role in Medicine, Politics, Science, and Culture. Sarasota: MAPS.
59. MacLean, K. A., Johnson, M. W., & Griffiths, R. R. (2011). Mystical Experiences Occasioned by the Hallucinogen Psilocybin Lead to Increases in the Personality Domain of Openness. *Journal of Psychopharmacology (Oxford, England)*, 25(11), 1453–1461.
60. www.botanicaldimensions.org
61. Luna, L.E. (1986) Vegetalismo: Shamanism Among the Mestizo Population of the Peruvian Amazon. Almqvist & Wiksell International. Stockholm, Sweden.
62. Luna, L.E. (1991) Ayahuasca Visions: The Religious Iconography of a Peruvian Shaman with Pablo Amaringo. North Atlantic Books, Berkley, CA, USA.
63. Luna, L.E. (2008) Inner Paths to Outer Space: Journeys to Alien Worlds through Psychedelics and Other Spiritual Technologies with Rick Strassman, Slawek Wojtowicz M.D Ede Frecska M.D.. Park Street Press, New York.
64. Johnson MW, Garcia-Romeu A, Cosimano MP, Griffiths RR3 (2014) Pilot study of the 5-HT2AR agonist psilocybin in the treatment of tobacco addiction. *J Psychopharmacol.* 28(11):983-92
65. Sessa, B. and Johnson, M. (2015) Is There a Role for Psychedelics in the Treatment of Drug Dependency? *British Journal of Psychiatry,* January 2015
66. Bogenschutz MP, Forcehimes AA, Pommy JA, Wilcox CE, Barbosa PC, Strassman RJ. (2015) Psilocybin-assisted treatment for alcohol dependence: a proof-of-concept study. J Psychopharmacol. 2015 Mar;29(3):289-99
67. Michael C. Mithoefer, Mark T. Wagner, Ann T. Mithoefer, Lisa Jerome and Rick Doblin (2010) 'The safety and efficacy of ±3,4-methylenedioxymetham-phetamine-assisted psychotherapy in subjects with chronic treatment-resistant posttraumatic stress disorder: the first randomised controlled pilot study.' *Journal of Psychopharmacology*, 19th July 2010
68. Mithoefer MC, Wagner MT, Mithoefer AT, Jerome L, Martin SF, Yazar-Klosinski B, Michel Y, Brewerton TD, Doblin R. (2013) Durability of improvement in post-traumatic stress disorder symptoms and absence

of harmful effects or drug dependence after 3,4-methylenedioxymeth-amphetamine-assisted psychotherapy: a prospective long-term follow-up study. *Journal of Psychopharmacology.* 27(1):28-39).

69. Stolaroff, Myron. (2004 / 1997) The Secret Chief Revealed: Conversations with a pioneer of the underground psychedelic therapy movement. Sarasota: MAPS.

70. Goldsmith, N. M. (2010) Psychedelic Healing: The Promise of Entheogens for Psychotherapy and Spiritual Development Kindle Edition Healing Arts Press, Rochester, USA).

71. Vayne, J. & Wyrd, N. (2012) The Book of Baphomet. Mandrake, Oxford, UK.

72. Gasser, P., Holstein, D., Michel, Y., Doblin, R., Yazar-Klosinski, B., Passie, T., & Brenneisen, R. (2014). Safety and Efficacy of Lysergic Acid Diethylamide-Assisted Psychotherapy for Anxiety Associated With Life-threatening Diseases.*The Journal of Nervous and Mental Disease, 202*(7), 513–520).

73. www.maps.org/research

74. Strassman RJ, Qualls C, Berg LM. (1996) 'Differential tolerance development to biological and subjective effects of four closely-spaced administrations of N,N-dimethyltryptamine in humans'. *Biological Psychiatry* 39:784-795

75. Strassman, Rick (2001) *DMT: The Spirit Molecule,* New York: Park Street Press.

76. *Luna, L.E. (2008) Inner Paths to Outer Space: Journeys to Alien Worlds through Psychedelics and Other Spiritual Technologies* with Rick Strassman, Slawek Wojtowicz M.D Ede Frecska M.D.. Park Street Press, New York.

77. Strassman, R. (2014) DMT and the Soul of Prophecy: A New Science of Spiritual Revelation in the Hebrew Bible. Park Street Press, New York, USA).

78. Yensen, R.; Di Leo, F. B.; Rhead, J. C.; Richards, W. A.; Soskin, R. A.; Turek, B.; Kurland, A. A. (1976). "MDA-assisted psychotherapy with neurotic outpatients: a pilot study". *The Journal of Nervous and Mental Disease.* **163** (4): 233–245)

79. Crockford, R.M. (2007) 'LSD in Prague: A Long-Term Follow-Up Study.' *MAPS Bulletin* - volume xvii - number 1 - spring/summer 2007

80. www.psypressuk.com

81. Forte, Robert (Editor) (1997) *Entheogens and the Future of Religion.* San Francisco: Council on Spiritual Practices.

82. Forte, R. (1999) Timothy Leary: *Outside Looking In.* Park Street Press, Rochester, Vermont, USA)

83. Hofmann, Albert., Wasson, G.R., Ruck, C. and Staples, B. (1998) *The Road to Eleusis: Unveiling the Secret of the Mysteries*. (Ed: Forte, R.) New Castle, PA: Hermes Press.

84. See Robin's multiple publications here: http://www.imperial.ac.uk/people/r.carhart-harris

85. See Roland's multiple publications here: www.heffter.org

86. Diamond PR[1], Farmery AD[2], Atkinson S[1], Haldar J[3], Williams N[4], Cowen PJ[5], Geddes JR[5], McShane R[6]. (2014) Ketamine infusions for treatment resistant depression: a series of 28 patients treated weekly or twice weekly in an ECT clinic. J Psychopharmacol. 2014 Jun;28(6):536-44

87. The Science Delusion (2012). Coronet Books, London, UK

88. Grof, S. (1975) Realms Of The Human Unconscious: Observations From LSD Research. Republished (2001), Souvenir Press, London.

89. Grof, S. & Halifax, J. (1977) The Human Encounter With Death. E.P. Dutton, New York.

90. Grof, S. (1980) LSD Psychotherapy. 3rd Edition (2001), MAPS, Sarasota.

91. Grof, S. (200) Holotropic Breathwork: A New Approach to Self-Exploration and Therapy (2010) State University of New York Press, New York.

92. Krippner, Stanley (1972) 'Mescaline psilocybin and creative artists.' In: Tart, Charles T., (ed), *Altered States of Consciousness*. New Jersey, USA: John Wiley and Sons.

93. Szara, S. (1956). "Dimethyltryptamin: its metabolism in man; the relation to its psychotic effect to the serotonin metabolism". *Experientia*. **12** (11): 441–2.

94. See Michael's multiple publications here: https://www.researchgate.net/profile/Michael_Winkelman2/publications

95. Winkelman, M. & Roberts, T. (2007) Psychedelic Medicine: New Evidence for Hallucinogenic Substances as Treatments 2 Vols: Praeger Perspectives, Westport, CO, USA.

96. Blackmore, S. (2000) The Meme Machine. Oxford University Press, Oxford, UK.

97. Krebs TS & Johansen P-Ø (2013) Psychedelics and Mental Health: A Population Study. PLoS ONE 8(8): e63972. doi:10.1371/journal.pone.0063972.)

98. Krebs, T.S and Johansen, P.O. (2012) Lysergic acid diethylamide (LSD) for alcoholism: a meta-analysis of randomized controlled trials. Journal of Psychopharmacology, 9 March 2012 DOI:10.1177/0269881112439253

99. www.muswellhillpress.co.uk

100. Roberts, Thomas B. (2006) *Psychedelic Horizons.* Charlottesville, VA: Imprint Academic.

101. Hintzen, A and Passie, T. (2010) *The Pharmacology of LSD: A critical review.* Oxford University Press, USA and Beckley Foundation, UK.

102. Sessa, Ben (2011) 'The Psychopharmacology of LSD by Annalie Hintzen and Torsten Passie. A Book Review' for *The British Journal of Psychiatry.* 199:258-259

103. See Val's multiple publications here: www.ucl.ac.uk/cpu/team/psychopharmacologyunit/valcurran

104. See Bill's multiple publications here: http://www.bpru.org/cancer-studies/about-usBill.html

Chapter 9: The Psychedelic Renaissance Part Two: Contemporary Research

1. Crockford, R.M. (2007) 'LSD in Prague: A Long-Term Follow-Up Study.' *MAPS Bulletin* - volume xvii - number 1 - spring/summer 2007

2. This might explain why the 2016 *Beyond Psychedelics* conference in Prague was such a resounding success. Check out this great video that came out a few weeks before the event: https://www.youtube.com/watch?v=JnYziUiwdi0

3. A cool video of that moment in history can be seen here: https://www.youtube.com/watch?v=LBTr2JEyfXU)

4. Dahlberg CC, Mechaneck R. & Feldstein S. (1968). "LSD research: the impact of lay publicity". Am J Psychiatry 125 (5): 685–9

5. Harrington, A. (2012) The fall of the schizophrenogenic mother. The Lancet, Volume 379, Issue 9823, Pages 1292 – 1293

6. Breakey, W. et al (1974) Halluconogenic Drugs as Precipitants of Schizophrenia Psychological Medicine. Vol. 4: 03; 255 – 261).

7. *Snyder*, S.H, Shailesh P. Banerjee, S.P., Yamamura, H.I. & David Greenberg (1974) Drugs, Neurotransmoitters and Schizophrenia. Science 21 June 1974: Vol. 184 no. 4143 pp. 1243-1253

8. McLellan AT, Woody GE & O'Brien Cl' (1979): Development of psychiatric illness in drug abusers. Possible role of drug preference. New Eng J Med 301:1310-1314

9. Sessa, B. (2010) Self-medication of LSD and MDMA to treat mental disorders: A case series – *Journal of Alternative Medicine Research.* Vol. 2, Issue 2.

10. Ng, R. (2008) *Drugs: From Discovery to Approval.* London: Wiley-Blackwell.

11. Michael C. Mithoefer, Mark T. Wagner, Ann T. Mithoefer, Lisa Jerome and Rick Doblin (2010) 'The safety and efficacy of ±3,4-methylene-

dioxymetham-phetamine-assisted psychotherapy in subjects with chronic treatment-resistant posttraumatic stress disorder: the first randomised controlled pilot study.' *Journal of Psychopharmacology*, 19th July 2010

12. Mithoefer MC, Wagner MT, Mithoefer AT, Jerome L, Martin SF, Yazar-Klosinski B, Michel Y, Brewerton TD, Doblin R. (2013) Durability of improvement in post-traumatic stress disorder symptoms and absence of harmful effects or drug dependence after 3,4-methylenedioxymeth-amphetamine-assisted psychotherapy: a prospective long-term follow-up study. *Journal of Psychopharmacology*. 27(1):28-39

13. Oehen P, Traber, R., Widmer, V., Schnyder, U. (2013) Pilot study of MDMA-assisted psychotherapy for treatment-resistant PTSD. *J Psychopharmacol*; 27(1): 40-52

14. Chabrol H. & Oehen, P. (2013) MDMA assisted psychotherapy found to have a large effect for chronic post-traumatic stress disorder. J Psychopharmacol; s27(9):865-6

15. Sessa Ben, Nutt David J. (2007) MDMA, politics and medical research: Have we thrown the baby out with the bathwater? *J Psychopharmacol* 21: 787-791

16. Holland, Julie (Editor) (2001) *Ecstasy: The Complete Guid : A Comprehensive Look at the Risks and Benefits of MDMA*. New York: Park Street Press.

17. Agarval,A.K.andAndrade,C(1997)'IndianPsychiatrists'AttitudesTowards Electroconvulsive Therapy.' *Indian Journal of Psychiatry. 1997, 39 (i) 54-66*

18. Danforth, A.L., Struble, C.M., Yazar-Klosinski, B. and Grob, C.S. (2016) MDMA-assisted therapy: A new treatment model for social anxiety in autistic adults. Progress in Neuro-Psychopharmacology and Biological Psychiatry. Volume 64, 4 January 2016, Pages 237–249

19. http://www.maps.org/videos/source2/video5.html

20. https://www.youtube.com/watch?v=UygZnBTWW0M

21. The NHS Information Centre. Statistics on alcohol 2010. http://www.ic.nhs. uk/pubs/alcohol10

22. Miller WR, Wilbourne PL. (2002) 'Mesa Grande: a methodological analysis of clinical trials of treatments for alcohol use disorders'. *Addiction*. Mar;97(3):265-77.

23. Mann K, Lehert K, Morgan M. (2004) 'The efficacy of acamprosate in the maintenance of abstinence in alcohol-dependent individuals: results of a meta-analysis.' *Alcohol Clin Exp Res*. 2004;28:51–63.

24. Srisurapanont et al (2005) 'Naltrexone for the treatment of alcoholism: a meta-analysis of Randomized Controlled Trials'. *Int J. Neuropsychopharma- cology;* 2005 Jun;8(2):267-80.

25. Anton, RF (2006) 'Combined pharmacotherapies and behavioral interventions for alcohol dependence.' *JAMA*. 2006 Oct 11;296(14):1727

26. Watson, L. and Beck, J. (1991) New Age Seekers: MDMA as an Adjunct to Spiritual Pursuit. Journal of Psychoactive Drugs. Vol 23(3)

27. Sumnall, H. R, Cole, J. and Jerome, L. (2006) The varieties of ecstatic experience: an exploration of the subjective experiences of ecstasy. *Journal of Psychopharmacology*. 20(5) (2006) 670–682

28. http://www.zendoproject.org/

29. http://www.kosmicareuk.org/

30. Gasser, P., Holstein, D., Michel, Y., Doblin, R., Yazar-Klosinski, B., Passie, T., & Brenneisen, R. (2014). Safety and Efficacy of Lysergic Acid Diethylamide-Assisted Psychotherapy for Anxiety Associated With Life-threatening Diseases.*The Journal of Nervous and Mental Disease, 202*(7), 513–520

31. Gasser, P., Kirchner. K, and Passie, T. (2015) LSD-assisted psychotherapyfor anxiety associated with a life-threatening disease: A qualitative study of acute and sustained subjective effects. Journal of Psychopharmaology. Vol. 29(1) 57–68).

32. Kast, Eric (1967). 'Attenuation of anticipation: a therapeutic use of lysergic acid diethylamide.' *Psychiat. Quart.* 41 (4): 646–57.

33. Sewell RA, Halpern JH, Pope HG Jr. (2006) 'Response of cluster headache to psilocybin and LSD.' *Neurology* 27; 66: 1920-1922.

34. Kurst,M., Bernateck, M., Passie, T. and Halpern, J. (2010) The non-hallucinogen 2-bromo-lysergic acid diethylamide as preventative treatment for cluster headache: An open, non-randomized case series. Cephalalgia 30: 1140-1144

35. http://ck-wissen.de/ckwiki/images/1/14/IHS_IHC_2009_BOL_Halpern.pdf

36. Carhart-Harris, Robin L.; Muthukumaraswamy, Suresh; Roseman, Leor; Kaelen, Mendel; Droog, Wouter; Murphy, Kevin; Tagliazucchi, Enzo; Schenberg, Eduardo E.; Nest, Timothy. "Neural correlates of the LSD experience revealed by multimodal neuroimaging". *Proceedings of the National Academy of Sciences*. doi:10.1073/pnas.1518377113

37. Moreno FA, Wiegand CB, Taitano EK, Delgado PL. (2006). 'Safety, tolerabil- ity, and efficacy of psilocybin in 9 patients with obsessive-compulsive disorder'. *Journal of Clinical Psychiatry* 67 (11): 1735–40

38. Grob Charles S., Danforth Alicia L., Chopra GS, Hagerty M, McKay CR, Halberstadt AL, Greer George R. (2011) Pilot study of psilocybin treatment for anxiety in patients with advanced-stage cancer. *Arch Gen Psychiatry*. 2011 Jan;68(1):71-8

39. Carhart-Harris RL, Bolstridge M, Rucker J, et al. Psilocybin with psychological support for treatment-resistant depression: an open-label

feasibility study. Lancet Psychiatry 2016; published online May 17. http://dx.doi.org/10.1016/S2215-0366(16)30065-7

40. Johnson MW, Garcia-Romeu A, Cosimano MP, Griffiths RR3 (2014) Pilot study of the 5-HT2AR agonist psilocybin in the treatment of tobacco addiction. *J Psychopharmacol.* 28(11):983-92

41. Krebs, T.S and Johansen, P.O. (2012) Lysergic acid diethylamide (LSD) for alcoholism: a meta-analysis of randomized controlled trials. Journal of Psychopharmacology, 9 March 2012 DOI:10.1177/0269881112439253

42. Bogenschutz, M. P. & Pommy, J. A. (2012) Re-Examining the Therapeutic Potential of Classical Hallucinogens in the Treatment of Addictions. Drug Testing and Analysis Drug Testing and Analysis 4 (7-8) 543-555

43. Michael P Bogenschutz, Alyssa A Forcehimes, Jessica A Pommy, Claire E Wilcox, PCR Barbosaand Rick J Strassman (2015) Psilocybin-assisted treatment for alcohol dependence: A proof-of-concept study J Psychopharmacol 0269881114565144, first published on January 13, 2015 doi:10.1177/0269881114565144

44. Sessa, B. and Johnson, M. (2015) Is There a Role for Psychedelics in the Treatment of Drug Dependency? *British Journal of Psychiatry,* January 2015

45. Griffiths, Roland R., Richards, William A., McCann, U, Jesse, Robert (2006) 'Psilocybin can occasion mystical experiences having substantial and sustained personal meaning and spiritual significance.' *Psychopharmacology (Berl)* 187: 268–283.

46. McClean, A., Johnson, W. and Griffiths, Roland. (2011) 'Mystical Experiences Occasioned by the Hallucinogen Psilocybin Lead to Increases in the Personality Domain of Openness.' *J Psychopharmacol* 26 (3)

47. Martin DA, Nichols CD, Psychedelics Recruit Multiple Cellular Types and Produce Complex Transcriptional Responses Within the Brain. (2016) EBioMedicine. 2016 Sep;11:262-277. doi: 10.1016/j.ebiom.2016.08.049. Epub 2016 Sep 3.

48. Preller KH, Pokorny T, Hock A, Kraehenmann R, Stämpfli P, Seifritz E, Scheidegger M, Vollenweider FX. Effects of serotonin 2A/1A receptor stimulation on social exclusion processing. (2016) Proc Natl Acad Sci U S A. May 3;113(18):5119-24. doi: 10.1073/pnas.1524187113. Epub 2016 Apr 18.,

49. Pokorny T, Preller KH, Kraehenmann R, Vollenweider FX. Modulatory effect of the 5-HT1A agonist buspirone and the mixed non-hallucinogenic 5-HT1A/2A agonist ergotamine on psilocybin-induced psychedelic experience. (2016) Eur Neuropsychopharmacol.

Apr;26(4):756-66. doi: 0.1016/j.euroneuro.2016.01.005. Epub 2016 Jan 22.

50. Kraehenmann R, Preller KH, Scheidegger M, Pokorny T, Bosch OG, Seifritz E, Vollenweider FX. Psilocybin-Induced Decrease in Amygdala Reactivity Correlates with Enhanced Positive Mood in Healthy Volunteers. (2015) Biol Psychiatry. Oct 15;78(8):572-81. doi: 10.1016/j.biopsych.2014.04.010. Epub 2014 Apr 26.

51. Kraehenmann R, Schmidt A, Friston K, Preller KH, Seifritz E, Vollenweider FX. The mixed serotonin receptor agonist psilocybin reduces threat-induced modulation of amygdala connectivity. (2015) Neuroimage Clin. Aug 22;11:53-60. doi: 10.1016/j.nicl.2015.08.009. eCollection 2016.

52. Kometer M, Pokorny T, Seifritz E, Volleinweider FX. Psilocybin-induced spiritual experiences and insightfulness are associated with synchronization of neuronal oscillations. (2015) Psychopharmacology (Berl). Oct;232(19):3663-76. doi: 10.1007/s00213-015-4026-7. Epub 2015 Aug 1.

53. Bernasconi F, Kometer M, Pokorny T, Seifritz E, Vollenweider FX. The electrophysiological effects of the serotonin 1A receptor agonist buspirone in emotional face processing. Eur Neuropsychopharmacol. 2015 Jan 17. pii: S0924-977X(15)00010-3. doi: 10.1016/j.euroneuro.2015.01.009.

54. Kraehenmann R, Preller KH, Scheidegger M, Pokorny T, Bosch OG, Seifritz E, Vollenweider FX. Psilocybin-Induced Decrease in Amygdala Reactivity Correlates with Enhanced Positive Mood in Healthy Volunteers. Biological Psychiatry, 2014 Apr 26. pii: S0006-3223(14)00275-3. doi: 10.1016/j.biopsych.2014.04.010.

55. Kometer M, Schmidt A, Jäncke L, Vollenweider FX. Activation of serotonin 2A receptors underlies the psilocybin-induced effects on α oscillations, N170 visual-evoked potentials, and visual hallucinations. Journal of Neuroscience, 2013 Jun 19;33(25):10544-51.)

56. Link to video of BRI mock scanner - https://www.youtube.com/watch?v=LBTr2JEyfXU

57. Carhart-Harris Robin L., Erritzoe D, Williams T, Stone JM, Read LJ, Colasanti A, et al. (2012) 'Neural correlates of the psychedelic state as determined by fMRI studies with psilocybin.' *Proc Natl Acad Sci* vol. 109 no. 6 2138-2143

58. Muthukumaraswamy, SD, Carhart-Harris, RL, Moran, RJ, Brookes, MJ, Williams, TM, Errtizoe, D, Sessa, B, Papadopoulos, A, Bolstridge, M, Singh, KD, Feilding, A, Friston, KJ & Nutt, DJ (2013) Cortical desynchronization underlies the human psychedelic state, *Journal of Neuroscience*. 09/2013; 33(38):15171-15183

59. Carhart-Harris, Robin. et al (2012) 'Implications for psychedelic-assisted psychotherapy: functional magnetic resonance imaging study with psilocybin.' *BJP* 200:238-244.
60. Carhart-Harris RL, Leech R, Hellyer PJ, Shanahan M, Feilding A, Tagliazucchi E, Chialvo DR, Nutt DJ. (2014) The entropic brain: A theory of conscious states informed by neuroimaging research with psychedelic drugs. Frontiers in Human Neuroscience. doi: 10.3389/fnhum.2014.00020.
61. Strassman RJ, Qualls C, Berg LM. (1996) 'Differential tolerance development to biological and subjective effects of four closely-spaced administrations of N,N-dimethyltryptamine in humans'. *Biological Psychiatry* 39:784-795
62. Daumann J, Heekeren K, Neukirch A, Thiel CM, Möller-Hartmann W, Gou- zoulis-Mayfrank E. (2008) Pharmacological modulation of the neural basis underlying inhibition of return (IOR) in the human 5-HT(2A) agonist and NMDA antagonist model of psychosis. *Psychopharmacology (Berl).* 2008 Nov;200(4):573-83. Epub2008 Jul 24.
63. Fontanilla et al., (2009) 'The Hallucinogen N,N-Dimethyltryptamine (DMT) Is an Endogenous Sigma-1 Receptor Regulator.' *Science.* 323 (5916): 934-941
64. Szabo, A., Kovacs, A., I., Riba, J., Frecska, E. (2016) The Endogenous Hallucinogen and Trace Amine N,N-Dimethyltryptamine (DMT) Displays Potent Protective Effects against Hypoxia via Sigma-1 Receptor Activation in Human Primary iPSC-Derived Cortical Neurons and Microglia- Like Immune Cells. Frontiers in Neuroscience 10(35)
65. http://www.ayahuasca.com/science/the-scientific-investigation-of-ayahuasca- a-review-of-past-and-current-research/
66. Hancock, Graham (2005). *Supernatural: Meetings with the Ancient Teachers of Mankind.* London: Century.
67. Metzner, R. (1999) Ayahuasca: Human Consciousness and the Spirits of Nature. Thinder's Mouth, New York.
68. Metzner, R. (2005) Sacred Vine of Spirits Park Street Press, South Paris,Maine, USA
69. Luis Eduardo Luna, L. E, & and White, S. (editors) (2000, 2016), 'Ayahuasca Reader: Encounters with the Amazon's Sacred Vine' Synergistic Press, Santa Fe, USA.
70. Pinto, J.P. (2010) Estudo sobre alterações neurofuncionais após ingestão de ayahuasca. Dissertação de Mestrado em Medicina. Universidade de São Paulo, Ribeirão Preto. (Available at: http://www.neip.info/html/objects/_downloadblob.php?cod_ blob=1003)

71. Dobkin de Rios, M.. and Grob, Charles S. (2005) 'Ayahuasca use in cross-cultural perspective: an introduction.' *Journal of Psychoactive Drugs* 37:119-121

72. Mabit, J (2007) Ayahuasca in the treatment of addiction. Chapter 6; In *Hallucinogens and Health : New Evidence for Psychedelic Substances as Treat- ment (Vol 2)* Ed. MJ. Winkelman & TB. Roberts; Westport, Connecticut: Greenwood Publishing Group; pp 87-105

73. Thomas G, Lucas P, Capler NR, Tupper KW, Martin G. (2013) Aya-huasca-assisted therapy for addiction: results from a preliminary observational study in Canada. Curr Drug Abuse Review; 6(1):30-42

74. Riba, J. et al. (2001) Subjective Effects and tolerability of the South American psychoactive beverage Ayahuasca in healthy volunteers. Psychopharmacology 154:85-95

75. Riba J., Rodriguez-Fornells A. & Barbanoj M (2002) Effects of aya-huasca on sensory and sensorimotor gating in humans as measured by P50 suppression and prepulse inhibition of the startle reflex, respec-tively. Psychopharmacology (Berl), 165: 18-28

76. Valle, M., Maqueda, A.E, Rabella, M., Rodríguez-Pujadas, A., Antoni-joan, R.M.,Romero, SA., Alonso, J. F., Mañanas, M.A., Barker, S., Friedlander, P., Feilding, A. and Riba. J. (2016) Inhibition of alpha oscillations through serotonin-2A receptor activation underlies the visual effects of ayahuasca in humans. European Neuropsychophar-macology, Volume 26, Issue 7, 1161 – 1175

77. Dos Santos RG[1], Balthazar FM[2], Bouso JC[3], Hallak JE[4]. (2016) The current state of research on ayahuasca: A systematic review of human studies assessing psychiatric symptoms, neuropsychological func-tioning, and neuroimaging. J Psychopharmacol. 2016 Jun 10. pii: 0269881116652578

78. Soler, J., Elices, M., Franquesa, A., Barker, S., Friedlander, P., Feild-ing, A., Pascual, J.C. and Riba, J. (2016) Exploring the therapeutic potential of Ayahuasca: acute intake increases mindfulness-related capacities. Psychopharmacology (2016) 233: 823

79. Bouso JC, Palhano-Fontes F, Rodríguez-Fornells A, Ribeiro S, Sanches R, Crippa JA, Hallak JE, de Araujo DB, Riba J. Long-term use of psy-chedelic drugs is associated with differences in brain structure and per-sonality in humans. European Neuropsychopharmacology, Volume 25, Issue 4, 483 – 492

80. Krupitsky EM, Grinenko AY (1997). 'Ketamine psychedelic therapy (KPT): a review of the results of ten years of research'. *Journal of Psychoactive Drugs* 29 (2): 165–183

81. Krupitsky EM, Burakov AM, Dunaevsky IV, Romanova TN, Slavina TY, Grinenko AY (March 2007). 'Single versus repeated sessions of

ketamine- assisted psychotherapy for people with heroin dependence'. *Journal of Psychoactive Drugs* 39 (1): 13–9

82. Jovaisa T, Laurinenas G, Vosylius S, Sipylaite J, Badaras R, Ivaskevicius J (2006). 'Effects of ketamine on precipitated opiate withdrawal'. *Medicina* 42 (8): 625–34.

83. D'Souza, D.C. et al (2012) 'Glycine Transporter Inhibitor Attenuates the Psychotomimetic Effects of Ketamine in Healthy Males: Preliminary Evidence.' *Neuropsychopharmacology* 37, 1036-1046

84. Correll GE, Futter GE (2006). 'Two case studies of patients with major depressive disorder given low-dose (subanesthetic) ketamine infusions'. *Pain Medi- cine* 7 (1): 92–5

85. Zarate CA, Singh JB, Carlson PJ, *et al.* (August 2006). 'A randomized trial of an N-methyl-D-aspartate antagonist in treatment-resistant major depression'. *Archives of General Psychiatry* 63 (8): 856–64.

86. Diamond PR, Farmery AD, Atkinson S, Haldar J, Williams N, Cowen PJ, Geddes JR, McShane R. (2014) Ketamine infusions for treatment resistant depression: a series of 28 patients treated weekly or twice weekly in an ECT clinic. J Psychopharmacol. 2014 Jun;28(6):536-44

87. Caddy C, Giaroli G, White TP, Shergill SS, Tracy DK. Ketamine as the prototype glutamatergic antidepressant: pharmacodynamic actions, and a systematic review and meta-analysis of efficacy. *Ther Adv Psychopharmacol.* 2014;4(2):75–99).

88. Kantrowitz JT[1], Halberstam B, Gangwisch J. (2015) Single-Dose Ketamine Followed by Daily D-Cycloserine in Treatment-Resistant Bipolar Depression. J Clin Psychiatry 2015;76(6):737–738

89. Lally N, Nugent AC, Luckenbaugh DA, Ameli R, Roiser JP, Zarate CA. (2014) Anti-anhedonic effect of ketamine and its neural correlates in treatment-resistant bipolar depression. Translational Psychiatry (2014) 4, e469; doi:10.1038/tp.2014.105 Published online 14 October 2014)

90. Rodriguez CI, Kegeles LS, Flood P, Simpson HB. Rapid resolution of obsessions after an infusion of intravenous ketamine in a patient with treatment-resistant obsessive-compulsive disorder. *J Clin Psychiatry.* 2011;72(4):567–569).

91. Bloch MH, Wasylink S, Landeros-Weisenberger A, et al. Effects of ketamine in treatment-refractory obsessive-compulsive disorder (2012). *Biol Psychiatry.* 2012; 72(11):964-970)

92. Rodriguez CI, Kegeles LS, Levinson A, et al. Randomized controlled crossover trial of ketamine in obsessive-compulsive disorder: proof-of-concept. *Neuropsychopharmacology.* 2013;38(12):2475-2483).

93. Alper, K.R., Beal, D. and Kaplan, C.D., (2001) 'A contemporary history of ibogaine in the United States and Europe. The Alkaloids'. *Chemistry and Biology* 56, 249-281

94. Alper,KR, Lotsof, HS, Frenken, GM, Luciano, DJ, Bastiaans, J. (1999). 'Treatment of Acute Opioid Withdrawal with Ibogaine'. *The American Journal on Addictions* 8 (3): 234–42.).
95. http://www.maps.org/research/ibogaine/
96. Mash, D. et al (2000) 'Ibogaine: Complex Pharmacokinetics, Concerns for Safety, and Preliminary Efficacy Measures. Neurobiological Mechanisms of Drugs of Abuse.' *Ann N Y Acad Sci* 2000;914: 394-401
97. Meisner, J. A., Wilcox, S. R., & Richards, J. B. (2016). Ibogaine-associated cardiac arrest and death: case report and review of the literature. *Therapeutic Advances in Psychopharmacology*, 6(2), 95–98
98. Scott, David Graham (2004) https://vimeo.com/25291673
99. Scott, David Graham (2014) https://vimeo.com/130630278

Chapter 10: Psychedelics Caught in the Crossfire of the War on Drugs

1. http://www.ncsl.org/research/health/state-medical-marijuana-laws.aspx
2. Institute of Alcohol Studies (2013) Marketing and Alcohol Factsheet, May 2013. http://www.ias.org.uk/uploads/pdf/Factsheets/Marketing%20and%20alcohol%20FS%20May%202013.pdf
3. One such hard-working organisation concerned with fighting against the War on Drugs is the international Students for Sensible Drug Policy. www.ssdp.org
4. www.beckleyfoundation.org
5. EMCDDA (2009) European Monitoring Centre for Drugs and Drug Addiction. Annual report on the state of the drugs problem in Europe, Lisbon.
6. Sessa, Ben and Nutt, David J. (2007) 'MDMA, Politics and Medical Research: Have we thrown the baby out with the bathwater?' *Journal of Psychopharmacology.* Vol. 21: 787-791.
7. United States Congress (1937) The Marijuana Tax Act. Effective: October 1st 1937.
8. Rothwell, V.L. (2011) The Boggs Act. In the *Encyclopedia of Drug Policy.* Edited by: Mark A. R. Kleiman & James E. Hawdon
9. Office of National Statistics (2014) – Alcohol Related Deaths in the United Kingdom: Registered in 2014
10. Health and Social Care Information Centre (2016) Statistics on Smoking: England, 2016 - Health and social care.
11. Halpern, John et al (2004). 'Residual neuropsychological effects of illicit 3,4-methylenedioxymethamphetamine (MDMA) in individuals

with minimal exposure to other drugs.' *Drug and Alcohol Dependence* 75 (2004) 135–147

12. Salvaraj, S. et al (2009) 'Brain serotonin transporter binding in former users of MDMA ('ecstasy').' *The British Journal of Psychiatry.* 194: 355-359

13. Huizink, A. et al (2006) 'Symptoms of anxiety and depression in childhood and use of MDMA: prospective, population based study.' *BMJ,* doi: 10.1136/ bmj.38743.539398.3A

14. Nutt, David J. et al (2007) 'The Development of a rational scale to assess the harm of drugs of potential misuse.' *The Lancet* Vol 369:1047-1053

15. http://www.drugscience.org.uk/

16. www.dancesafe.org

17. http://www.maps.org/news-letters/v18n3/v18n3-39to44.pdf

18. Marlatt, G. Alan (2002). *Highlights of Harm Reduction. Harm Reduction: Pragmatic Strategies for Managing High-Risk Behaviors.* London: Guilford Press.

19. Gable, R. S. (2006). 'Acute toxicity of drugs versus regulatory status'. In J. M. Fish (Ed.),*Drugs and Society:* U.S. Public Policy, pp.149-162, Lanham, MD: Rowman & Littlefield Publishers.

20. http://niu.academia.edu/ThomasRoberts/Talks/66495/Looking_Forward_ Campus and_a_Company_powerpoints. Roberts, Thomas B. (2006) Psychedelic Horizons. Charlottesville: Imprint

Bibliography and Further Reading

The books with an asterisk are my favourite texts for an introduction on the subject of psychedelic drugs.

Arthur, James (2003) Mushrooms and Mankind: The Impact of Mushrooms on Human Consciousness and Religion. San Diego: The Book Tree.

Ball, M. (2007) Sage Spirit: Salvia Divinorum and the Entheogenic Experience. Oregon: Kyandara Publishing

Burroughs, William. (1963) The Yage Letters. San Francisco: City Lights.

Castaneda, Carlos (1968) The Teachings of Don Juan: A Yaqui Way of Knowledge. Berkeley: University of California Press.

Dobkin de Rios, and M, Janiger, (2003) LSD, Spirituality and the Creative Process. Rochester, Vermont: Park Street Press.

*Doblin, Rick and Burge, Brad (Editors) (2014) Manifesting Minds: A Review of Psychedelics in Science, Medicine, Sex, and Spirituality. Evolver Editions, USA.

*Ellens, Harold and Roberts, Thomas (Editors) (2015) The Psychedelic Policy Quagmire: Health, Law, Freedom, and Society (Psychology, Religion, and Spirituality) Preager, USA.

Eliade, Mircea (1951) Shamanism: Archaic Techniques of Ecstasy. Princeton: Princeton University Press.

Evans Schultes, Hofmann, Albert and Ratsch, Christian (1998) Plants of the Gods. New York: Healing Arts Press.

Fielding, Leaf. (2011) To Live Outside The Law. London: Serpents Tail. Foucault, M. (1964) Madness and Civilisation. New York: Pantheon Books.

Goffman, I. (1961) Asylums: Essays on the Social Situation of Mental Patients and Other Inmates. New York: Anchor Books.

Gottlieb, Adam. (1977) Peyote and other psychoactive cacti. New York: Ronin.

Greenfield, Robert. (2006) Timothy Leary. A Biography. Boston: Houghton Mifflin Harcourt

*Grinspoon, Lester. and Bakalar, J. (1979) Psychedelic Drugs Reconsidered. New York: The Lindesmith Center.

*Grob, Charles – Editor (2002) Hallucinogens: A Reader. New York: Tarcher-Putnam.

*Grof, Stanislav (2001). LSD Psychotherapy (3rd ed.). Sarasota: MAPS. Hancock, Graham (2005). Supernatural: Meetings with the Ancient Teachers of Mankind. London: Century.

Harner, Michael, The Way of the Shaman: A Guide to Power and Healing, New York: Harper & Row.

*Hofmann, A. (1979 / 2005) LSD My Problem Child: Reflections on Sacred Drugs, Mysticism, and Science. Sarasota: MAPS.

Hofmann, A., Wasson, G.R., Ruck, C. and Staples, B. (1998) The Road to Eleusis: Unveiling the Secret of the Mysteries. New Castle, PA: Hermes Press.

*Holland, Julie. (Editor) (2001) Ecstasy: The Complete Guide : A Comprehensive Look at the Risks and Benefits of MDMA. New York: Park Street Press.

Holland, Julie. (Editor) (2010) The Pot Book: A Complete Guide to Cannabis: Its Role in Medicine, Politics, Science, and Culture. Sarasota: MAPS. Hollingshead, Michael (1973) The Man Who Turned On the World. New York: Abelard-Schuman.

*Huxley, Aldous. (1954) The Doors of Perception. London: Chatto and Windus.

*Huxley, Aldous. (1962) Island. New York: Harper and Brothers.

*Huxley, Aldous (Edited by Michael Horowitz and Cynthia Palmer) (1999) Moksha: Aldous Huxley's Classic Writings on Psychedelics and the Visionary Experience. New York: Park Street Press.

James, William. (1902) The Varieties of Religious Experience. Harlow, UK: Longmans, Green and Co.

Jansen, Karl. (2004) Ketamine: Dreams and Realities. Sarasota: MAPS.

Kehoe, Alice (2000) Shamans and Religion: An Anthropological Exploration in Critical Thinking. Long Grove: Waveland Press.

Kerouac, Jack. (1957) On The Road. New York: Viking Press.

Kesey, Ken. (1962) One Flew Over The Cuckoo's Nest. New York: Viking Press. Laing, Adrian (1997) R.D. Laing: A Biography. London: Harper Collins.

Laing, RD (1963) The Divided Self. London: Penguin. Leary, Timothy. (1968) High Priest. The New American Library Inc. New York.

*Leary, Timothy; Ralph Metzner, and Richard Alpert (1963/1992). The Psychedelic Experience: A Manual Based on the Tibetan Book of the Dead (paperback ed.). New York: Citadel Press.

*Lee, MA and Shalin, B (1992) Acid Dreams. The complete social history of LSD: The CIA, the sixties and beyond. New York: Grove Press.

Lesh, Phil. (2005) Searching for the Sound: My Life with the Grateful Dead. New York: Little, Brown and Company.

*Letcher, Andy. (2007) Shroom: A Cultural History of the Magic Mushroom. London: Ecco.

Lilly John. (1972) The Center of the Cyclone. London: Bantam Books.

*Masters, R.L. and Houston, J. (1966). The Varieties of Psychedelic Experience. Rochester, Vermont: Park Street Press.

McKenna, Terence. (1993) True Hallucinations. San Francisco: Harper *McKenna, Terence. (1982) Food of the Gods. London, Bantam Press.

Merkur, D. (2000) The mystery of manna: the psychedelic sacrament of the Bible. New York: Inner Traditions / Bear and Co.

Metzner, Ralph. (2005) Sacred Vine of Spirits: Ayahuasca. New York: Park Street Press.

Miles, Barry. (2005) Hippie. London: Cassell Illustrated /Octopus Publishing Ltd.

Moore, M. (1978) Journeys into the Bright World. Rockport: Para Research Inc

Morgan, Bill. (2006) I Celebrate Myself: The Somewhat Private Life of Allen Ginsberg. London: Viking / Penguin.

Neville, R. (2012) Hippie Hippie Shake. New York: Overlook TP. Perry, Charles. (2005) The Haight-Ashbury. New York: Wenner Books.

*Roberts, Andy (2008) Albion Dreaming: A popular history of LSD in Britain. London: Marshall Cavendish.

*Roberts, Andy (2016) Acid Drops. Strange Attractor Press, Totnes, UK

*Roberts, Thomas B. (2006) Psychedelic Horizons. Charlottesville: Imprint Academic.

Samorini, G. (2000) Animals and Psychedelics. Rochester, Vermont: Park Street Press.

Schultes, Richard Evans; and Albert Hofmann (1980). The Botany and Chemistry of Hallucinogens (2nd ed. ed.). Springfield, Ill.: Thomas.

Sessa, B. (2015) To Fathom Hell or Soar Angelic. Psychedelic Press UK, St. Ives, UK.

*Shulgin, Alexander and Shulgin, Anne. (1991) PIHKAL: Phenethylamines I Have Known And Loved – A Chemical Love Story. Berkley: Transform Press.

*Shulgin, Alexander and Shulgin, Anne. (1997) TIHKAL: Tryptamines I Have Known And Loved – A Chemical Love Story. Berkley: Transform Press.

Stafford, Peter. (1993) Psychedelics Encyclopedia. New York: Ronin Publishing.

*Stevens, Jay. (1987) Storming Heaven: LSD and the American Dream. New York: Grove Press.

Stolaroff, Myron. (1994) Thanatos to Eros – Thirty-Five years of psychedelic exploration. Berlin: VWB.

*Stolaroff, Myron. (2004 / 1997) The Secret Chief Revealed: Conversations with a pioneer of the underground psychedelic therapy movement. Sarasota: MAPS.

*Strassman, Rick (2001) DMT: The Spirit Molecule. New York: Park Street Press. Szasz, Thomas. (1961) The Myth of Mental Illness. New York: Harper and Row.

Strassman, Rick (2014) DMT and the Soul of Prophecy: A New Science of Spiritual Revelation in the Hebrew Bible. Park Strett Press, UK.

Tendler, S. and May, D (1984) Brotherhood of Eternal Love. London: Harper Collins. White, Timothy. (2006) Catch a Fire: The Life of Bob Marley. London: Omnibus Press.

Wolfe, Thomas. (1968) The Electric Kool-Aid Acid Test. New York: Farrar, Strous and Giroux.

Zaehner, R.C. (1972) Drugs, Mysticism and Make Believe. London: Collins.

Index